Urinalysis and Body Fluids

Urinalysis and Body Fluids

Fourth Edition

Susan King Strasinger, D.A., M.T.(A.S.C.P.)
Visiting Assistant Professor
The University of West Florida
Pensacola, Florida

Marjorie Schaub Di Lorenzo, M.T.(A.S.C.P.) SH
Adjunct Instructor
Division of Medical Technology
School of Allied Health Professionals
University of Nebraska Medical Center
Omaha, Nebraska
Phlebotomy Program Coordinator
Continuing Education
Methodist College
Omaha, Nebraska

PHOTOGRAPHY BY:
BO WANG, M.D.
DONNA L. CANTERBURY, B.A., M.T.(A.S.C.P.) SH
JOANNE M. DAVIS, B.S., M.T.(A.S.C.P.) SH
M. PAULA NEUMANN, M.D.
GREGORY J. SWEDO, M.D.

ILLUSTRATIONS BY:
SHERMAN BONOMELLI, M.S.
Medical Technology Program
The University of West Florida

F. A. Davis Company • Philadelphia

F. A. Davis Company
1915 Arch Street
Philadelphia, PA 19103
www.fadavis.com

Printed in the United States of America

Last digit indicates print number: 10 9 8 7 6 5 4 3 2 1

Publisher: Margaret M. Biblis
Associate Editor: Christa Fratantoro
Production Editor: Nwakaego Fletcher-Perry
Cover Designer: Louis Forgione

Library of Congress Cataloging-in-Publication Data

Strasinger, Susan King.
Urinalysis and body fluids / Susan King Strasinger, Marjorie Schaub Di Lorenzo ; Photography by Bo Wang . . . [et al.] ; illustrations by Sherman Bonomelli.— 4th ed.
p. cm.
Includes bibliographical references and index.
ISBN 0–8036–0793–8 (pbk.)
1. Urine—Analysis. 2. Body fluids—Analysis. I. Di Lorenzo, Marjorie Schaub, 1953-
II. Title.

RB53 .S87 2001
616.07′566—dc21

To Harry, my Editor-in-Chief

SKS

To my husband, Scott, and my children,
Michael, Christopher, and Lauren

MSD

Preface

As will be apparent to the readers, the fourth edition of Urinalysis and Body Fluids has been substantially revised and enhanced. However, the objective of the text—to provide concise, comprehensive, and carefully structured instruction in the analysis of nonblood body fluids—remains the same.

This fourth edition has been redesigned to meet the changes occurring in both laboratory medicine and instructional methodology.

To meet the expanding technical information required by students in laboratory medicine, additional chapters have been added and previous chapters expanded. Chapter 1 is devoted to overall laboratory safety and the precautions relating to urine and body fluid analysis. Chapter 7 addresses quality assurance and management in the urinalysis laboratory. Preanalytical, analytical, and postanalytical factors, procedure manuals, current regulatory issues, and methods for continuous quality improvement are stressed. In Chapter 8 the most frequently encountered diseases of glomerular, tubular, interstitial, and vascular origin are related to their associated laboratory tests. To accommodate advances in laboratory testing of seminal, synovial, serous, and amniotic fluids, individual chapters have been added for each of these fluids. Appendix A provides coverage of the ever-increasing variety of automated instrumentation available to the urinalysis laboratory.

This fourth edition has been redesigned to include not only color, but also a larger variety of instructional aids. In response to the reader's suggestions, the number of color slides has been significantly increased and they have been included within the text to increase user-friendliness. The text has been extensively supplemented with tables, summaries, and procedure boxes and many figures are now in full color. The multiple-choice format of study questions at the end of each chapter has been revised to require students to consider more in-depth responses. Case studies in the traditional format and clinical situations relating to technical considerations are included at the end of the chapters. Answers to the study questions, case studies, and clinical situations are also included at the end of the book. Highlighted terms and abbreviations in the text are included in the glossary and abbreviations appendices. Additional support is provided to adopting instructors in the form of accompanying test-generating software.

We have given consideration to the suggestions of our previous readers and believe these valuable suggestions have enabled us to produce a text to meet the needs of all users.

SUSAN KING STRASINGER

MARJORIE SCHAUB DI LORENZO

Acknowledgements

Many people deserve credit for the help and encouragement they have provided us in the preparation of this fourth edition. Our continued appreciation is also extended to all of the people who have been instrumental in the preparation of previous editions.

The color illustrations would not have been possible without the expertise of Sherman Bonomelli, M.S. from the University of West Florida.

New color plates of urine sediment constituents were very skillfully photographed by Bo Wang, M.D. from the Creighton University School of Medicine. Persons assisting in collection of sediments include: Ulrike Otten, M.T.(A.S.C.P.)SC, Darlene Waters, M.T.(A.S.C.P.), Karen Keller, M.T.(A.S.C.P.)SH, Valerie Henry, M.T.(A.S.C.P.), and Katherine Swanson, M.T.(A.S.C.P.)SC from the University of Nebraska Medical Center.

Laboratory personnel in Omaha were extremely helpful in providing us with procedures, forms, and information. We extend our thanks to Linda Fell, M.S., M.T.(A.S.C.P.)SH and Carol Larson, M.S., M.T.(A.S.C.P.) from the University of Nebraska Medical Center, Julie Richards, M.P.A., M.T.(A.S.C.P.)BB from Methodist Hospital, and Patricia Studts, M.T.(A.S.C.P.)NRCC-TC and Susan Wilwerding, M.T.(A.S.C.P.) from St. Joseph Hospital.

We would like to thank Michael Di Lorenzo for using his computer skills to provide the basis for many of the color tables, charts, and procedure boxes.

The valuable suggestions from previous readers and the support from our colleagues at The University of West Florida, Northern Virginia Community College, The University of Nebraska Medical Center, Methodist Hospital, and St. Joseph Hospital have been a great asset to us in production of this new edition. We thank each and every one of you.

Reviewers

Ellen P. Digan, MA, MT(ASCP)
Professor of Biology
Coordinator of Medical Laboratory Technology Program
Manchester Community Tech College
Department of Math, Science, and Health Careers
Manchester, Connecticut

Cynthia A. Martine, MEd, MT(ASCP)
Assistant Professor
Department of Clinical Laboratory Sciences
University of Texas Medical Branch
School of Allied Health
Galveston, Texas

Contents

CHAPTER 1

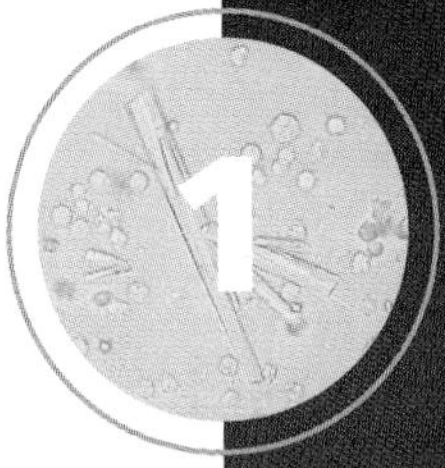
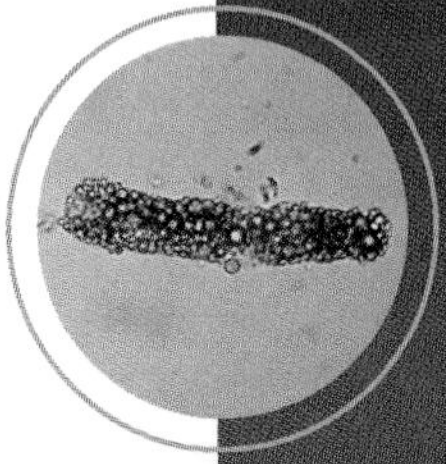
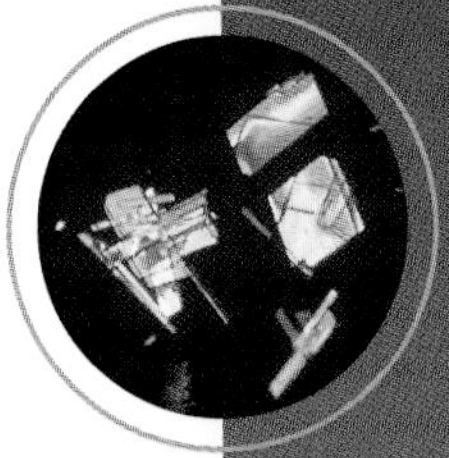
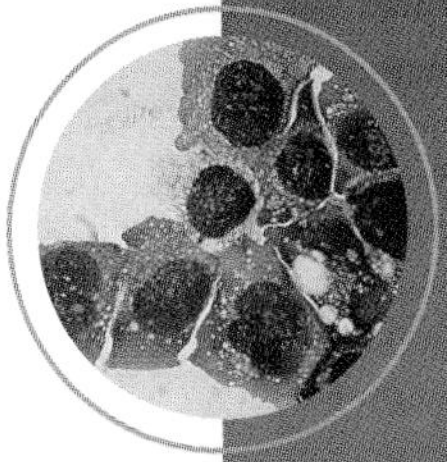
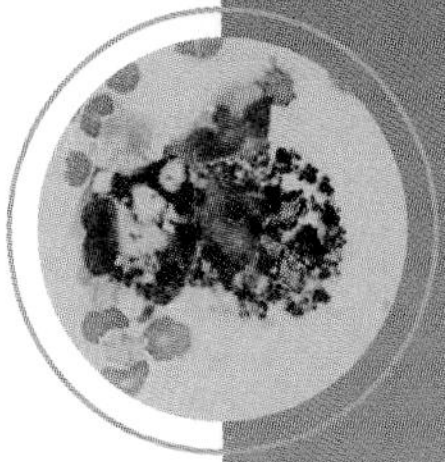

Safety in the Clinical Laboratory

LEARNING OBJECTIVES

Upon completion of this chapter, the reader will be able to:

1. List the components of the chain of infection and the laboratory safety precautions that break the chain.
2. Differentiate among and state the precautions addressed by Universal Precautions, body substance isolation, and Standard Precautions.
3. State the specifics of the Blood-Borne Pathogens Standard.
4. Describe the types of personal protective equipment that laboratory personnel wear, including when, how, and why each article is used.
5. Correctly perform routine handwashing.
6. Describe the acceptable methods for disposing of biological waste in the urinalysis laboratory.
7. Discuss the components and purpose of Chemical Hygiene Plans and Material Safety Data Sheets.
8. State the components of the National Fire Protection Association hazardous material labeling system.
9. Describe precautions that laboratory personnel should take with regard to radioactive and electrical hazards.
10. Explain the RACE actions to be taken when a fire is discovered.
11. Differentiate among class A, B, C, and D fires with regard to material involved and methods of extinguishing each type.
12. Recognize standard hazard warning symbols.

KEY TERMS

biohazardous
body substance isolation
chain of infection
Chemical Hygiene Plan
Material Safety Data Sheet
Occupational Safety and Health Administration
personal protective equipment
radioisotope
Standard Precautions
Universal Precautions

The clinical laboratory contains a variety of safety hazards, many of which are capable of producing serious injury or life-threatening disease. To work safely in this environment, laboratory personnel must learn what hazards exist, the basic safety precautions associated with them, and finally to apply the basic rules of common sense required for everyday safety. As can be seen in Table 1–1, some hazards are unique to the health-care environment, and others are encountered routinely throughout life.

Biological Hazards

BIOHAZARD

The health-care setting provides abundant sources of potentially harmful microorganisms. These microorganisms are frequently present in the specimens received in the clinical laboratory. Understanding how microorganisms are transmitted (***chain of infection***) is essential to preventing infection. The chain of infection requires a continuous link between a source, a method of transmission, and a susceptible host. The source is the location of potentially harmful microorganisms, such as a contaminated clinical specimen or an infected patient. Microorganisms from the source are transmitted to the host. This may occur by direct contact (e.g., the host touches the patient, specimen, or a contaminated object), inhalation of infected material (e.g., **aerosol** droplets from a patient or an uncapped centrifuge tube), ingestion of contaminated food and water, or an animal or insect vector. Once the chain of infection is complete, the infected host then becomes another source able to transmit the microorganisms to others.

In the clinical laboratory, the most direct contact with the source of infection is through contact with patient specimens, although contact with patients and infected objects also occurs. Preventing completion of the chain of infection is a primary objective of biological safety. Figure 1–1 uses the universal symbol for ***biohazardous*** material to demonstrate how following prescribed safety practices can break the chain of infection. Figure 1–1 places particular emphasis on laboratory practices.

Proper handwashing and the wearing of ***personal protective equipment*** (PPE) are of major importance in the laboratory. Concern over exposure to blood-borne pathogens, primarily hepatitis B virus (**HBV**) and human immunodeficiency virus (**HIV**), resulted in the drafting of guidelines and regulations by the Centers for Disease Control and Prevention (**CDC**) and the ***Occupational Safety and Health Administration*** (OSHA) to prevent exposure. In 1987, the CDC instituted ***Universal Precautions*** (UP). Under UP, all patients are considered to be possible carriers of bloodborne pathogens. The guideline recommends wearing gloves when collecting or handling blood and body fluids contaminated with blood, wearing face shields when there is danger of blood splashing on mucous membranes, and disposing of all needles and sharp objects in puncture-resistant containers. The CDC excluded urine and body fluids not visibly contaminated by blood from UP, although many specimens can contain a considerable amount of blood before the blood becomes visible. The modification of UP to ***body substance isolation*** (BSI) helped to alleviate this concern. BSI is not limited to bloodborne pathogens and considers all body fluids and moist body substances to be potentially infectious. According to BSI, personnel should wear gloves at all times when encountering moist body substances. A major disadvantage of the BSI guideline is that it does not recommend handwashing following the removal of gloves unless visual contamination is present.

In 1996, the CDC combined the major features of UP and BSI and called the new guidelines ***Standard Precautions***. Although Standard Precautions, as described below, stress patient contact, the principles most certainly can also be applied to patient specimens.[1]

Standard Precautions are as follows:

1. **Handwashing:** Wash hands after touching blood, body fluids, secretions, excretions, and contaminated items, whether or not gloves are worn. Wash hands immediately after gloves are removed, between patient contacts, and when otherwise indicated, to avoid transfer of microorganisms to other patients or environments. Washing hands may be necessary between tasks and procedures on the same patient to prevent cross-contamination of different body sites.
2. **Gloves:** Wear gloves (clean, nonsterile gloves are adequate) when touching blood, body fluids, secretions, excretions, and contaminated items. Put on gloves just before touching mucous membranes and nonintact skin. Change gloves between tasks and procedures on the same patient after contact with material that may contain a high concentration of microorganisms. Remove gloves promptly after use,

TABLE 1–1 **Types of Safety Hazards**

Type	Source	Possible Injury
Biological	Infectious agents	Bacterial, fungal, viral, or parasitic infections
Sharp	Needles, lancets, and broken glass	Cuts, punctures, or bloodborne pathogen exposure
Chemical	Preservatives and reagents	Exposure to toxic, carcinogenic, or caustic agents
Radioactive	Equipment and radioisotopes	Radiation exposure
Electrical	Ungrounded or wet equipment and frayed cords	Burns or shock
Fire/explosive	Bunsen burners and organic chemicals	Burns or dismemberment
Physical	Wet floors, heavy boxes, and patients	Falls, sprains, or strains

From Strasinger and DiLorenzo,[5] p 62, with permission.

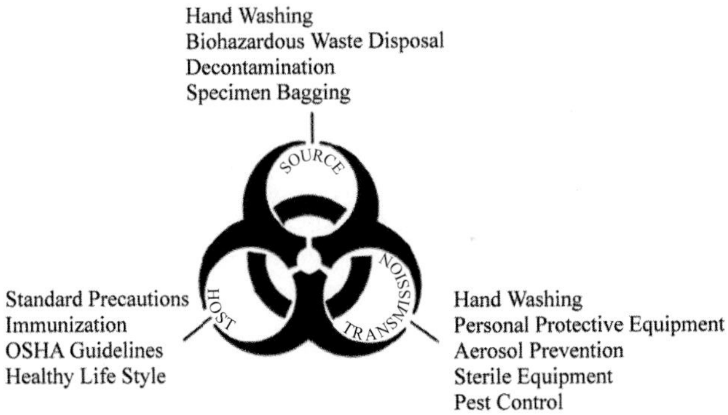

FIGURE 1–1 Chain of infection and safety practices related to the biohazard symbol. (Adapted from Strasinger and DiLorenzo,[5] p 63.)

before touching noncontaminated items and environmental surfaces, and before going to another patient, and wash hands immediately to avoid transfer of microorganisms to other patients or environments.

3. **Mask, eye protection, and face shield:** Wear a mask and eye protection or a face shield to protect mucous membranes of the eyes, nose, and mouth during procedures and patient-care activities that are likely to generate splashes or sprays of blood, body fluids, secretions, and excretions.
4. **Gown:** Wear a gown (a clean, nonsterile gown is adequate) to protect skin and to prevent soiling of clothing during procedures and patient-care activities that are likely to generate splashes or sprays of blood, body fluids, secretions, or excretions. Select a gown that is appropriate for the activity and the amount of fluid likely to be encountered. Remove a soiled gown as promptly as possible and wash hands to avoid the transfer of microorganisms to other patients or environments.
5. **Patient-care equipment:** Handle used patient-care equipment soiled with blood, body fluids, secretions, and excretions in a manner that prevents skin and mucous membrane exposures, contamination of clothing, and transfer of microorganisms to other patients or environments. Ensure that reusable equipment is not used for the care of another patient until it has been cleaned and reprocessed appropriately. Ensure that single-use items are discarded properly.
6. **Environmental control:** Ensure that the hospital has adequate procedures for the routine care, cleaning, and disinfection of environmental surfaces, beds, bedrails, bedside equipment, and other frequently touched surfaces and ensure that these procedures are being followed.
7. **Linen:** Handle, transport, and process linen soiled with blood, body fluids, secretions, and excretions in a manner that prevents skin and mucous membrane exposures and contamination of clothing and that avoids the transfer of microorganisms to other patients and environments.
8. **Occupational health and bloodborne pathogens:** Take care to prevent injuries when using needles, scalpels, and other sharp instruments or devices; when handling sharp instruments after procedures; when cleaning used instruments; and when disposing of used needles. Never recap used needles, or otherwise manipulate them using both hands, or use any other technique that involves directing the point of a needle toward any part of the body; rather, use either a one-handed "scoop" technique or a mechanical device designed for holding the needle sheath. Do not remove used needles from disposable syringes by hand, and do not bend, break, or otherwise manipulate used needles by hand. Place used disposable syringes and needles, scalpel blades, and other sharp items in appropriate puncture-resistant containers, which are located as close as practical to the area in which the items were used, and place reusable syringes and needles in a puncture-resistance container for transport to the reprocessing area. Use mouthpieces, resuscitation bags, or other ventilation devices as an alternative to mouth-to-mouth resuscitation methods in areas where the need for resuscitation is predictable.
9. **Patient placement:** Place a patient who contaminates the environment or who does not (or cannot be expected to) assist in maintaining appropriate hygiene or environment control in a private room. If a private room is not available, consult with infection control professionals regarding patient placement or other alternatives.

The Occupational Exposure to Blood-Borne Pathogens Standard is a law monitored and enforced by OSHA.[3] Specific requirements of this OSHA standard include the following:

1. Requiring all employees to practice UP/Standard Precautions
2. Providing laboratory coats, gowns, face and respiratory protection, and gloves to employees, and laundry facilities for nondisposable protective clothing
3. Providing sharps disposal containers and prohibiting recapping of needles
4. Prohibiting eating, drinking, and smoking, and applying cosmetics in the work area
5. Labeling all biohazardous material and containers
6. Providing free immunization for HBV
7. Establishing a daily disinfection protocol for work surfaces. The **disinfectant** of choice for bloodborne pathogens is sodium hypochlorite (household bleach diluted 1:10).
8. Providing medical follow-up for employees who have been accidentally exposed to bloodborne pathogens
9. Documenting regular training in safety standards for employees

PERSONAL PROTECTIVE EQUIPMENT

PPE used in the laboratory includes gloves, fluid-resistant gowns, eye and face shields, and Plexiglas countertop shields. Gloves should be worn when in contact with patients, specimens, and laboratory equipment or fixtures.

When specimens are collected, gloves must be changed between every patient. In the laboratory, they are changed whenever they become noticeably contaminated or damaged and are always removed when leaving the work area. Wearing gloves is not a substitute for handwashing, and hands must be washed after gloves are removed. A variety of gloves are available, including sterile and nonsterile, powdered and unpowdered, and latex and nonlatex. Allergy to latex is increasing among health-care workers, and laboratory workers should be alert for any allergy symptoms, such as redness or a rash after removing gloves. Should allergy symptoms occur, use of latex products must be avoided in the future.

Fluid-resistant laboratory coats with wrist cuffs are worn to protect clothing and skin from exposure to patients' body substances. They should always be completely buttoned, and gloves should be pulled over the cuffs. Coats are worn at all times when working with patient specimens and are removed prior to leaving the work area. They are changed when they become visibly soiled. Disposable coats are placed in containers for biohazardous waste and nondisposable coats in designated laundry receptacles.

The mucous membranes of the eyes, nose, and mouth must be protected from specimen splashes and aerosols. A variety of protective equipment is available, including goggles, full-face plastic shields, and Plexiglas countertop

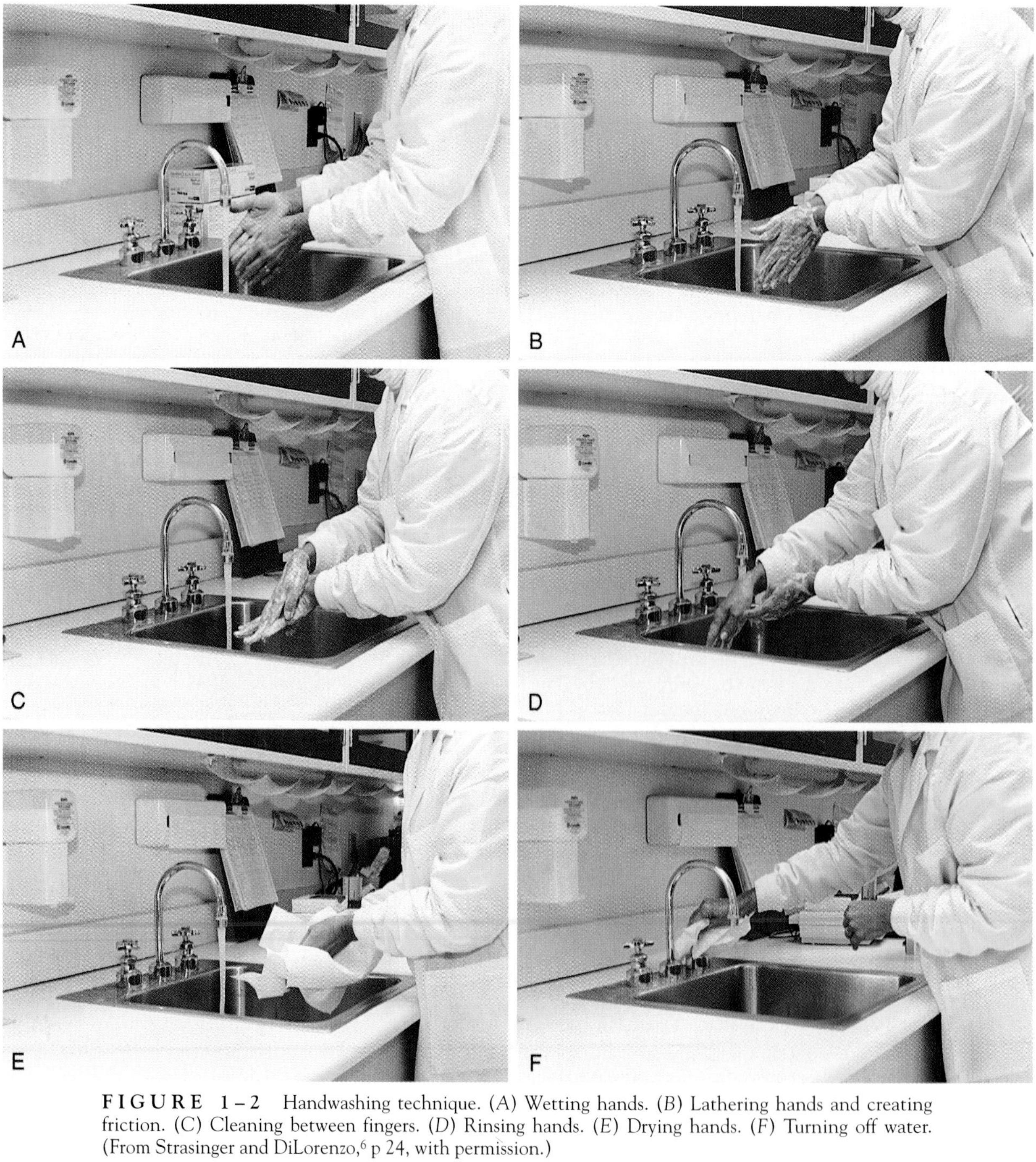

FIGURE 1–2 Handwashing technique. (*A*) Wetting hands. (*B*) Lathering hands and creating friction. (*C*) Cleaning between fingers. (*D*) Rinsing hands. (*E*) Drying hands. (*F*) Turning off water. (From Strasinger and DiLorenzo,[6] p 24, with permission.)

shields. Particular care should be taken to avoid splashes and aerosols when removing container tops, pouring specimens, and centrifuging specimens. Specimens must never be centrifuged in uncapped tubes or in uncovered centrifuges. Special precautions, which may include specimen rejection, must be taken when specimens are received in containers with contaminated exteriors.

HANDWASHING

Handwashing is emphasized in Figure 1–1 and in the Standard Precautions guidelines. Hand contact is the number-one method of infection transmission. Laboratory personnel must always wash hands after gloves are removed, prior to leaving the work area, at any time when hands have been knowingly contaminated, and before going to designated break areas, as well as before and after using bathroom facilities.

Correct handwashing technique is shown in Figure 1–2 and includes the following steps:

1. Wet hands with warm water.
2. Apply antimicrobial soap.
3. Rub to form a lather, create friction, and loosen debris.
4. Thoroughly clean between fingers, under fingernails and rings, and up to the wrist for at least 15 seconds.
5. Rinse hands in a downward position.
6. Dry with a paper towel.
7. Turn off faucets with the used paper towel to prevent recontamination.

DISPOSAL OF BIOLOGICAL WASTE

All biological waste, except urine, must be placed in appropriate containers labeled with the biohazard symbol (see Fig. 1–1). This includes not only specimens, but also the materials with which the specimens come in contact. The waste is then decontaminated following institutional policy: incineration, autoclaving, or pickup by a certified hazardous waste company.

Urine may be discarded by pouring it into a laboratory sink. Care must be taken to avoid splashing and the sink should be flushed with water after specimens are discarded. Disinfection of the sink using a 1:5 or 1:10 dilution of sodium hypochlorite should be performed on a daily basis. Sodium hypochlorite dilutions are effective for 1 week after preparation. The same solution also can be used for routinely disinfecting countertops and when accidental spills occur. Absorbent materials used for cleaning countertops and removing spills must be discarded in biohazard containers.

Sharp Hazards

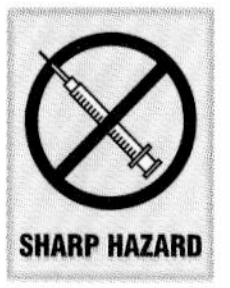

Sharp objects in the laboratory, including needles, lancets, and broken glassware, present a serious biological hazard, particularly for the transmission of bloodborne pathogens. All sharp objects must be disposed of in puncture-resistant containers, such as those shown in Figure 1–3. Puncture-resistant containers should be conveniently located within the work area.

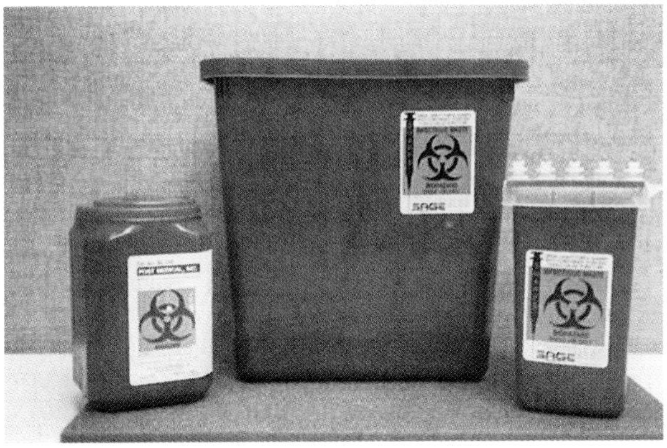

FIGURE 1–3 Examples of puncture-resistant containers. (From Strasinger and DiLorenzo,[5] p 67, with permission.)

Chemical Hazards

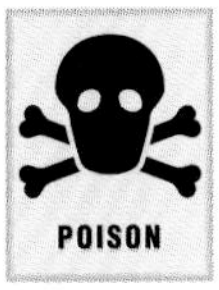

The same general rules for handling biohazardous materials apply to chemically hazardous materials; that is, to avoid getting these materials in or on bodies, clothes, or work area. Every chemical in the work place should be presumed hazardous.

CHEMICAL SPILLS

When skin contact occurs, the best first aid is to flush the area with large amounts of water. For this reason, all laboratory personnel should know the location of emergency showers and eye wash stations. Contaminated clothing should be removed as soon as possible. No attempt should be made to neutralize chemicals that come in contact with the skin. Chemical spill kits containing protective apparel, nonreactive absorbent material, and bags for disposal of contaminated materials should be available for cleaning up spills.

CHEMICAL HANDLING

Chemicals should never be mixed together, unless specific instructions are followed, and they must be added in the order specified. This is particularly important when combining acid and water; acid should always be added to water to avoid the possibility of sudden splashing. Wearing goggles and preparing reagents under a fume hood is a recommended safety precaution. Chemicals should be used from containers that are of an easily manageable size. Pipetting by mouth is unacceptable in the laboratory. State and federal regulations are in place for the disposal of chemicals and should be consulted.

CHEMICAL HYGIENE PLAN

OSHA also requires all facilities that use hazardous chemicals to have a written ***Chemical Hygiene Plan*** (CHP) available to employees.[4] The purpose of the plan is to detail the following:

1. Appropriate work practices
2. Standard operating procedures
3. Personal protective equipment

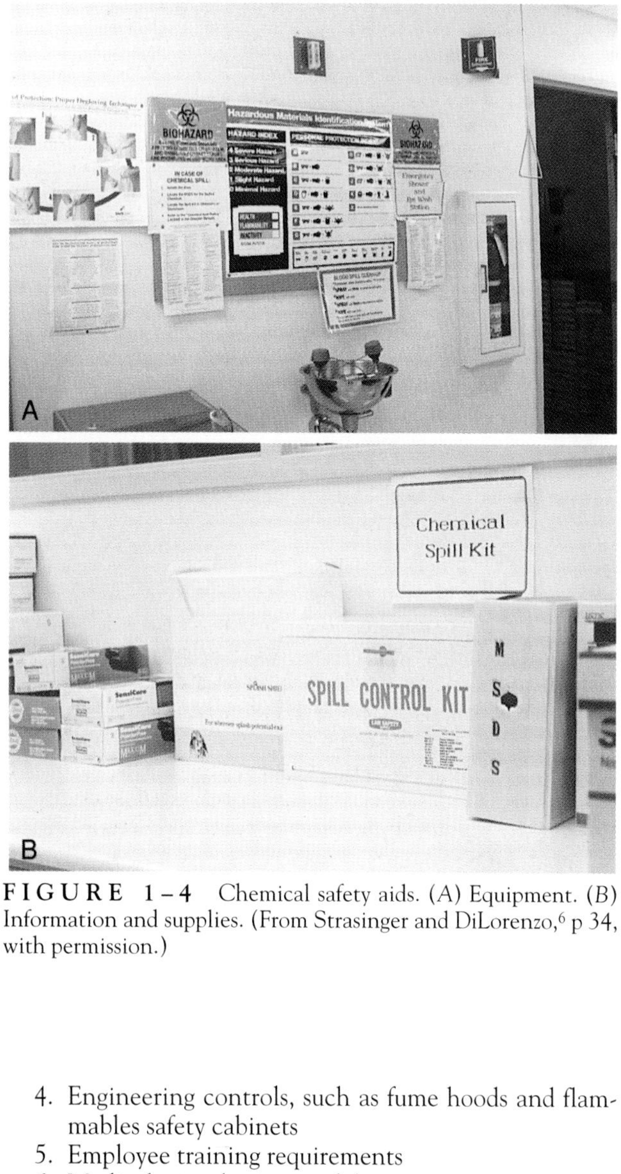

FIGURE 1–4 Chemical safety aids. (*A*) Equipment. (*B*) Information and supplies. (From Strasinger and DiLorenzo,[6] p 34, with permission.)

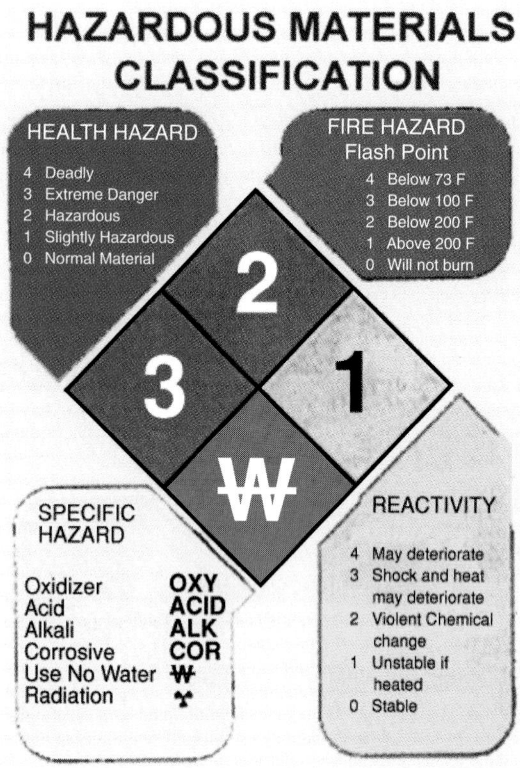

FIGURE 1–5 NFPA Hazardous material symbols.

4. Engineering controls, such as fume hoods and flammables safety cabinets
5. Employee training requirements
6. Medical consultation guidelines

Each facility must appoint a chemical hygiene officer, who is responsible for implementing and documenting compliance with the plan. Examples of required safety equipment and information are shown in Figure 1–4.

CHEMICAL LABELING

Hazardous chemicals should be labeled with a description of their particular hazard, such as poisonous, corrosive, or **carcinogenic**. The National Fire Protection Association (**NFPA**) has developed the Standard System for the Identification of the Fire Hazards of Materials, NFPA 704.[2] This symbol system is used to inform fire fighters of the hazards they may encounter with fires in a particular area. The diamond-shaped, color-coded symbol contains information relating to health, flammability, reactivity, and personal protection/special precautions. Each category is graded on a scale of 0 to 4, based on the degree of concern. These symbols are placed on doors, cabinets, and containers. An example of this system is shown in Figure 1–5.

MATERIAL DATA SAFETY SHEETS

The OSHA Federal Hazard Communication Standard requires that all employees have a right to know about all chemical hazards present in their workplace. The information is provided in the form of ***Material Safety Data Sheets*** **(MSDSs)** on file in the workplace. By law, vendors are required to provide these sheets to purchasers; however, the facility itself is responsible for obtaining and making MSDSs available to employees. Information contained in an MSDS includes the following:

1. Physical and chemical characteristics
2. Fire and explosion potential
3. Reactivity potential
4. Health hazards
5. Methods for safe handling

Radioactive Hazards

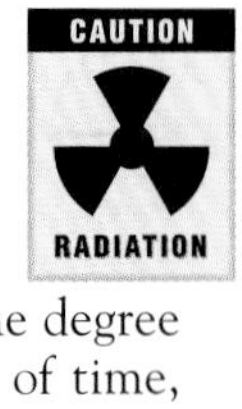

Radioactivity is encountered in the clinical laboratory when procedures using ***radioisotopes*** are performed. The amount of radioactivity present in the clinical laboratory is very small and represents little danger; however, the effects of radiation are cumulative related to the amount of exposure. The degree of radiation exposure is related to a combination of time,

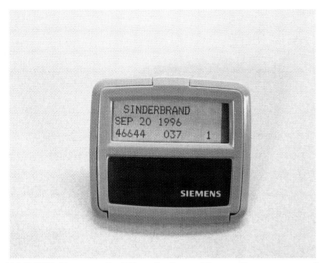

FIGURE 1–6 Film badge. (From Strasinger and DiLorenzo,[6] p 436, with permission.)

distance, and shielding. Persons working in a radioactive environment are required to wear measuring devices to determine the amount of radiation they are accumulating (Fig. 1–6).

Laboratory personnel should be familiar with the radioactive hazard symbol in the margin. This symbol must be displayed on the doors of all areas where radioactive material is present. Exposure to radiation during pregnancy presents a danger to the fetus; personnel who are pregnant, or think they may be, should avoid areas with this symbol.

Electrical Hazards

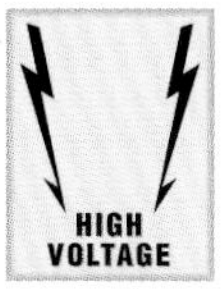

The laboratory setting contains a large amount of electrical equipment with which workers have frequent contact. The same general rules of electrical safety observed outside the workplace apply. The danger of water or fluid coming in contact with equipment is greater in the laboratory setting. Equipment should not be operated with wet hands. Designated hospital personnel closely monitor electrical equipment; however, laboratory personnel should continually observe for any dangerous conditions, such as frayed cords and overloaded circuits, and report them to the appropriate persons. Equipment that has become wet should be unplugged and allowed to dry completely before reusing. Equipment also should be unplugged before cleaning. All electrical equipment must be grounded with three-pronged plugs.

When an accident involving electrical shock occurs, the electrical source must be immediately removed. This must be done without touching the person or the equipment involved to avoid transference of the current to you. Turning off the circuit breaker, unplugging the equipment, or moving the equipment using a nonconductive glass or wood object are safe procedures to follow.

Fire/Explosive Hazards

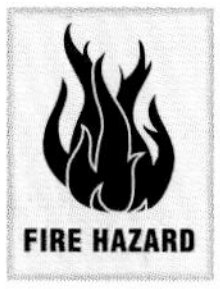

The Joint Commission on Accreditation of Healthcare Organizations **(JCAHO)** requires that all health-care institutions post evacuation routes and detailed plans to follow in the event of a fire. Laboratory personnel should be familiar with these procedures. When a fire is discovered, all employees are expected to take the actions outlined in the mnemonic RACE.

Rescue—rescue anyone in immediate danger.

Alarm—activate the institutional fire alarm system.

Contain—close all doors to potentially affected areas.

Extinguish—attempt to extinguish the fire, if possible.

As discussed previously, laboratory workers often use potentially volatile or explosive chemicals that require special procedures for their handling and storage. Flammable chemicals should be stored in safety cabinets and explosion-proof refrigerators, and cylinders of compressed gas should be located away from heat and securely fastened to a stationary device to prevent accidental capsizing. Fire blankets must be present in the laboratory. Persons with burning clothes should be wrapped in the blanket to smother the flames.

The NFPA classifies fires with regard to the type of burning material. It also classifies the type of fire extinguisher that is used to control them. This information is summarized in Table 1–2. The multipurpose ABC fire extinguishers are the most common, but the label should always be checked before using.

TABLE 1–2 Types of Fires and Fire Extinguishers

Fire Type	Composition of Fire	Type of Fire Extinguisher	Extinguishing Material
Class A	Wood, paper, or clothing	Class A	Water
Class B	Flammable organic chemicals	Class B	Dry chemicals, carbon dioxide, foam, or halon
Class C	Electrical	Class C	Dry chemicals, carbon dioxide, or halon
Class D	Combustible metals	None	Sand or dry powder
		Class ABC	Dry chemicals

From Strasinger and DiLorenzo,[5] p 70, with permission.

Physical Hazards

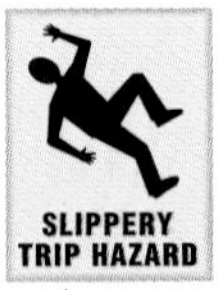

Physical hazards are not unique to the laboratory, and routine precautions observed outside the workplace apply. General precautions to consider are to avoid running in rooms and hallways, watch for wet floors, bend the knees when lifting heavy objects, keep long hair pulled back, avoid dangling jewelry, and maintain a clean, organized work area. Closed-toe shoes that provide maximum support are essential for safety and comfort.

REFERENCES

1. Centers for Disease Control and Prevention: Guideline for Isolation Precautions in Hospitals, Parts I and II. Available at: http://www.cdc.gov.
2. National Fire Protection Association: Hazardous Chemical Data, No. 49. Boston, NFPA, 1991.
3. Occupational Exposure to Blood-Borne Pathogens, Final Rule. Federal Register 29 (Dec 6), 1991.
4. Occupational Exposure to Hazardous Chemicals in Laboratories, Final Rule. Federal Register 55 (Jan 31), 1990.
5. Strasinger, SK, and DiLorenzo, MA: Phlebotomy Workbook for the Multiskilled Healthcare Professional. FA Davis, Philadelphia, 1996.
6. Strasinger, SK, and DiLorenzo, MA: Skills for the Patient Care Technician. FA Davis, Philadelphia, 1999.

STUDY QUESTIONS

1. List an example of each of the following health-care hazards that can be found in the clinical laboratory: biological, sharp, chemical, radioactive, electrical, fire/explosive, and physical.
2. List the three components of the chain of infection and give an example of each that could be found in the urinalysis laboratory.
3. What was the primary purpose for the CDC Universal Precautions guideline?
4. Which of the following guidelines provides the least protection for a person performing urinalysis? Why?
   a. Body substance isolation
   b. Universal Precautions
   c. Standard Precautions
5. A laboratory that fails to provide its employees with an adequate supply of gloves is in danger of being fined by ______________________________.
6. A laboratory worker notices a red rash on the hands after removing his or her gloves. Should the worker be concerned? Why or why not?
7. What is the purpose of a Plexiglas shield on the urinalysis laboratory counter?
8. For what two purposes is a paper towel used when washing the hands?
9. Name a biological waste that does not have to be discarded in a biohazard container.
10. A urine specimen is accidentally overturned on the countertop. Where should the towels used to absorb the spill be discarded? Describe an acceptable disinfectant.
11. What is the correct way to dispose of a glass cylinder that is broken while being cleaned?
12. When a caustic solution such as phenol is spilled on the skin, what is the recommended first aid?
13. When preparing a 1:10 dilution of hydrochloric acid, in what order should the hydrochloric acid and water be added? Why?
14. How can an employee learn the carcinogenic potential of phenol?
15. What are the locations of the following: MSDS, Chemical Hygiene Plan, and NFPA symbols.
16. What is the significance of an NFPA symbol labeled: 4 - 4 - 4 - ~~W~~?
17. When should a laboratory worker avoid performing tests using radioisotopes?
18. List three ways to remove the source of an electrical shock.
19. State the RACE actions to be performed when a fire is discovered.
20. What type of fire can be extinguished using water?

CHAPTER 2

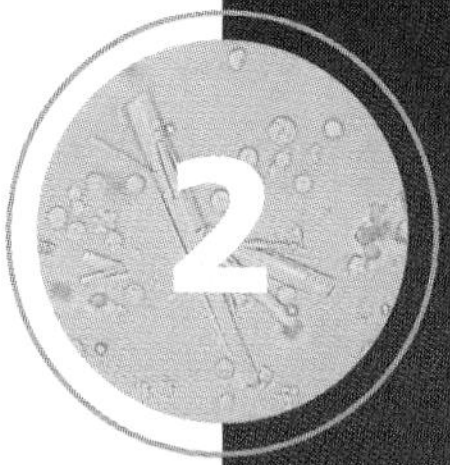

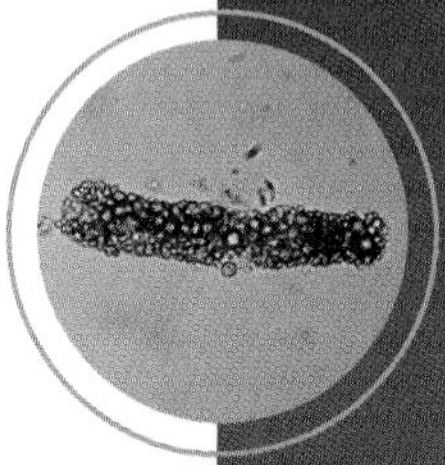

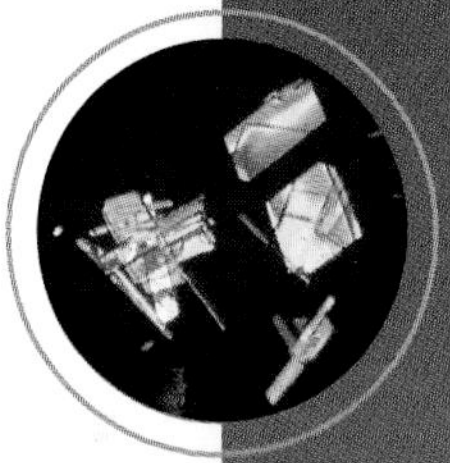

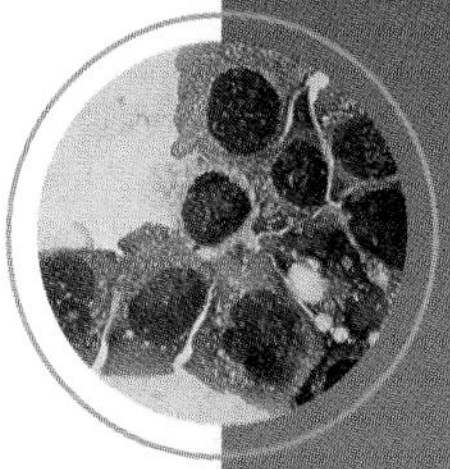

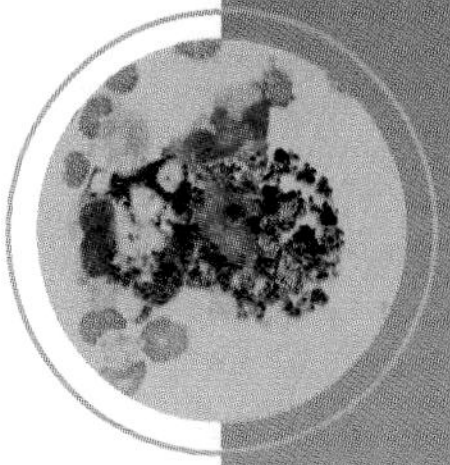

Renal Function

LEARNING OBJECTIVES

Upon completion of this chapter, the reader will be able to:

1 Identify the components of the nephron, kidney, and excretory system.
2 Trace the flow of blood through the nephron, and state the physiologic functions that occur.
3 Describe the process of glomerular ultrafiltration.
4 Discuss the functions and regulation of the renin-angiotensin-aldosterone system.
5 Differentiate between active and passive transport in relation to renal concentration.
6 Explain the function of antidiuretic hormone in the concentration of urine.
7 Describe the role of tubular secretion in maintaining acid-base balance.
8 Identify the laboratory procedures used to evaluate glomerular filtration, tubular reabsorption and secretion, and renal blood flow.
9 Discuss the advantages and disadvantages in using urea, inulin, creatinine, $beta_2$ microglobulin, and radionucleotides to measure glomerular filtration.
10 Given hypothetic laboratory data, calculate a creatinine clearance and determine whether the result is normal.
11 Discuss the clinical significance of the creatinine clearance test.
12 Define osmolarity and discuss its relationship to urine concentration.
13 Describe the basic principles of clinical osmometers.
14 Given hypothetic laboratory data, calculate a free-water clearance and interpret the result.
15 Given hypothetic laboratory data, calculate a PAH clearance and relate this result to renal blood flow.
16 Describe the relationship of urinary ammonia and titratable acidity to the production of an acidic urine.

KEY TERMS

active transport
aldosterone
maximal reabsorptive capacity
osmolarity
passive transport
podocytes
renal threshold
renal tubular acidosis
renin
renin-angiotension-aldosterone system
titratable acidity
tubular reabsorption
tubular secretion
vasopressin

This chapter reviews nephron anatomy and physiology and discusses its relationship to urinalysis and renal function testing. A section on laboratory assessment of renal function follows.

Renal Physiology

Each kidney contains approximately 1 to 1.5 million functional units called **nephrons**. As shown in Figure 2–1, the human kidney contains two types of nephrons. Cortical nephrons, which make up approximately 85% of nephrons, are situated primarily in the cortex of the kidney. Juxtamedullary nephrons have longer Henle's loops that extend deep into the medulla of the kidney.

The ability of the kidneys to selectively clear waste products from the blood and simultaneously maintain the body's essential water and electrolyte balances is controlled in the nephron by the following renal functions: renal blood flow, glomerular filtration, ***tubular reabsorption***, and ***tubular secretion***. The physiology, laboratory testing, and associated pathology of these four functions are discussed in this chapter.

RENAL BLOOD FLOW

The renal artery supplies blood to the kidney. Blood enters the capillaries of the nephron through the **afferent arteriole**. It then flows through the glomerulus and into the **efferent arteriole**. The varying sizes of these arterioles help to create the hydrostatic pressure differential important for glomerular filtration and also to maintain consistency of glomerular capillary pressure and renal blood flow within the glomerulus. Notice the smaller size of the efferent arteriole in Figure 2–2. This increases the glomerular capillary pressure.

Before returning to the renal vein, blood from the efferent arteriole enters the **peritubular capillaries** and the **vasa recta** and flows slowly through the cortex and medulla of the kidney close to the tubules. The peritubular capillaries surround the proximal and distal convoluted tubules, providing for the immediate reabsorption of essential substances from the fluid in the **proximal convoluted tubule** and final adjustment of the urinary composition in the **distal convoluted tubule**. The vasa recta are located adjacent to the ascending and descending **loop of Henle** in juxtamedullary nephrons. In this area, the major exchanges of water and salts take place between the blood and the **medullary interstitium**. The exchange of water and salts between the blood in the vasa recta and the medullary interstitium maintains the **osmotic gradient** (salt concentration) in the medulla that is necessary for renal concentration.

Based on an average body size of 1.73 m^2 of surface, the total renal blood flow is approximately 1200 mL/min and the total **renal plasma flow** ranges from 600 to 700 mL/min. Normal values for renal blood flow and renal function tests depend on body size. When dealing with sizes that vary greatly from the average 1.73 m^2 of body surface, a correction must be calculated to determine whether

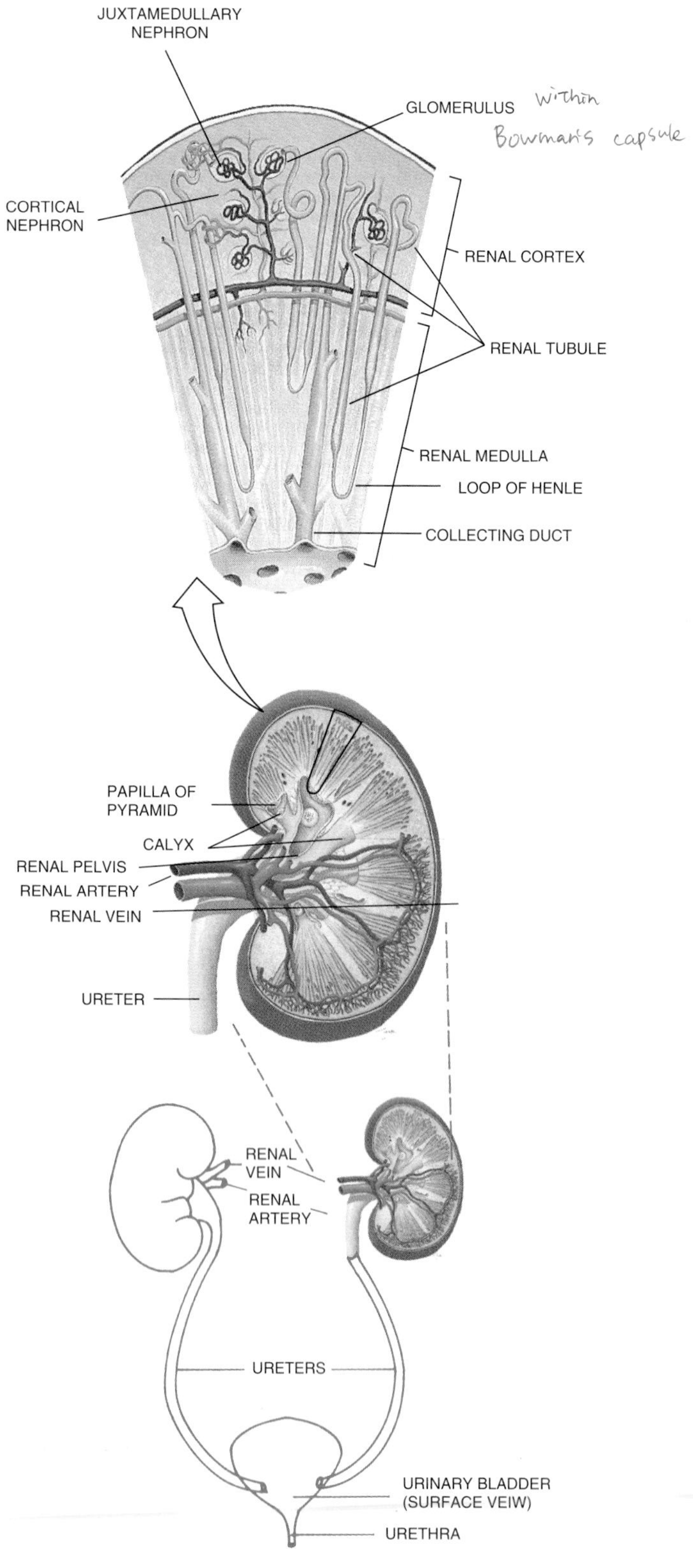

FIGURE 2–1 The relationship of the nephron to the kidney and excretory system. (From Scanlon, VC, and Sanders, T: Essentials of Anatomy and Physiology, ed 3. FA Davis, Philadelphia, 1999, p 405, with permission.)

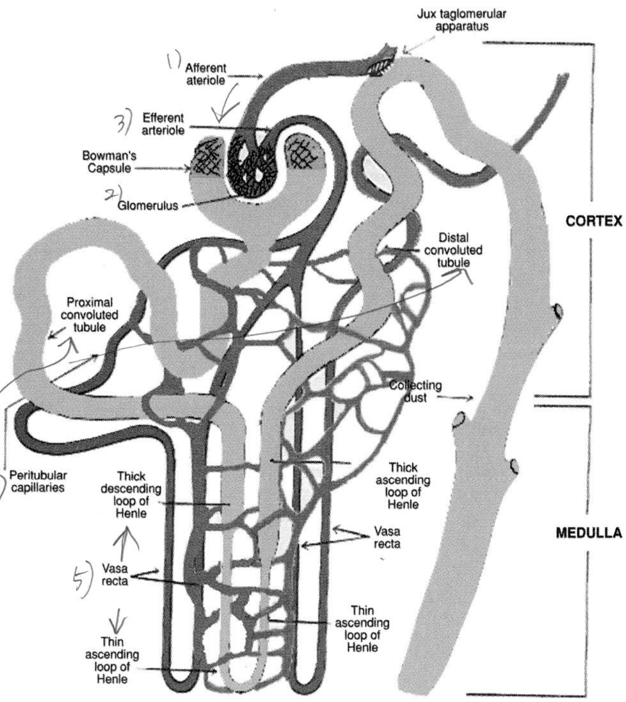

FIGURE 2–2 The nephron and its component parts.

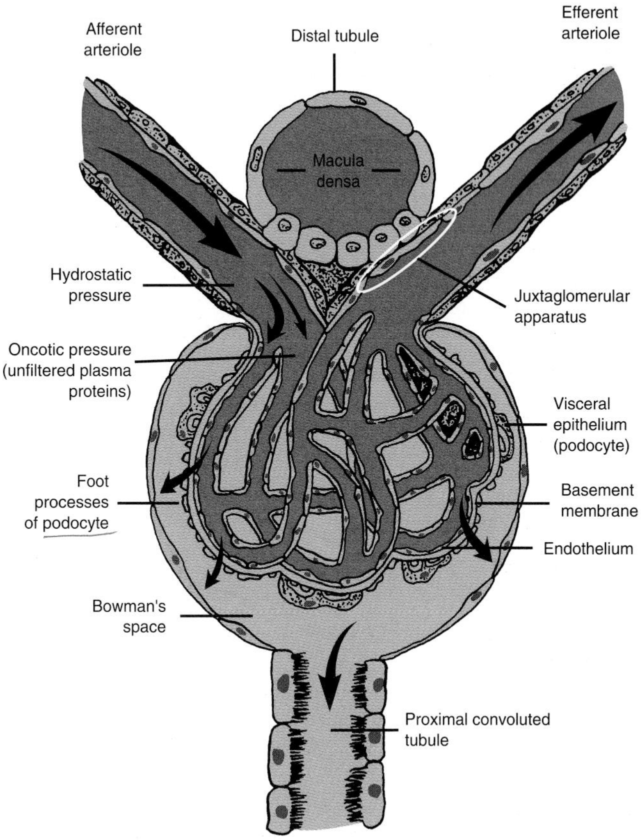

FIGURE 2–3 Factors affecting glomerular filtration in the renal corpuscle.

the observed measurements represent normal function. This calculation is covered in the discussion on tests for **glomerular filtration rate** later in this chapter. Variations in normal values also have been published for different age groups and should be considered when evaluating renal function studies.

GLOMERULAR FILTRATION

The **glomerulus** consists of a coil of approximately eight capillary lobes referred to collectively as the capillary tuft. It is located within **Bowman's capsule** and forms the beginning of the renal tubule. Although the glomerulus serves as a nonselective filter of plasma substances with molecular weights of less than 70,000, several factors influence the actual filtration process. These include the cellular structure of the capillary walls and Bowman's capsule, **hydrostatic** and **oncotic pressures**, and the feedback mechanisms of the ***renin-angiotensin-aldosterone system***. Figure 2–3 provides a diagrammatic view of the glomerular areas influenced by these factors.

Plasma filtrate must pass through three cellular layers: the capillary wall membrane, the basement membrane (basal lamina), and the visceral epithelium of Bowman's capsule. The endothelial cells of the capillary wall differ from those in other capillaries by containing pores and are referred to as fenestrated. The pores increase capillary permeability but do not allow the passage of large molecules and blood cells. Further restriction of large molecules occurs as the filtrate passes through the basement membrane and the thin membranes covering the filtration slits formed by the intertwining foot processes of the ***podocytes*** of the inner layer of Bowman's capsule (see Fig. 2–3).

As mentioned previously, the presence of hydrostatic pressure resulting from the smaller size of the efferent arteriole and the glomerular capillaries enhances filtration. This pressure is necessary to overcome the opposition of pressures from the fluid within Bowman's capsule and the oncotic pressure of unfiltered plasma proteins in the glomerular capillaries. By increasing or decreasing the size of the afferent arteriole, an autoregulatory mechanism within the kidney maintains the glomerular blood pressure at a relatively constant rate regardless of fluctuations in systemic blood pressure. Dilation of the afferent arterioles when blood pressure drops prevents a marked decrease in blood flowing through the kidney, thus preventing an increase in the blood level of toxic waste products.

The renin-angiotensin-aldosterone system controls the regulation of the flow of blood to and within the kidney. The system responds to changes in blood pressure and plasma sodium content that are monitored by the **juxtaglomerular apparatus**, which consists of the juxtaglomerular cells in the afferent arteriole and the **macula densa** of the distal convoluted tubule (see Fig. 2–2). Low plasma sodium content decreases water retention within the circulatory system, resulting in a decreased overall blood volume

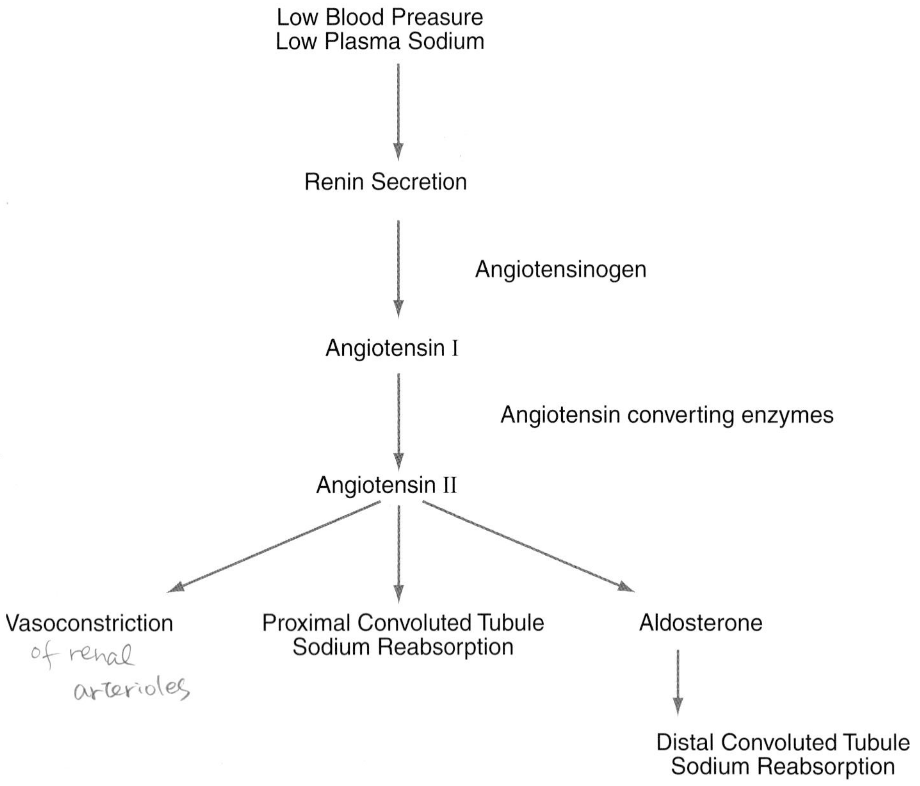

FIGURE 2–4 Actions of the renin-angiotensin-aldosterone system.

and subsequent decrease in blood pressure. When the juxtaglomerular apparatus senses such changes, a cascade of reactions within the renin-angiotensin-aldosterone system occurs (Figure 2–4). ***Renin***, an enzyme produced by the juxtaglomerular apparatus, is secreted and reacts with the bloodborne substrate angiotensinogen to produce the inert hormone angiotensin I. As angiotensin I passes through the lungs, converting enzymes change it to the active form angiotensin II. Angiotensin II corrects renal blood flow in the following three ways: causing vasoconstriction of the renal arterioles, stimulating reabsorption of sodium in the proximal convoluted tubule, and triggering the release of the sodium-retaining hormone ***aldosterone*** from the adrenal cortex. As systemic blood pressure and plasma sodium content increase, the secretion of renin decreases. Therefore, the actions of angiotensin II produce a constant pressure within the nephron.

As a result of the above glomerular mechanisms, every minute approximately 2 to 3 million glomeruli filter approximately 120 mL of water-containing low-molecular-weight substances. Because this filtration is nonselective, the only difference between the compositions of the filtrate and the plasma is the absence of plasma protein, any protein-bound substances, and cells. Analysis of the fluid as it leaves the glomerulus shows the filtrate to have a specific gravity of 1.010 and confirms that it is chemically an ultrafiltrate of plasma. This information provides a useful baseline for evaluating the renal mechanisms involved in converting the plasma ultrafiltrate into the final urinary product.

TUBULAR REABSORPTION

The body cannot lose 120 mL of water-containing essential substances every minute. Therefore, when the plasma ultrafiltrate enters the proximal convoluted tubule, the kidney, through cellular transport mechanisms, begins reabsorbing these essential substances and water (Table 2–1).

The cellular mechanisms involved in tubular reabsorption are termed ***active*** and ***passive transport***. For active transport to occur, the substance to be reabsorbed must combine with a carrier protein contained in the membranes of the renal tubular cells. The electrochemical energy created by this interaction transfers the substance across the cell membranes and back into the bloodstream. Active transport is responsible for the reabsorption of glucose, amino acids, and salts in the proximal convoluted tubule and the reabsorption of chloride in the ascending loop of Henle and sodium in the distal convoluted tubule.

Passive transport is the movement of molecules across a membrane as a result of differences in their concentration or electrical potential on opposite sides of the membrane. These physical differences are called gradients. Passive reabsorption of water takes place in all parts of the nephron except the ascending loop of Henle, the walls of which are impermeable to water. Urea is passively reabsorbed in the proximal convoluted tubule and the ascending loop of Henle, and passive reabsorption of sodium accompanies the active transport of chloride in the ascending loop of Henle.

TABLE 2–1 **Tubular Reabsorption**

	Substance	Location
Active transport	Glucose, amino acids, and salts	Proximal convoluted tubule
	Chloride	Ascending loop of Henle
	Sodium	Distal convoluted tubule
Passive transport	Water	Proximal convoluted tubule, descending loop of Henle, and collecting tubules
	Urea	Proximal convoluted tubule and ascending loop of Henle
	Sodium	Ascending loop of Henle

Active transport, like passive transport, can be influenced by the concentration of the substance being transported. When the plasma concentration of a substance that is normally completely reabsorbed reaches an abnormally high level, the filtrate concentration exceeds the ***maximal reabsorptive capacity*** **(Tm)** of the tubules, and the substance begins appearing in the urine. The plasma concentration at which active transport stops is termed the ***renal threshold***. For glucose, the renal threshold is 160 to 180 mg/dL, and glucose appears in the urine when the plasma concentration reaches this level. Knowledge of the renal threshold and the plasma concentration can be used to distinguish between excess solute filtration and renal tubular damage. For example, glucose appearing in the urine of a person with a normal blood glucose level is the result of tubular damage and not diabetes mellitus.

Active transport of more than two-thirds of the filtered sodium out of the proximal convoluted tubule is accompanied by the passive reabsorption of an equal amount of water. Therefore, as can be seen in Figure 2–5, the fluid leaving the proximal convoluted tubule still maintains the same concentration as the ultrafiltrate.

Renal concentration begins in the descending and ascending loop of Henle, where the filtrate is exposed to the high osmotic gradient of the renal medulla. Water is removed by osmosis in the descending loop of Henle, and sodium and chloride are reabsorbed in the ascending loop of Henle. Excessive reabsorption of water as the filtrate passes through the highly concentrated medulla is prevented by the water-impermeable walls of the ascending loop. This selective reabsorption process is called the **countercurrent mechanism** and serves to maintain the osmotic gradient of the medulla. The sodium and chloride leaving the filtrate in the ascending loop prevent dilution of the medullary interstitium by the water reabsorbed from the descending loop. Maintenance of this osmotic gradient is essential for the final concentration of the filtrate when it reaches the **collecting duct**.

In Figure 2–5, the actual concentration of the filtrate leaving the ascending loop of Henle is quite low owing to the reabsorption of salt and not water in that part of the tubule. Reabsorption of sodium continues in the distal convoluted tubule, but it is now under the control of the hormone aldosterone, which regulates reabsorption in response to the body's need for sodium.

The final concentration of the filtrate through the reabsorption of water begins in the late distal convoluted tubule and continues in the collecting duct. Reabsorption depends on the osmotic gradient in the medulla and the hormone ***vasopressin*** (antidiuretic hormone **[ADH]**). One would expect that as the dilute filtrate in the collecting duct comes in contact with the higher osmotic concentration of the medullary interstitium, passive reabsorption of water would occur. However, the process is controlled by the presence or absence of ADH, which renders the walls of the distal convoluted tubule and collecting duct permeable or impermeable to water. A high level of ADH increases permeability, resulting in increased reabsorption of water and a low-volume, concentrated urine. Likewise, absence of ADH renders the walls impermeable to water, resulting in a large volume of dilute urine. Just as the production of aldosterone is controlled by the body's sodium concentration, production of ADH is determined by the state of body hydration. Therefore, the chemical balance in the body is actually the final determinant of urine volume and concentration. The concept of ADH control can be summarized in the following manner:

↑Body Hydration = ↓ADH = ↑Urine Volume
↓Body Hydration = ↑ADH = ↓Urine Volume

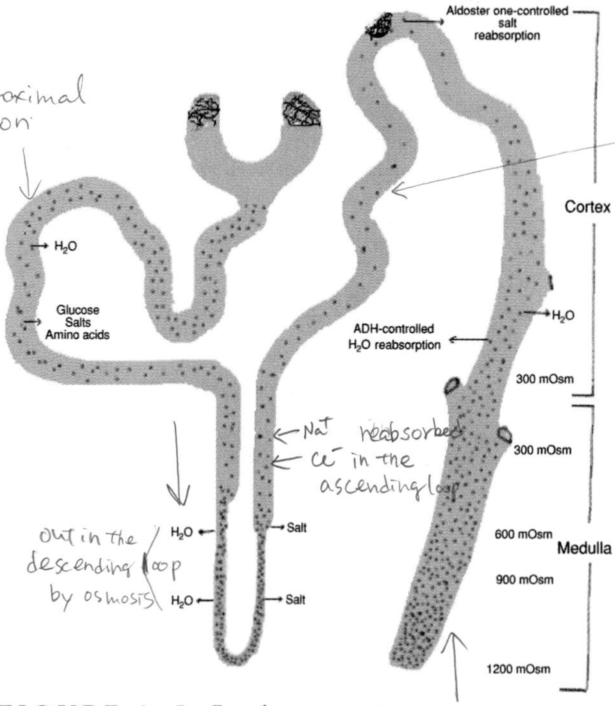

FIGURE 2–5 Renal concentration.

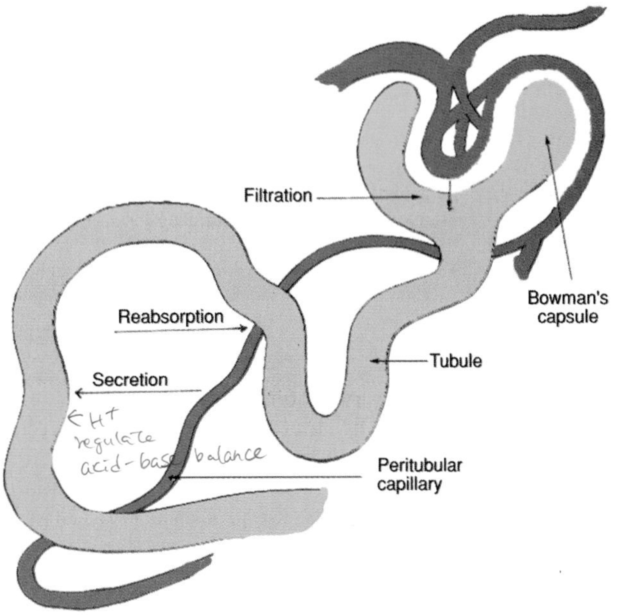

FIGURE 2-6 The movement of substances in the nephron.

TUBULAR SECRETION

In contrast to tubular reabsorption, in which substances are removed from the glomerular filtrate and returned to the blood, tubular secretion involves the passage of substances from the blood in the peritubular capillaries to the tubular filtrate (Figure 2–6). Tubular secretion serves two major functions: elimination of waste products not filtered by the glomerulus and regulation of the acid-base balance in the body through the secretion of hydrogen ions.

Many foreign substances, such as medications, cannot be filtered by the glomerulus because they are bound to plasma proteins. However, when these protein-bound substances enter the peritubular capillaries, they develop a strong affinity for the tubular cells and dissociate from their carrier proteins, which results in their transport into the filtrate by the tubular cells. The major site for removal of these nonfiltered substances is the proximal convoluted tubule.

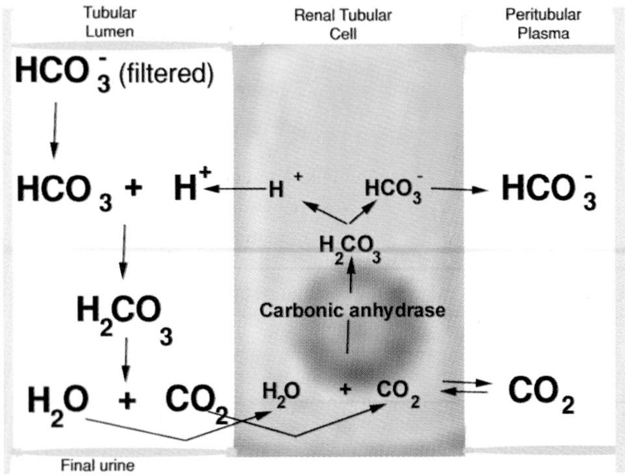

FIGURE 2-7 Reabsorption of filtered bicarbonate.

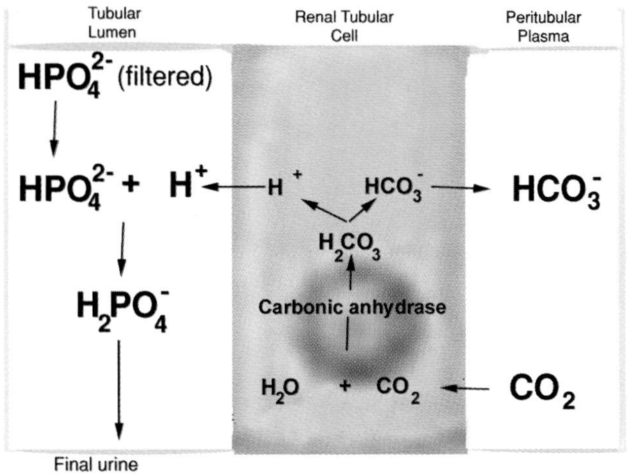

FIGURE 2-8 Excretion of secreted hydrogen ions combined with phosphate.

To maintain the normal blood pH of 7.4, the blood must buffer and eliminate the excess acid formed by dietary intake and body metabolism. The buffering capacity of the blood depends on bicarbonate (HCO_3^-) ions, which are readily filtered by the glomerulus and must be expediently returned to the blood to maintain the proper pH. As shown in Figure 2–7, the secretion of hydrogen ions by the renal tubular cells into the filtrate prevents the filtered bicarbonate from being excreted in the urine and causes the return of a bicarbonate ion to the plasma. This process provides for almost 100 percent reabsorption of filtered bicarbonate and occurs primarily in the proximal convoluted tubule.

The actual excretion of excess hydrogen ions also depends on tubular secretion. Figures 2–8 and 2–9 are diagrams of the two primary methods for hydrogen ion excretion in the urine. In Figure 2–8, the secreted hydrogen ion combines with a filtered phosphate ion instead of a bicarbonate ion and is excreted rather than reabsorbed. Additional excretion of hydrogen ions is accomplished through their reaction with ammonia produced and secreted by the cells of the distal convoluted tubule (see Fig. 2–9). The resulting ammonium ion is excreted in the urine.

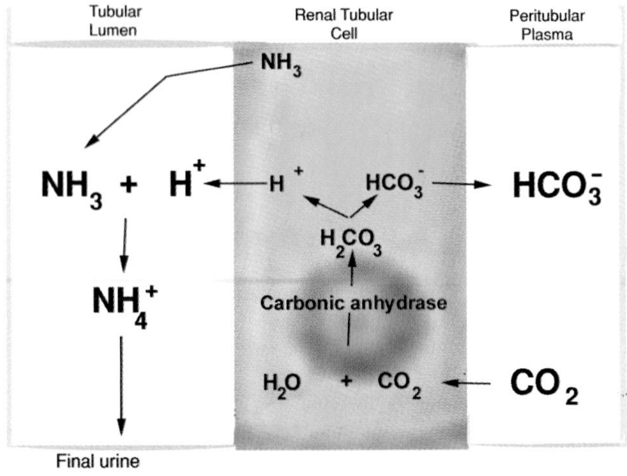

FIGURE 2-9 Excretion of secreted hydrogen ions combined with ammonia produced by the tubules.

All three of these processes are occurring simultaneously at rates determined by the acid-base balance in the body. A disruption in these secretory functions can result in **metabolic acidosis** or ***renal tubular acidosis***, the inability to produce an acid urine.

Renal Function Tests

This brief review of renal physiology shows that there are many metabolic functions and chemical interactions to be evaluated through laboratory tests of renal function. In Figure 2–10, the parts of the nephron are related to the laboratory tests used to assess their function.

GLOMERULAR FILTRATION TESTS

The standard test used to measure the filtering capacity of the glomeruli is the clearance test. As its name implies, a clearance test measures the rate at which the kidneys are able to remove (to clear) a filterable substance from the blood. To ensure that glomerular filtration is being accurately measured, the substance analyzed must be one that is neither reabsorbed nor secreted by the tubules. Other factors to consider in the selection of a clearance test substance include the stability of the substance in urine during a possible 24-hour collection period, the consistency of the plasma level, the substance's availability to the body, and the availability of tests for chemical analysis of the substance.

Clearance Tests

The earliest glomerular filtration tests measured urea because of its presence in all urine specimens and the existence of routinely used methods of chemical analysis. Because approximately 40 percent of the filtered urea is reabsorbed, normal values were adjusted to reflect the reabsorption, and patients were hydrated to produce a urine flow of 2 mL/min to ensure that no more than 40 percent of the urea was reabsorbed. At present, the use of urea as a test substance for glomerular filtration has been replaced by the measurement of either **creatinine**, **inulin**, **beta$_2$ microglobulin**, or radioisotopes.

Inulin, a polymer of fructose, is an extremely stable substance that is not reabsorbed or secreted by the tubules. It is not a normal body constituent, however, and must be infused at a constant rate throughout the testing period. A test that requires an infused substance is termed an **exogenous procedure** and is seldom the method of choice if a suitable test substance is already present in the body (**endogenous procedure**). Therefore, inulin has not been routinely used for glomerular filtration testing.

The development of simplified procedures measuring the plasma disappearance of infused substances, thereby eliminating the need for urine collection, has enhanced interest in exogenous procedures.[3,17] Injection of radionucleotides provides not only a method for determining glomerular filtration through the plasma disappearance of the radioactive material but also enables visualization of the filtration in one or both kidneys.[4]

Good correlation between the glomerular filtration rate and plasma levels of beta$_2$ microglobulin has been demonstrated. Beta$_2$ microglobulin (molecular weight 11,800) dissociates from human leukocyte antigens at a constant rate and is rapidly removed from the plasma by glomerular filtration. Sensitive methods using radioimmunoassay and enzyme immunoassay are available for the measurement of beta$_2$ microglobulin.[14] A rise in the plasma level of beta$_2$ microglobulin has been shown to be a more sensitive indicator of a decrease in glomerular filtration rate than the **creatinine clearance**. However, the test is not reliable in patients who have a history of immunologic disorders or malignancy.[13]

Currently, routine laboratory measurements of glomerular filtration rate employ creatinine as the test substance. Creatinine, a waste product of muscle metabolism that is normally found at a relatively constant level in the blood, provides the laboratory with an endogenous procedure for evaluating glomerular function. The use of creatinine has several disadvantages not found with inulin, and careful consideration should be given to them. Disadvantages are as follows:

1. Some creatinine is secreted by the tubules, and secretion increases as blood levels rise.
2. Chromogens present in human plasma react in the chemical analysis. Their presence, however, may help counteract the falsely elevated rates caused by tubular secretion.
3. Bacteria will break down urinary creatinine if specimens are kept at room temperature for extended periods.[15]
4. A diet heavy in meat consumed during collection of a 24-hour urine specimen will influence the results if the plasma specimen is drawn prior to the collection period.[11]

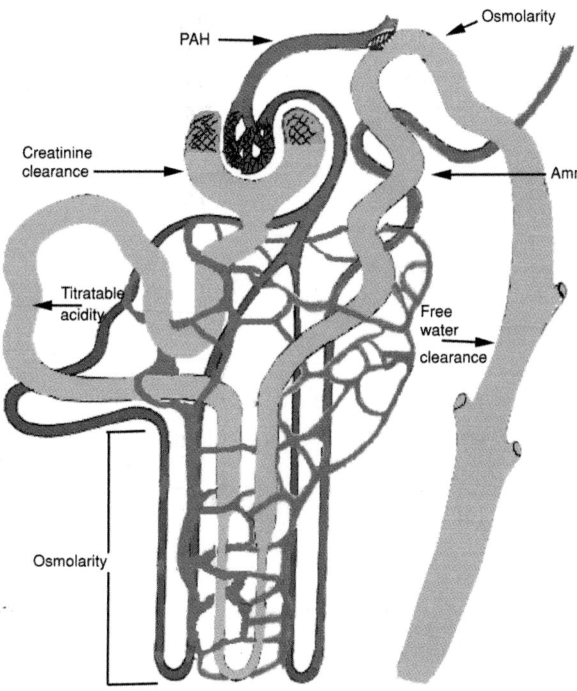

FIGURE 2–10 The relationship of nephron areas to renal function tests.

5. Measurement of creatinine clearance is not a reliable indicator in patients suffering from muscle-wasting diseases.[16]

Because of these drawbacks, abnormal results may be followed up with more sophisticated tests, but the creatinine clearance test can provide the routine clinical laboratory with a method to screen the glomerular filtration rate.

Calculations

By far the greatest source of error in any clearance procedure is the use of improperly timed urine specimens. The importance of using an accurately timed specimen (see Chap. 3) will become evident in the following discussion of the calculations involved in converting isolated laboratory measurements to glomerular filtration rate. The glomerular filtration rate is reported in milliliters per minute; therefore, determining the number of milliliters of plasma from which the clearance substance (creatinine) is completely removed during 1 minute is necessary. To calculate this information, one must know urine volume in milliliters per minute (V), urine creatinine concentration in milligrams per deciliter (U), and plasma creatinine concentration in milligrams per deciliter (P).

The urine volume is calculated by dividing the number of milliliters in the specimen by the number of minutes used to collect the specimen.

EXAMPLE

Calculate the urine volume (V) for a 2-hour specimen measuring 240 mL:

$$2 \text{ hours} \times 60 \text{ minutes} = 120 \text{ minutes}$$

$$\frac{240 \text{ mL}}{120 \text{ minutes}} = 2 \text{ mL/min} \quad V = 2 \text{ mL/min}$$

The plasma and urine concentrations are determined by chemical testing. The standard formula used to calculate the milliliters of plasma cleared per minute (C) is:

$$C = \frac{UV}{P}$$

This formula is derived as follows. The milliliters of plasma cleared per minute (C) times the milligrams per deciliter of plasma creatinine (P) must equal the milligrams per deciliter of urine creatinine (U) times the urine volume in milliliters per minute (V), because all of the filtered creatinine will appear in the urine. Therefore,

$$CP = UV \text{ and } C = \frac{UV}{P}$$

EXAMPLE

Using urine creatinine of 120 mg/dL (U), plasma creatinine of 1.0 mg/dL (P), and urine volume of 1440 mL obtained from a 24-hour specimen (V), calculate the glomerular filtration rate.

$$V = \frac{1440 \text{ mL}}{60 \text{ minutes} \times 24 = 1440 \text{ minutes}} = 1 \text{ mL/min}$$

$$C = \frac{120 \text{ mg/dL (U)} \times 1 \text{ mL/min (V)}}{1.0 \text{ mg/dL (P)}} = 120 \text{ mL/min}$$

By analyzing this calculation and referring to Figure 2–11, one can see that at a 1 mg/dL concentration, each milliliter of plasma contains 0.01 mg creatinine. Therefore, to arrive at a urine concentration of 120 mg/dL (1.2 mg/mL), it would be necessary to clear 120 mL of plasma. Although the filtrate volume is reduced, the amount of creatinine in the filtrate does not change.

Knowing that in the average person (1.73 m^2 body surface) the approximate amount of plasma filtrate produced per minute is 120 mL, it is not surprising that normal creatinine clearance values approach 120 mL/min (men, 107 to 139 mL/min; women, 87 to 107 mL/min). The normal plasma creatinine is 0.5 to 1.5 mg/dL. These normal values take into account variations in size and muscle mass. Values are considerably lower in older people, however, and an adjustment also may have to be made to the calculation when dealing with body sizes that deviate greatly from 1.73 m^2 of surface, such as in children. To adjust a clearance for body size, the formula is:

$$C = \frac{UV}{P} \times \frac{1.73}{A}$$

with A being the actual body size in square meters of surface. The actual body size may be calculated as:

$$\log A = (0.425 \times \log \text{weight}) + (0.725 \times \log \text{height}) - 2.144$$

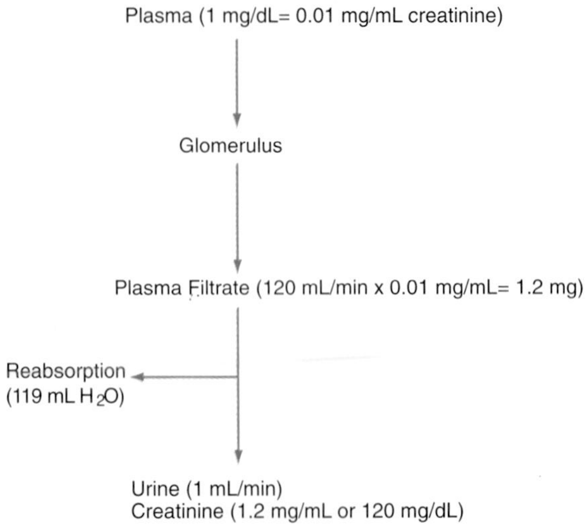

FIGURE 2–11 A diagram representing creatinine filtration and excretion.

or it may be obtained from the nomogram shown in Figure 2–12.

Clinical Significance

When interpreting the results of a creatinine clearance test, one must keep in mind that the glomerular filtration rate is determined not only by the number of functioning nephrons but also by the functional capacity of these nephrons. In other words, even though one-half of the available nephrons may be nonfunctional, a change in the glomerular filtration rate will not occur if the remaining nephrons double their filtering capacity. This is evidenced by those persons who lead normal lives with only one kidney. Therefore, although the creatinine clearance is a frequently requested laboratory procedure, its value does not lie in the detection of early renal disease. Instead, it is used to determine the extent of nephron damage in known cases of renal disease, to monitor the effectiveness of treatment designed to prevent further nephron damage, and to determine the feasibility of administering medications, which can build up to dangerous blood levels if the glomerular filtration rate is markedly reduced.

When medications need to be prescribed prior to waiting for collection of a 24-hour urine specimen, formulas have been developed to predict the creatinine clearance from the serum creatinine. Variables included in the formulas are age, sex, and weight. The most frequently used formula is by Cockcroft and Gault:[6]

$$C_{cr} = \frac{(140 - \text{age})(\text{weight in kilograms})}{72 \times \text{serum creatinine in milligrams per deciliter}}$$

Because the average male weight is approximately 72 kg, the formula can be simplified to:

$$C_{cr} = \frac{140 - \text{age}}{\text{serum creatinine in milligrams per deciliter}}$$

The results are multiplied by 0.85 for female patients. Figures in the formula were obtained by regression analysis of performed and calculated creatinine clearances on 249 male subjects ranging in age from 18 to 92 years.

EXAMPLE

A 50-year-old man has a serum creatinine of 1.1 mg/dL. Calculate his creatinine clearance.

$$\frac{140 - 50}{1.1} = \frac{90}{1.1} = 81.8 \text{ mL/min}$$

This is a reasonable clearance for someone 50 years of age.

TUBULAR REABSORPTION TESTS

Whereas measurement of the glomerular filtration rate is not a useful indication of early renal disease, the loss of tubular reabsorption capability is often the first function affected in renal disease. This is not surprising when one considers the complexity of the tubular reabsorption process.

Tests to determine the ability of the tubules to reabsorb the essential salts and water that have been nonselectively filtered by the glomerulus are collectively termed concentration tests. As mentioned previously, the ultrafiltrate that enters the tubules has a specific gravity of 1.010; therefore, after reabsorption one would expect the final urine product to be more concentrated. However, from our experience in performing routine urinalysis, we know that many specimens do not have a specific gravity higher than 1.010, yet no renal disease is present. This is because urine concentration is largely determined by the body's state of hydration, and the normal kidney will reabsorb only the amount of

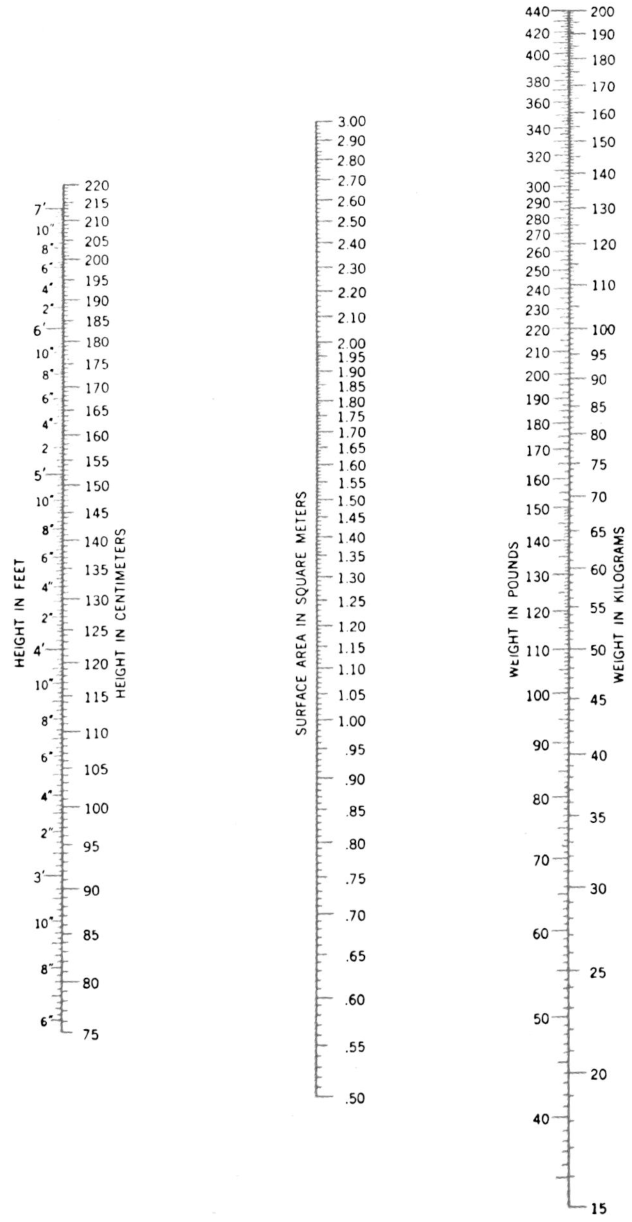

FIGURE 2–12 A nomogram for the determination of body surface area. (From Boothby, WM, and Sandiford, RB: Nomogram for determination of body surface area. N Engl J Med 185:227, 1921, with permission.)

water necessary to preserve an adequate supply of body water.

As can be seen in Figure 2–13, both specimens contain the same amount of solute; however, the urine density (specific gravity) of patient A will be higher. Therefore, control of fluid intake must be incorporated into laboratory tests that measure the concentrating ability of the kidney.

Throughout the years, various methods have been used to produce water deprivation, including the Fishberg and Mosenthal concentration tests that measured specific gravity. In the Fishberg test, patients were deprived of fluids for 24 hours prior to measuring specific gravity. The Mosenthal test compared the volume and specific gravity of day and night urine samples to evaluate concentrating ability. Neither test is in use today because the information provided by specific gravity measurements is most useful as a screening procedure and quantitative measurement of renal concentrating ability is best assessed through osmometry. However, persons with normal concentrating ability should have a specific gravity of 1.025 when deprived of fluids for 16 hours. Following overnight water deprivation a urine ***osmolarity*** of 800 mOsm or above indicates normal concentrating ability. Osmometry is particularly essential when evaluating neonates.[1,2]

Osmolarity

Specific gravity depends on the number of particles present in a solution and the density of these particles, whereas osmolarity is affected only by the number of particles present. When evaluating renal concentration ability, the substances of interest are small molecules, primarily sodium (molecular weight, 23) and chloride (molecular weight, 35.5). However, urea (molecular weight, 60), which is of no importance to this evaluation, will contribute more to the specific gravity than will the sodium and chloride molecules. Because all three molecules contribute equally to the osmolarity of the specimen, a more representative measure of renal concentrating ability can be obtained by measuring osmolarity.

An osmole is defined as 1 g molecular weight of a substance divided by the number of particles into which it dissociates. A nonionizing substance such as glucose (molecular weight, 180) contains 180 g per osmole, whereas sodium chloride (**NaCl**) (molecular weight, 58.5), if completely dissociated, contains 29.25 g per osmole. Just as we have the terms molality and molarity, we also have osmolality and osmolarity. An osmolal solution of glucose has 180 g of glucose dissolved in 1 kg of solvent, and an osmolar solution has 180 g of glucose dissolved in 1 L of solvent. In the clinical laboratory, the terms are used interchangeably, inasmuch as the difference under normal temperature conditions with water as the solvent is minimal. The unit of measure used in the clinical laboratory is the milliosmole (**mOsm**), because it is not practical when dealing with body fluids to use a measurement as large as the osmole (23 g of sodium per liter or kilogram).

The osmolarity of a solution can be determined by measuring a property that is mathematically related to the number of particles in the solution (colligative property) and comparing this value with the value obtained from the pure solvent. Solute dissolved in solvent causes the following changes in colligative properties: lower freezing point, higher boiling point, increased osmotic pressure, and lower vapor pressure.

Because water is the solvent in both urine and plasma, the number of particles present in a sample can be determined by comparing a colligative property value of the sample with that of pure water. Clinical laboratory instruments are available to measure freezing point depression and vapor pressure depression.

Freezing Point Osmometers

Measurement of freezing point depression was the first principle incorporated into clinical osmometers, and many

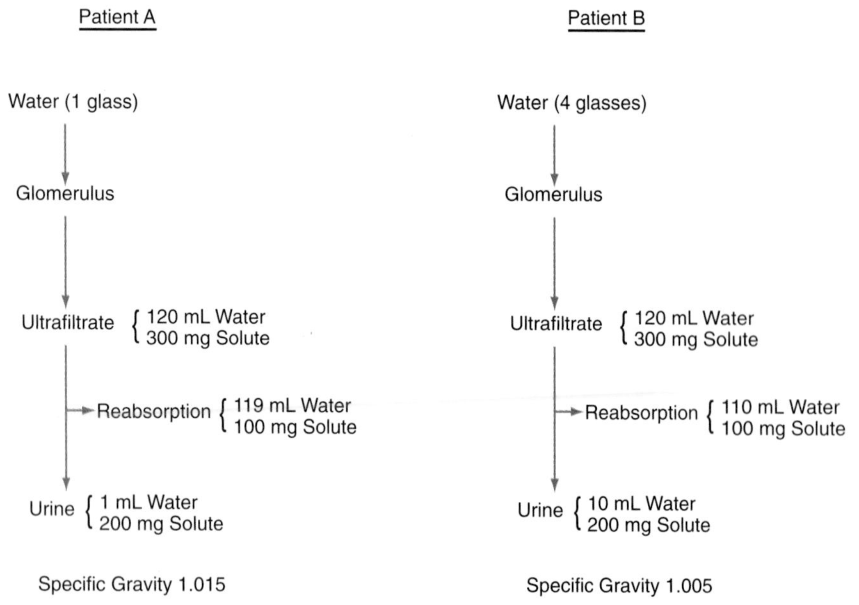

FIGURE 2–13 The effect of hydration on specific gravity.

instruments employing this technique are available. These osmometers determine the freezing point of a solution by supercooling a measured amount of sample to approximately −7°C. The supercooled sample is then vibrated to produce crystallization of water in the solution. The heat of fusion produced by the crystallizing water temporarily raises the temperature of the solution to its freezing point. A temperature-sensitive probe measures this temperature increase, which corresponds to the freezing point of the solution, and the information is converted into milliosmoles. Conversion is made possible by the fact that 1 mol (1000 mOsm) of a nonionizing substance dissolved in 1 kg of water is known to lower the freezing point 1.86°C. Therefore, by comparing the freezing point depression of an unknown solution to that of a known molal solution, the osmolarity of the unknown solution can be calculated. Clinical osmometers use solutions of known NaCl concentration as their reference standards because a solution of partially ionized substances is more representative of urine and plasma composition.

Vapor Pressure Osmometers

The other instrument used in clinical osmometry is called the vapor pressure osmometer; however, the actual measurement performed is the dew point (temperature at which water vapor condenses to a liquid). The depression of dew point temperature by solute parallels the decrease in vapor pressure, thereby providing a measure of this colligative property.

Samples are absorbed into small filter paper disks that are placed in a sealed chamber containing a temperature-sensitive thermocoupler. The sample evaporates in the chamber, forming a vapor. When the temperature in the chamber is lowered, water condenses in the chamber and on the thermocoupler. The heat of condensation produced raises the temperature of the thermocoupler to the dew point temperature. This dew point temperature is proportional to the vapor pressure from the evaporating sample. Temperatures are compared with those of the NaCl standards and converted into milliosmoles. The vapor pressure osmometer uses microsamples of less than 0.01 mL; therefore, care must be taken to prevent any evaporation of the sample prior to testing. Correlation studies have shown more variation with vapor pressure osmometers, stressing the necessity of careful technique.

Technical Factors

Factors to consider because of their influence on true osmolarity readings include lipemic serum and the presence of lactic acid or volatile substances, such as ethanol, in the specimen. In lipemic serum, the displacement of serum water by insoluble lipids produces erroneous results with both vapor pressure and freezing point osmometers. Falsely elevated values owing to the formation of lactic acid also will occur with both methods if serum samples are not separated or refrigerated within 20 minutes.[12] Vapor pressure osmometers will not detect the presence of volatile substances, inasmuch as they become part of the solvent phase; however, measurements performed on similar specimens using freezing point osmometers will be elevated. Comparisons of serum osmolarities run on cryoscopic and vapor pressure osmometers can be used as a method for rapid screening of comatose patients for alcohol ingestion.[8]

Clinical Significance

Major clinical uses of osmolarity include initially evaluating renal concentrating ability, monitoring the course of renal disease, monitoring fluid and electrolyte therapy, establishing the differential diagnosis of **hypernatremia** and **hyponatremia**, and evaluating the secretion of and renal response to ADH. These evaluations may require determination of serum in addition to urine osmolarity.

Normal serum osmolarity values are between 275 and 300 mOsm. Normal values for urine osmolarity are difficult to establish, because factors such as fluid intake and exercise can greatly influence the urine concentration. Values can range between 50 and 1400 mOsm.[15] Determining the ratio of urine to serum osmolarity can provide a more accurate evaluation. Under normal random conditions, the ratio of urine to serum osmolarity should be at least 1:1; after controlled fluid intake, it should reach 3:1.

The urine-to-serum osmolarity ratio, in conjunction with procedures such as controlled fluid intake and injection of ADH, is used to differentiate whether diabetes insipidus is caused by decreased ADH production or inability of the renal tubules to respond to ADH. Failure to achieve a urine to serum osmolarity ratio of 3:1 following injection of ADH indicates that the collecting duct does not have functional ADH receptors. In contrast, if concentration takes place following ADH injection, an inability to produce adequate ADH is indicated. Tests to measure the ADH concentration in plasma and urine directly are available for difficult diagnostic cases.[7]

Free Water Clearance

The urine-to-serum osmolarity ratio can be further expanded by performing the analyses using water deprivation and a timed urine specimen and calculating the **free water clearance**. The free water clearance is determined by first calculating the **osmolar clearance** using the standard clearance formula of

$$C_{osm} = \frac{U_{osm} \times V}{P_{osm}}$$

and then subtracting the osmolar clearance value from the urine volume in milliliters per minute.

EXAMPLE

Using a urine osmolarity of 600 mOsm (U), a urine volume of 2 mL/min (V), and a plasma osmolarity of 300 mOsm (P), calculate the free water clearance:

$$C_{osm} = \frac{600\ (U) \times 2\ (V)}{300\ (P)} = 4.0\ \text{mL/min}$$

$$C_{H_2O} = 2\ (V) - 4.0\ (C_{osm}) = -2.0$$

Calculation of the osmolar clearance tells how much water must be cleared each minute to produce a urine with the same osmolarity as the plasma. The ultrafiltrate contains the same osmolarity as the plasma; therefore, the osmotic differences found in the urine are the result of renal concentrating and diluting mechanisms. By comparing the osmolar clearance with the actual urine volume excreted per minute, it can be determined whether the water being excreted is more or less than the amount needed to maintain an osmolarity the same as that of the ultrafiltrate.

The above calculation shows a free water clearance of −2.0, indicating that less than the necessary amount of water is being excreted, indicating a possible state of dehydration. If the value had been 0, no renal concentration or dilution would be taking place; likewise, if the value had been +2.0, excess water would have been excreted, indicating decreased production of or response to ADH.[15] Therefore, calculation of the free water clearance can be used to determine the ability of the kidney to respond to the state of body hydration.

TUBULAR SECRETION AND RENAL BLOOD FLOW TESTS

Tests to measure tubular secretion of nonfiltered substances and renal blood flow are closely related in that total renal blood flow through the nephron must be measured by a substance that is secreted rather than filtered through the glomerulus. Impaired tubular secretory ability or inadequate presentation of the substance to the capillaries owing to decreased renal blood flow may cause an abnormal result. Therefore, an understanding of the principles and limitations of the tests and correlation with other clinical data are important in test interpretation.

The test most commonly associated with tubular secretion and renal blood flow is the *p*-aminohippuric acid **(PAH)** test. Historically excretion of the dye phenolsulfonphthalein **(PSP)** was used to evaluate these functions. Standardization and interpretation of PSP results are difficult, however, because of interference by medications and elevated waste products in patients' serum and the necessity to obtain several very accurately timed urine specimens. Therefore, the PSP test is not currently performed.

PAH Test

To measure the exact amount of blood flowing through the kidney, it is necessary to use a substance that is completely removed from the blood (plasma) each time it comes in contact with functional renal tissue. The principle is the same as in the clearance test for glomerular filtration. However, to ensure measurement of the blood flow through the entire nephron, the substance must be removed from the blood primarily in the peritubular capillaries rather than being removed when the blood reaches the glomerulus.

Although it has the disadvantage of being exogenous, the chemical PAH meets the criteria needed to measure renal blood flow. This nontoxic substance does not bind strongly to plasma proteins, which permits its complete removal as the blood passes through the peritubular capillaries. Except for a small amount of PAH contained in plasma that does not come in contact with functional renal tissue, all the plasma PAH is secreted by the proximal convoluted tubule. Therefore, the volume of plasma flowing through the kidneys determines the amount of PAH excreted in the urine. The standard clearance formula

$$C_{PAH}\,(\text{mL/min}) = \frac{U\,(\text{mg/dL PAH}) \times V\,(\text{mL/min urine})}{P\,(\text{mg/dL PAH})}$$

can be used to calculate the effective renal plasma flow. Based on normal hematocrit readings, normal values for the effective renal plasma flow range from 600 to 700 mL/min, making the average renal blood flow about 1200 mL/min. The actual measurement is renal plasma flow rather than renal blood flow, because the PAH is contained only in the plasma portion of the blood. Also, the term "effective" is included because approximately 8 percent of the renal blood flow does not come into contact with the functional renal tissue.[9]

The amount of PAH infused must be carefully monitored to ensure accurate results; therefore, the test is usually performed by specialized renal laboratories. Nuclear medicine procedures using radioactive hippurate can determine renal blood flow by measuring the plasma disappearance of a single radioactive injection and at the same time provide visualization of the blood flowing through the kidneys.[4,17]

Titratable Acidity and Urinary Ammonia

As discussed previously, the ability of the kidney to produce an acid urine depends on the tubular secretion of hydrogen ions and production and secretion of ammonia by the cells of the distal convoluted tubule. A normal person excretes approximately 70 mEq/day of acid in the form of either titratable acid **(H^+)** or ammonium ions **(NH_4^+)**. In normal persons, a diurnal variation in urine acidity consisting of alkaline tides appears shortly after arising and postprandially at approximately 2 PM and 8 PM. The lowest pH is found at night.[10]

The inability to produce an acid urine in the presence of metabolic acidosis is called renal tubular acidosis. This condition may result from impaired tubular secretion of hydrogen ions associated with the proximal convoluted tubule or defects in ammonia secretion associated with the distal convoluted tubule.

Measurement of urine pH, ***titratable acidity***, and urinary ammonia can be used to determine the defective function. The tests can be run simultaneously on either fresh or toluene-preserved urine specimens collected at 2-hour intervals from patients who have been primed with an acid load consisting of oral ammonium chloride. By titrating the amount of free H^+ (titratable acidity) and then the total acidity of the specimen, the ammonium concentration can be calculated as the difference between the titratable acidity and the total acidity.[5]

REFERENCES

1. Assadi, F, and Fornell, L: Estimation of urine specific gravity in neonates with a reagent strip. J Pediatr 108(6):995–996, 1986.

2. Benitez, O, et al: Inaccuracy in neonatal measurement of urine concentration with a refractometer. J Pediatr 108(4):613–616, 1986.
3. Bianchi, C: Noninvasive methods for the measurement of renal function. In Duart, C (ed): Renal Function Tests: Clinical Laboratory Procedures and Diagnosis. Little, Brown & Co., Boston, 1980.
4. Chachati, A, et al: Rapid method for the measurement of differential renal function. Validation. J Nucl Med 28(5):829–836, 1987.
5. Chan, J: Renal acidosis. In Duart, C (ed): Renal Function Tests: Clinical Laboratory Procedures and Diagnosis. Little, Brown & Co, Boston, 1980.
6. Cockcroft, DW, and Gault, HH: Prediction of creatinine clearance from serum creatinine. N Engl J Med 281:1405–1415, 1969.
7. Daves, BB, and Zenser, TV: Evaluation of renal concentrating and diluting ability. Clin Lab Med 13(1):131–134, 1993.
8. Draviam, EJ, Custer, EM, and Schoen, I: Vapor pressure and freezing point osmolality measurements applied to a volatile screen. Am J Clin Pathol 82(6):706–709, 1984.
9. Duston, H, and Corcoran, A: Functional interpretation of renal tests. Med Clin North Am 39:947–956, 1955.
10. Elliot, JS, Sharp, RF, and Lewis, L: Urinary pH. J Urol 81(2):339, 1959.
11. Jacobsen, FK, et al: Evaluation of kidney function after meals. Lancet i(8163):319–320, 1980.
12. Mercier, DE, Feld, RD, and Witte, DI: Comparison of dewpoint and freezing point osmometry. Am J Med Technol 44(11):1066–1069, 1978.
13. Murray, B, and Ferris, TF: Blood and urinary chemistries in the evaluation of renal function. Semin Nephrol 5(3):208–221, 1985.
14. Peterson, L: β_2 microglobulin. Clin Chem News 14(1):6, 1988.
15. Pincus, MR, Preuss, HG, and Henry, JB: Evaluation of renal function and water, electrolyte and acid-base balance. In Henry, JB (ed): Clinical Diagnosis and Management by Laboratory Methods. WB Saunders, Philadelphia, 1996.
16. Price, JD, and Durnford, J: Laboratory test for kidney function: Urea or creatinine? Lancet ii(8140):420–422, 1979.
17. Schnurr, E, Lahme, W, and Kuppers, H: Measurement of renal clearance of inulin and PAH in the steady state without urine collection. Clin Nephrol 13(1):26–29, 1980.

STUDY QUESTIONS

1. State two major processes associated with the peritubular capillaries.
2. Why is the glomerulus referred to as a nonselective filter?
3. How do the capillary endothelial cells in the glomerulus differ from other capillary endothelial cells?
4. When is the kidney stimulated to produce renin? What is the primary chemical affected by the renin-angiotensin-aldosterone system?
5. Define the term ultrafiltrate of plasma.
6. List four substances reabsorbed by active transport and two substances reabsorbed by passive transport.
7. When will a substance that is usually completely reabsorbed by active transport appear in the urine?
8. How does reabsorption in the descending loop of Henle differ from reabsorption in the ascending loop? What is the primary reason for this difference?
9. Why is water not always reabsorbed from the collecting duct when it passes through the medulla?
10. When the body is dehydrated, is the production of ADH increased or decreased?
11. If a waste product is not filtered at the glomerulus, how can it be removed from the blood?
12. Name a chemical that is filtered by the glomerulus and reabsorbed and secreted by the tubules.
13. How does tubular secretion maintain the buffering capacity of the blood?
14. How will failure of the distal convoluted tubule to produce ammonia affect urine pH?
15. State whether the following are endogenous or exogenous test substances: urea, inulin, creatinine, $beta_2$ microglobulin, and radionucleotides.
16. How will bacterial breakdown of urine creatinine, increased plasma chromogens, and an incomplete urine collection affect the results of a creatinine clearance test?
17. Given the following information, calculate the creatinine clearance: 24-hour urine volume = 720 mL, plasma creatinine = 1.5 mg/dL, and urine creatinine = 300 mg/dL.
18. When calculating creatinine clearance tests performed on children, are any additional calculations required? Why or why not?
19. Why is the creatinine clearance test not useful for detecting early renal disease?
20. Why do tests for renal concentrating ability incorporate water deprivation?
21. Why is urine osmolarity more representative of urine concentration than specific gravity?
22. State the two colligative properties measured by clinical osmometers.
23. With which clinical osmometer is specimen evaporation of greatest concern?
24. A random urine sample has a urine osmolarity of 305 mOsm and a serum omolarity of 295 mOsm. Is this normal or abnormal?
25. Given the following information, calculate the free water clearance and interpret the result: Urine volume = 720 mL in 6 hours, urine osmolarity = 75 mOsm, and plasma osmolarity = 300 mOsm.
26. Explain the relationship of tubular secretion to tests for renal blood flow.
27. Given the following information, calculate the effective renal plasma flow: Urine volume = 240 mL in 2 hours, urine PAH = 150 mg/dL, and plasma PAH = 0.5 mg/dL.
28. Why is the result obtained in Study Question #27 called effective renal plasma flow rather than renal blood flow?
29. Define the term renal tubular acidosis.

30. Following administration of ammonium chloride to a normal person, will the levels of titratable acidity and urinary ammonia be decreased or increased?

CASE STUDIES AND CLINICAL SITUATIONS

1. A 44-year-old man diagnosed with acute tubular necrosis has a blood urea nitrogen of 60 mg/dL and a blood glucose level of 100 mg/dL. Urinalysis results are as follows:

COLOR: Dark yellow	KETONES: Negative
CLARITY: Hazy	BLOOD: Moderate
SPECIFIC GRAVITY: 1.020	BILIRUBIN: Negative
PH: 6.0	UROBILINOGEN: Normal
PROTEIN: 2+	NITRITE: Negative
GLUCOSE: 2+	LEUKOCYTE ESTERASE: Trace

a. State the renal threshold for glucose.
b. What is the significance of the positive urine glucose and normal blood glucose?
c. Considering the diagnosis, what specific gravity result would be expected?
d. What could be causing this discrepancy?
e. How could a more representative measure of urine concentration be obtained?

2. A patient develops a sudden drop in blood pressure.
a. Diagram the reactions that take place to ensure adequate blood pressure within the nephrons.
b. How do these reactions increase blood volume?
c. When blood pressure returns to normal, how does the kidney respond?

3. A physician would like to prescribe a nephrotoxic antibiotic for a 60-year-old man with a temperature of 102°F. The patient has a serum creatinine level of 1.0 mg/dL.
a. How can the physician determine whether it is safe to prescribe this medication before the patient leaves the office?
b. Can the medication be prescribed to this patient with a reasonable assurance of safety?

4. A laboratory is obtaining erratic serum osmolarity results on a patient who is being monitored at 6 AM, 12 PM, 6 PM, and 12 AM. Osmolarities are not performed on the night shift; therefore, the midnight specimen is run at the same time as the 6 AM specimen.
a. What two reasons could account for these discrepancies?
b. If the laboratory is using a freezing point osmometer, would these discrepancies still be encountered? Why or why not?
c. If a friend was secretly bringing the patient a pint of whiskey every night, would this affect the results? Explain your answer.

5. Following overnight (6 PM to 8 AM) fluid deprivation, the urine-to-serum osmolarity ratio in a patient who is exhibiting polyuria and polydipsia is 1:1. The ratio remains the same when a second specimen is tested at 10 AM. Vasopressin is then administered subcutaneously to the patient, and the fluid deprivation is continued until 2 PM when another specimen is tested.
a. What disorder do these symptoms and initial laboratory results indicate?
b. If the urine to serum osmolarity ratio on the 2 PM specimen is 3:1, what is the underlying cause of the patient's disorder?
c. If the urine to serum osmolarity ratio on the 2 PM specimen remains 1:1, what is the underlying cause of the patient's disorder?

CHAPTER 3

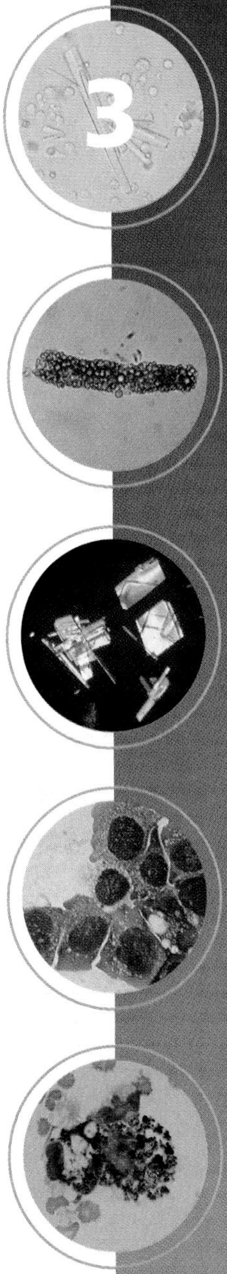

Introduction to Urinalysis

LEARNING OBJECTIVES

Upon completion of this chapter, the reader will be able to:

1. List three major organic and three major inorganic chemical constituents of urine.
2. Describe a method for determining whether a questionable fluid is urine.
3. Recognize normal and abnormal daily urine volumes.
4. Describe the characteristics of the recommended urine specimen containers.
5. Describe the correct methodology for labeling urine specimens.
6. State four possible reasons why a laboratory would reject a urine specimen.
7. List 10 changes that may take place in a urine specimen that remains at room temperature for more than 2 hours.
8. Discuss the actions of bacteria on an unpreserved urine specimen.
9. Briefly discuss five methods for preserving urine specimens, including their advantages and disadvantages.
10. Instruct a patient in the correct procedure for collecting a timed urine specimen and a midstream clean-catch specimen.
11. Describe the type of specimen needed to obtain optimal results when a specific urinalysis procedure is requested.

KEY TERMS

anuria
catheterized specimen
chain of custody
fasting specimen
first morning specimen
2-hour postprandial specimen
midstream clean-catch specimen
nocturia
oliguria
polyuria
suprapubic aspiration
three-glass collection
timed specimen

History and Importance

The analysis of urine was actually the beginning of laboratory medicine. References to the study of urine can be found in the drawings of cavemen and in Egyptian hieroglyphics, such as the Edwin Smith Surgical Papyrus. Pictures of early physicians commonly showed them examining a bladder-shaped flask of urine (Figure 3–1). Often these physicians never saw the patient, only the patient's urine. Although these physicians lacked the sophisticated testing mechanisms now available, they were able to obtain diagnostic information from such basic observations as color, turbidity, odor, volume, viscosity, and even sweetness (by noting that certain specimens attracted ants). These same urine characteristics are still reported by laboratory personnel today. However, modern urinalysis has expanded its scope to include not only the physical examination of urine but also the chemical analysis and microscopic examination of the urinary sediment.

Many well-known names in the history of medicine are associated with the study of urine, including Hippocrates, who in the 5th century BC wrote a book on "uroscopy." During the Middle Ages, physicians concentrated their efforts very heavily on the art of "uroscopy," with physicians receiving instruction in urine examination as part of their training (Figure 3–2). By 1140 AD, color charts had been developed that described the significance of 20 different colors (Figure 3–3). Chemical testing progressed from "ant testing" and "taste testing" for glucose to Frederik Dekkers' discovery in 1694 of **albuminuria** by boiling urine.[5]

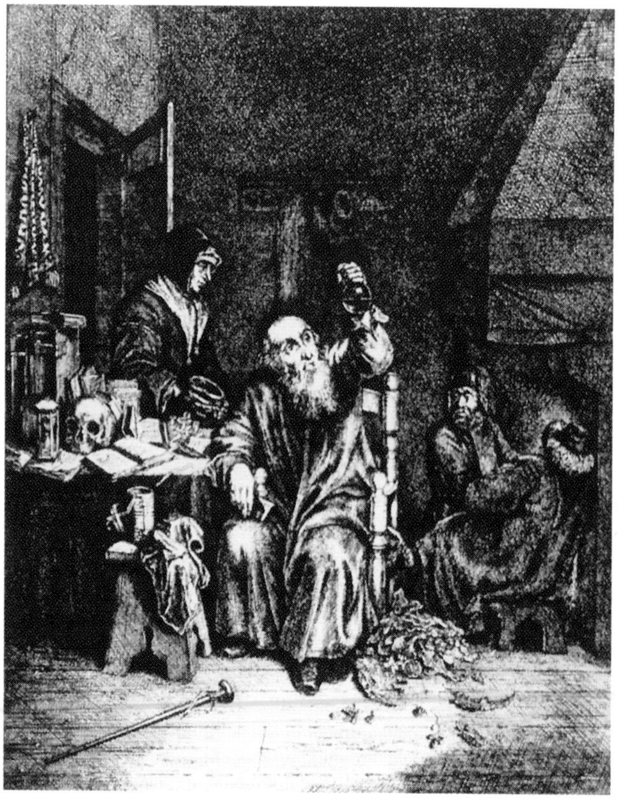

FIGURE 3–1 Physician examines urine flask. (Courtesy of the National Library of Medicine.)

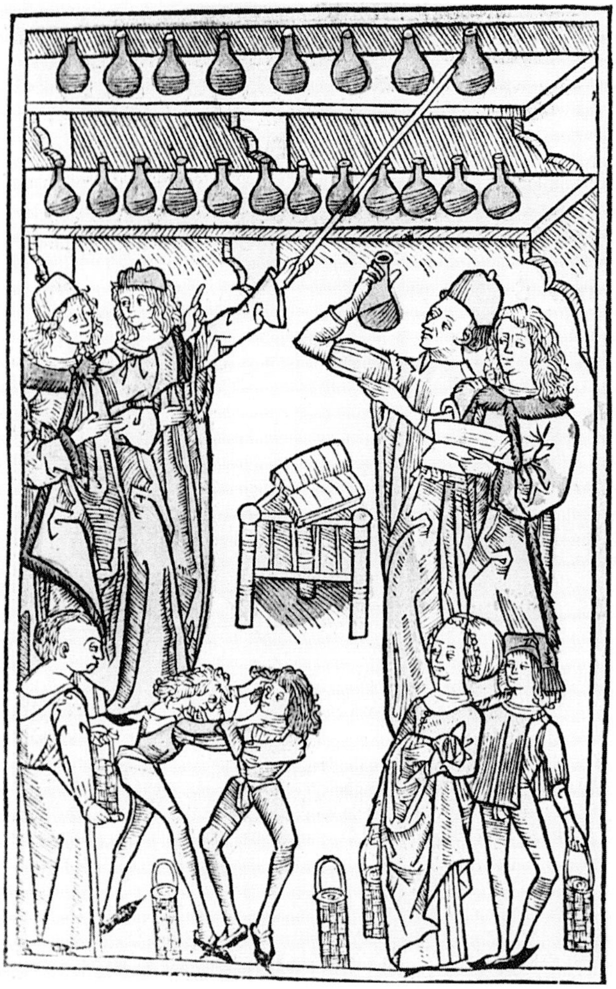

FIGURE 3–2 Instruction in urine examination. (Courtesy of the National Library of Medicine.)

The credibility of the urinalysis became compromised when charlatans without medical credentials began offering their predictions to the public for a healthy fee. These charlatans, called "pisse prophets," became the subject of a book published by Thomas Bryant in 1627. The revelations in this book inspired the passing of the first medical licensure laws in England—another contribution of urinalysis to the field of medicine!

The invention of the microscope in the 17th century led to the examination of urinary sediment and to the development by Thomas Addis of methods for quantitating the microscopic sediment. Richard Bright introduced the concept of urinalysis as part of a doctor's routine patient examination in 1827. By the 1930s, however, the number and complexity of the tests performed in a urinalysis had reached a point of impracticality, and the urinalysis began to disappear from routine examinations. Fortunately, the development of modern testing techniques rescued the routine urinalysis, which has remained an integral part of the patient examination.

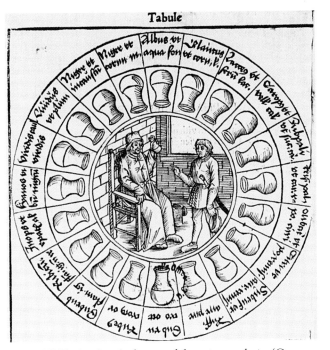

FIGURE 3–3 A chart used for urine analysis. (Courtesy of the National Library of Medicine.)

Two unique characteristics of a urine specimen can account for this continued popularity:

1. Urine is a readily available and easily collected specimen.
2. Urine contains information about many of the body's major metabolic functions, and this information can be obtained by inexpensive laboratory tests.

These characteristics fit in well with the current trends toward preventive medicine and lower medical costs. In fact, the National Committee for Clinical Laboratory Standards (**NCCLS**) defines urinalysis as "the testing of urine with procedures commonly performed in an expeditious, reliable, accurate, safe, and cost-effective manner." Reasons for performing the urinalysis identified by NCCLS include aiding in the diagnosis of disease, screening asymptomatic populations for undetected disorders, and monitoring the progress of disease and the effectiveness of therapy.[7]

Urine Formation

As detailed in Chapter 2, the kidneys continuously form urine as an ultrafiltrate of plasma. Reabsorption of water and filtered substances essential to body function converts approximately 170,000 mL of filtered plasma to the average daily urine output of 1200 mL.

Urine Composition

In general, urine consists of urea and other organic and inorganic chemicals dissolved in water. Considerable variations in the concentrations of these substances can occur owing to the influence of factors such as dietary intake, physical activity, body metabolism, endocrine functions, and even body position. Urea, a metabolic waste product produced in the liver from the breakdown of protein and amino acids, accounts for nearly half of the total dissolved solids in urine. Other organic substances include primarily creatinine and uric acid. The major inorganic solid dissolved in urine is chloride, followed by sodium and potassium. Small or trace amounts of many additional inorganic chemicals are also present in urine (Table 3–1). Dietary intake greatly influences the concentrations of these inorganic compounds, making it difficult to establish normal levels. Other substances found in urine include hormones, vitamins, and medications. Although not a part of the original plasma filtrate, the urine also may contain formed elements, such as cells, casts, crystals, mucus, and bacteria. Increased amounts of these formed elements are often indicative of disease.

Should it be necessary to determine whether a particular fluid is actually urine, the specimen can be tested for its urea and creatinine content. Since both of these substances are present in much higher concentrations in urine than in other body fluids, a high urea and creatinine content can identify a fluid as urine.

Urine Volume

Urine volume depends on the amount of water that the kidneys excrete. Water is a major body constituent; therefore, the amount excreted is usually determined by the body's state of hydration. Factors that influence urine volume include fluid intake, fluid loss from nonrenal sources, variations in the secretion of antidiuretic hormone, and the necessity to excrete increased amounts of dissolved solids, such as glucose or salts. Taking these factors into consideration, it can be seen that although the normal daily urine output is usually 1200 to 1500 mL, a range of 600 to 2000 mL may be considered normal.[4]

Oliguria, a decrease in the normal daily urine volume, is commonly seen when the body enters a state of dehydration as a result of excessive water loss from vomiting, diarrhea, perspiration, or severe burns. Oliguria leading to ***anuria***, cessation of urine flow, may result from any serious damage to the kidneys or from a decrease in the flow of blood to the kidneys. The kidneys excrete two to three times more urine during the day than during the night. An increase in the nocturnal excretion of urine is termed ***nocturia***. ***Polyuria***, an increase in daily urine volume, is often associated with diabetes mellitus and diabetes insipidus; however, it also may be artificially induced by the use of diuretics, caffeine, or alcohol, all of which suppress the secretion of antidiuretic hormone.

Diabetes mellitus and diabetes insipidus produce polyuria for different reasons, and analysis of the urine is an important step in the differential diagnosis (Figure 3–4). Diabetes mellitus is caused by a defect either in the pancreatic production of insulin or in the function of insulin that results in an increased body glucose concentration. The kidneys do not reabsorb excess glucose, necessitating the

TABLE 3–1 Composition of Urine Collected for 24 Hours

Component	Amount	Remark
Organic		
Urea	25.0–35.0 g	60–90% of nitrogenous material; derived from the metabolism of amino acids into ammonia
Creatinine	1.5 g	Derived from creatine, a nitrogenous substance in muscle tissue
Uric acid	0.4–1.0 g	Common component of kidney stones; derived from the catabolism of nucleic acid in food and cell destruction
Hippuric acid	0.7 g	Benzoic acid is eliminated from the body in this form; increases with high-vegetable diets
Other substances	2.9 g	Carbohydrates, pigments, fatty acids, mucin, enzymes, and hormones; may be present in small amounts depending on diet and health
Inorganic		
Sodium chloride (NaCl)	15.0 g	Principal salt; varies with intake
Potassium (K^+)	3.3 g	Occurs as chloride, sulfate, and phosphate salts
Sulfate (SO_4^{2-})	2.5 g	Derived from amino acids
Phosphate (PO_4^{3-})	2.5 g	Occurs primarily as sodium compounds that serve as buffers in the blood
Ammonium (NH_4^+)	0.7 g	Derived from protein metabolism and from glutamine in kidneys; amount varies depending on blood and tissue fluid acidity
Magnesium (Mg^{2+})	0.1 g	Occurs as chloride, sulfate, and phosphate salts
Calcium (Ca^{2+})	0.3 g	Occurs as chloride, sulfate, and phosphate salts

Adapted from Tortora, GJ, and Anagnostakos, NP: Principles of Anatomy and Physiology, ed 6, Harper & Row, New York, 1990, p. 51.

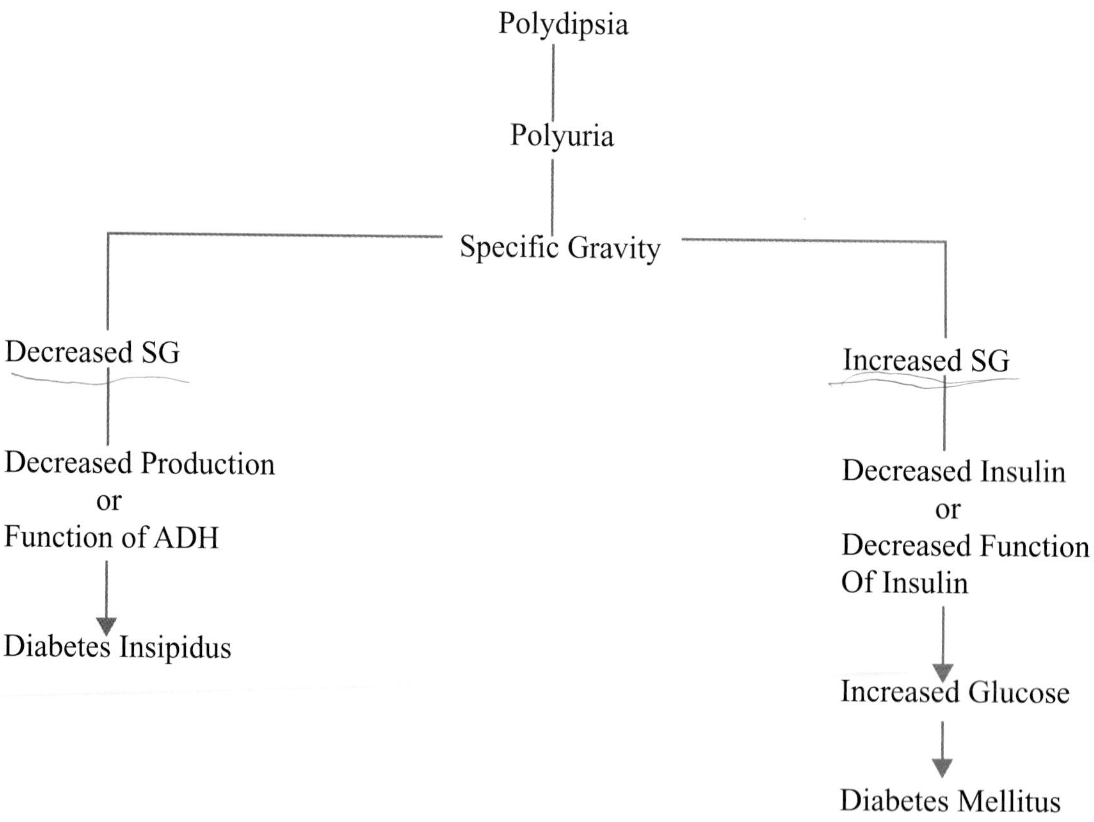

FIGURE 3–4 Differentiation between diabetes mellitus and diabetes insipidus.

excretion of increased amounts of water to remove the dissolved glucose from the body. Although appearing to be dilute, a urine specimen from a patient with diabetes mellitus will have a high specific gravity because of the increased glucose content.

Diabetes insipidus results from a decrease in the production or function of antidiuretic hormone; thus, the water necessary for adequate body hydration is not reabsorbed from the plasma filtrate. In this condition, the urine will be truly dilute and will have a low specific gravity. Fluid loss in both diseases is compensated for by increased ingestion of water (**polydipsia**), producing an even greater urine volume. Polyuria accompanied by increased fluid intake is often the first symptom of either disease.

Specimen Collection

As discussed in Chapter 1, urine is a biohazardous substance that requires the observance of Standard Precautions. Gloves should be worn at all times when in contact with the specimen.

Specimens must be collected in clean, dry, leak-proof containers. Disposable containers are recommended because they eliminate the chance of contamination due to improper washing. These disposable containers are available in a variety of sizes and shapes, including bags with adhesive for the collection of pediatric specimens and large containers for 24-hour specimens. Properly applied screw-top lids are less likely to leak than are snap-on lids.

Containers for routine urinalysis should have a wide mouth to facilitate collections from female patients and a wide, flat bottom to prevent overturning. They should be made of a clear material to allow for determination of color and clarity. The recommended capacity of the container is 50 mL, which will allow collection of the 12 mL of specimen needed for microscopic analysis, additional specimen for repeat analysis, and enough room for the specimen to be mixed by swirling the container.

All specimens must be properly labeled with the patient's name and identification number, the date and time of collection, and additional information, such as the patient's age and location and the physician's name, as required by institutional protocol. Labels must be attached to the container, not to the lid, and should not become detached if the container is refrigerated.

A requisition form (manual or computerized) must accompany specimens delivered to the laboratory. The information on the form must match the information on the specimen label. Additional information present on the requisition form can include method of collection or type of specimen, possible interfering medications, and the patient's clinical information. The time the specimen is received in the laboratory should be recorded on the form.

Improperly labeled and collected specimens should be rejected by the laboratory, and appropriate personnel should be notified to collect a new specimen. Examples of unacceptable specimens include those in unlabeled containers, nonmatching labels and requisition forms, specimens contaminated with feces or toilet paper, containers with contaminated exteriors, specimens of insufficient quantity, and specimens that have been improperly transported. Laboratories should have a written policy detailing their conditions for specimen rejection (see Chap. 7).

Specimen Handling

The fact that a urine specimen is so readily available and easily collected often leads to laxity in the treatment of the specimen after its collection. Changes in urine composition take place not only in vivo but also in vitro, thus necessitating correct handling procedures after the specimen is collected.

SPECIMEN INTEGRITY

Following collection, specimens should be delivered to the laboratory promptly and tested within 2 hours. A specimen that cannot be delivered and tested within 2 hours should be refrigerated or have an appropriate chemical preservative added. Table 3–2 describes the 11 most significant changes that may occur in a specimen allowed to remain unpreserved at room temperature for longer than 2 hours. Notice that most of the changes are related to the presence and growth of bacteria.

These variations are discussed again under the individual test procedures. At this point it is important to realize that improper preservation can seriously affect the results of a routine urinalysis.

TABLE 3–2 **Changes in Unpreserved Urine**

Analyte	Change	Cause
Color	Modified/ Darkened	Oxidation or reduction of metabolites
Clarity	Decreased	Bacterial growth and precipitation of amorphous material
Odor	Increased	Multiplication of bacteria or bacterial breakdown of urea to ammonia
pH	Increased	Breakdown of urea to ammonia by urease-producing bacteria/loss of CO_2
Glucose	Decreased	Glycolysis and bacterial use
Ketones	Decreased	Volatilization and bacterial metabolism
Bilirubin	Decreased	Exposure to light/photo oxidation to biliverdin
Urobilinogen	Decreased	Oxidation to urobilin
Nitrite	Increased	Multiplication of nitrate-reducing bacteria
Red and white blood cells and casts	Decreased	Disintegration in dilute alkaline urine
Bacteria	Increased	Multiplication

SPECIMEN PRESERVATION

The most routinely used method of preservation is refrigeration at 2°C to 8°C, which decreases bacterial growth and metabolism. Refrigeration of the specimen can increase the specific gravity when measured by urinometer and the precipitation of amorphous phosphates and urates, which may obscure the microscopic sediment analysis. Allowing the specimen to return to room temperature prior to performing chemical testing by reagent strips is required. This will correct the specific gravity and may dissolve some of the amorphous urates.

When a specimen must be transported over a long distance and refrigeration is impossible, chemical preservatives may be added. The ideal preservative should be bactericidal, inhibit urease, and preserve formed elements in the sediment. At the same time, it should not interfere with chemical tests. Unfortunately, as can be seen in Table 3–3, the ideal preservative does not currently exist; therefore, a preservative that best suits the needs of the required analysis should be chosen.

Types of Specimens

To obtain a specimen that is truly representative of a patient's metabolic state, regulation of certain aspects of specimen collection often is necessary. These special conditions may include time, length, and method of collection and the patient's dietary and medicinal intake. It is important to instruct patients when they must follow special collection procedures. Frequently encountered specimens are listed in Table 3–4.

RANDOM SPECIMEN

This is the most commonly received specimen because of its ease of collection and convenience for the patient. The **random specimen** is useful for routine screening tests to detect obvious abnormalities. However, it may also produce erroneous results caused by dietary intake or physical activity just prior to the collection of the specimen. The patient

TABLE 3–3 **Urine Preservatives**

Preservatives	Advantages	Disadvantages	Additional Information
Refrigeration	Does not interfere with chemical tests	Raises specific gravity by hydrometer Precipitates amorphous phosphates and urates	Prevents bacterial growth for 24 h[2]
Thymol	Preserves glucose and sediments well	Interferes with acid precipitation tests for protein	
Boric acid	Preserves protein and formed elements well Does not interfere with routine analyses other than pH	May precipitate crystals when used in large amounts	Keeps pH at about 6.0 Is bacteriostatic (not bactericidal) at 18 g/L; can be used for culture transport Interferes with drug and hormone analyses[9]
Formalin (formaldehyde)	Is an excellent sediment preservative	Acts as a reducing agent interfering with chemical tests for glucose, blood, leukocyte esterase, and copper reduction	Rinse specimen container with formalin to preserve cells and casts
Toluene	Does not interfere with routine tests	Floats on the surface of specimens and clings to pipettes and testing materials	
Sodium fluoride	Prevents glycolysis Is a good preservative for drug analyses[11]	Inhibits reagent strip tests for glucose, blood, and leukocytes	May use sodium benzoate instead of fluoride for reagent strip testing[8]
Phenol	Does not interfere with routine tests	Causes an odor change	Use 1 drop per ounce of specimen
Commercial preservative tablets	Are convenient when refrigeration is not possible Have controlled concentration to minimize interference	May contain one or more of the above preservatives including sodium fluoride	Check tablet composition to determine possible effects on desired tests
Urine C + S Transport Kit (Becton Dickinson, Rutherford, NJ)	Can run urinalysis and culture on the same specimen[6,10]	Decreases pH	Preservative is boric acid
Saccomanno's Fixative	Preserves cellular elements		Used for cytology studies

TABLE 3–4 **Types of Urine Specimens**

Type of Specimen	Purpose
Random	Routine screening
First morning	Routine screening Pregnancy tests Orthostatic protein
Fasting (second morning)	Diabetic screening/monitoring
2-h postprandial	Diabetic monitoring
Glucose tolerance test	Accompaniment to blood samples in glucose tolerance test
24-h (or timed)	Quantitative chemical tests
Catheterized	Bacterial culture
Midstream clean-catch	Routine screening Bacterial culture
Suprapubic aspiration	Bladder urine for bacterial culture Cytology
Three-glass collection	Prostatic infection

will then be requested to collect additional specimens under more controlled conditions.

FIRST MORNING SPECIMEN

Although it may require the patient to make an additional trip to the laboratory, this is the ideal screening specimen. It is also essential for preventing false-negative pregnancy tests and for evaluating orthostatic **proteinuria**. The ***first morning specimen*** is a concentrated specimen, thereby assuring detection of chemicals and formed elements that may not be present in a dilute random specimen. The patient should be instructed to collect the specimen immediately upon arising and to deliver it to the laboratory within 2 hours.

FASTING SPECIMEN (SECOND MORNING)

A ***fasting specimen*** differs from a first morning specimen by being the second voided specimen after a period of fasting. This specimen will not contain any metabolites from food ingested prior to the beginning of the fasting period. It is recommended for glucose monitoring.[3]

2-HOUR POSTPRANDIAL SPECIMEN

With this specimen, the patient is instructed to void shortly before consuming a routine meal and to collect a specimen 2 hours after eating. The specimen is tested for glucose, and the results are used primarily for monitoring insulin therapy in persons with diabetes mellitus. A more comprehensive evaluation of the patient's status can be obtained if the results of the ***2-hour postprandial specimen*** are compared with those of a fasting specimen and corresponding blood glucose tests.

GLUCOSE TOLERANCE SPECIMENS

Glucose tolerance specimens are sometimes collected to correspond with the blood samples drawn during a glucose tolerance test (GTT). The number of specimens varies with the length of the test. GTTs may include fasting, ½-hour, 1-hour, 2-hour, and 3-hour specimens, and possibly 4-hour, 5-hour, and 6-hour specimens. The urine is tested for glucose and ketones, and the results are reported with the blood test results as an aid to interpreting the patient's ability to metabolize a measured amount of glucose and are correlated with the renal threshold for glucose.

24-HOUR (OR TIMED) SPECIMEN

Often measuring the exact amount of a urine chemical is necessary rather than just reporting its presence or absence. A carefully ***timed specimen*** must be used to produce accurate quantitative results. When the concentration of the substance to be measured varies with daily activities such as exercise, meals, and body metabolism, 24-hour collection is required. If the concentration of a particular substance remains constant, the specimen may be collected over a shorter period. Care must be taken, however, to keep the patient adequately hydrated during short collection periods. Patients must be explicitly instructed on the procedure for collecting a timed specimen. To obtain an accurately timed specimen, the patient must begin and end the collection period with an empty bladder. Keep in mind that the concentration of a substance in a particular time period must be calculated from the urine volume produced during that time. Addition of urine formed prior to the start of the collection period or failure to include urine produced at the end of the collection period will produce inaccurate results.

Upon its arrival in the laboratory, a 24-hour specimen must be thoroughly mixed and the volume accurately measured and recorded. If only an aliquot is needed for testing, the amount saved must be adequate to permit repeat or additional testing. If a specimen is collected in two containers, the contents of the two containers should be combined and thoroughly mixed prior to aliquoting. Consideration also must be given to the preservation of specimens col-

PROCEDURE

24-Hour (Timed) Specimen Collection Procedure

- Provide patient with written instructions and explain the collection procedure.
- Issue the proper collection container and preservative.
- Day 1—7 AM Patient voids and discards specimen. Patient collects all urine for the next 24 hours.
- Day 2—7 AM Patient voids and adds this urine to the previously collected urine.
- Upon arrival in the laboratory, the entire 24-hour specimen is thoroughly mixed, and the volume accurately measured and recorded.
- An aliquot is saved for testing and additional or repeat testing. Discard remaining urine.

lected over extended periods. All specimens should be refrigerated or kept on ice during the collection period and also may require the addition of a chemical preservative. The preservative chosen must be nontoxic to the patient and should not interfere with the tests to be performed. Appropriate collection information is included with test procedures and should be referred to before issuing a container and instructions to the patient. To ensure the accuracy of a 24-hour specimen, a known quantity of a nontoxic chemical marker, such as 4-aminobenzoic acid, may be given to the patient at the start of the collection period. The concentration of excreted marker in the specimen is measured to determine the completeness of the collection.[1] Use of an injected inert marker, the concentration of which can be controlled, is recommended over measurement of endogenous urine creatinine, which varies with dietary intake and body mass.

CATHETERIZED SPECIMEN

This specimen is collected under sterile conditions by passing a hollow tube (catheter) through the urethra into the bladder. The most commonly requested test on a ***catheterized specimen*** is a bacterial culture. If a routine urinalysis is also requested, the culture should be performed first to prevent contamination of the specimen.

A less frequently encountered type of catheterized specimen is used to measure functions in the individual kidneys. Specimens from the right and left kidneys are collected separately by passing catheters through the ureters of the respective kidneys.

MIDSTREAM CLEAN-CATCH SPECIMEN

As an alternative to the catheterized specimen, the ***midstream clean-catch specimen*** provides a safer, less traumatic method for obtaining urine for bacterial culture and routine urinalysis. It provides a specimen that is less contaminated by epithelial cells and bacteria and, therefore, more representative of the actual urine than the routinely voided specimen. Patients must be provided with appropriate cleansing materials, a sterile container, and instructions for cleansing and voiding. Strong bacterial agents such as hexachlorophene or povidone-iodine should not be used as cleansing agents. Mild antiseptic towelettes are recommended. Patients are instructed to wash their hands prior to beginning the collection. Male patients should clean the **glans** beginning at the urethra and withdrawing the foreskin, if necessary. Female patients should separate the **labia** and clean the **urinary meatus** and surrounding area. When cleansing is complete, patients are to void first into the toilet, then collect an adequate amount of urine in the sterile container, and finish voiding into the toilet. Care should be taken not to contaminate the specimen container.

SUPRAPUBIC ASPIRATION

Occasionally urine may be collected by external introduction of a needle through the abdomen into the bladder. Because the bladder is sterile under normal conditions, ***suprapubic aspiration*** provides a sample for bacterial culture that is completely free of extraneous contamination. The specimen also can be used for cytologic examination.

THREE-GLASS COLLECTION

Similar to the midstream clean-catch collection, the ***three-glass collection*** procedure is used to determine prostatic infection. Instead of discarding the first urine passed, it is collected in a sterile container. Next the midstream portion is collected in another sterile container. The prostate is then massaged so that prostate fluid will be passed with the remaining urine into a third sterile container. Quantitative cultures are performed on all specimens, and the first and third specimens are examined microscopically. In prostatic infection, the third specimen will have a white blood cell/high-power field count and a bacterial count 10 times that of the first specimen. Macrophages containing lipids also may be present. The second specimen is used as a control for bladder and kidney infection. If it is positive, the results from the third specimen are invalid because infected urine has contaminated the specimen.[12]

PEDIATRIC SPECIMEN

Collection of pediatric specimens can present a challenge. Soft, clear plastic bags with adhesive to attach to the genital area of both boys and girls are available for collecting routine specimens. Sterile specimens may be obtained by catheterization or by suprapubic aspiration. Specimens for culture also may be obtained using a clean-catch cleansing procedure and a sterile collection bag. Care must be taken not to touch the inside of the bag when applying it. For quantitative testing, bags are available that allow a tube to be attached and excess urine transferred to a larger container.

DRUG SPECIMEN COLLECTION

Urine specimen collection is the most vulnerable part of a drug-testing program. Correct collection procedures and documentation are necessary to ensure that the drug testing results are those of the specific individual submitting the specimen. The ***chain of custody*** (COC) is the process that provides this documentation of proper sample identification from the time of collection to the receipt of laboratory results. The COC is a standardized form that must document and accompany every step of drug testing, from collector to courier to laboratory to medical review officer to employer.

For urine specimens to withstand legal scrutiny, it is necessary to prove that no tampering of the specimen took place, such as substitution, adulteration, or dilution of the urine. All personnel handling the specimen must be noted. The specimen must be handled securely with a guarantee that no unauthorized access to the specimen was possible. Proper identification of the individual whose information is indicated on the label is required. Acceptable identification includes photo identification or identification by an employer representative with photo ID who can positively identify the donor.

PROCEDURE

Urine Drug Specimen Collection Procedure[13,14]

1 The collector washes hands and wears gloves.
2 The collector adds bluing agent (dye) to the toilet water reservoir to prevent an adulterated specimen.
3 The collector eliminates any source of water other than toilet by taping the toilet lid and faucet handles.
4 The donor provides photo identification or positive identification from employer representative.
5 The collector completes step 1 of the Chain of Custody (COC) form and has the donor sign the form.
6 The donor leaves his or her coat, briefcase, and/or purse outside the collection area to avoid the possibility of concealed substances contaminating the urine.
7 The donor washes his or her hands and receives a specimen cup.
8 The collector remains in the restroom, but outside the stall, listening for unauthorized water use, unless a witnessed collection is requested.
9 The donor hands specimen cup to the collector. Transfer is documented.
10 The collector checks the urine for abnormal color and for the required amount (30–45 mL).
11 The collector checks that the temperature strip on the specimen cup reads between 32.5–37.7°C. The collector records the in-range temperature on the COC form (COC step 2). If the specimen temperature is out of range or the specimen is suspected to have been diluted or adulterated, a new specimen must be collected and a supervisor notified.
12 The specimen must remain in the sight of the donor and collector at all times.
13 With the donor watching, the collector peels off the specimen identification strips from the COC form (COC step 3) and puts them on the capped bottle covering both sides of the cap.
14 The donor initials the specimen bottle seals.
15 The date and time are written on the seals.
16 The donor completes step 4 on the COC form.
17 The collector completes step 5 on the COC form.
18 Each time the specimen is handled, transferred, or placed in storage, every individual must be identified and the date and purpose of the change recorded.
19 The collector follows laboratory-specific instructions for packaging the specimen bottles and laboratory copies of the COC form.
20 The collector distributes the COC copies to appropriate personnel.

Urine specimen collections may be "witnessed" or "unwitnessed." The decision to obtain a witnessed collection is indicated when it is suspected that the donor may alter or substitute the specimen or it is the policy of the client ordering the test. If a witnessed specimen collection is ordered, a same-gender collector will observe the collection of 30 to 45 mL of urine. Witnessed and unwitnessed collections should be immediately handed to the collector.

The urine temperature must be taken within 4 minutes from the time of collection to confirm the specimen has not been adulterated. The temperature should read within the range of 32.5°C to 37.7°C. If the specimen temperature is not within range, the specimen temperature should be recorded and the supervisor or employer contacted immediately. Urine temperatures outside of the recommended range may indicate specimen contamination. Recollection of a second specimen as soon as possible will be necessary. The urine color is inspected to identify any signs of contaminants. The specimen is labeled, packaged, and transported following laboratory-specific instructions.

REFERENCES

1. Bingham, S, and Cummings, JH: The use of 4-aminobenzoic acid as a marker to validate the completeness of 24 hour urine collections in man. Clin Sci 64(6):629–635, 1984.
2. Culhane, JK: Delayed analysis of urine. J Fam Pract 30(4):473–474, 1990.
3. Guthrie, D, Hinnen, D, and Guthrie, R: Single-voided vs. double-voided urine testing. Diabetes Care 2(3):269–271, 1979.
4. Henry, JB, Lauzon, RB, and Schumann, GB: Basic Examination of Urine. In Henry, JB (ed): Clinical Diagnosis and Management by Laboratory Methods. WB Saunders, Philadelphia, 1996.
5. Herman, JR: Urology: A View Through the Retrospectroscope. Harper & Row, Hagerstown, MD, 1973.
6. Meers, PD, and Chow, CK: Bacteriostatic and bactericidal actions of boric acid against bacteria and fungi commonly found in urine. J Clin Pathol 43:484–487, 1990.
7. National Committee for Clinical Laboratory Standards Approved Guideline GP16-A: Urinalysis and Collection, Transportation, and Preservation of Urine Specimens. NCCLS, Villanova, PA, 1995.
8. Onstad, J, Hancock, D, and Wolf, P: Inhibitory effect of fluoride on glucose tests with glucose oxidase strips. Clin Chem 21:898–899, 1975.
9. Porter, IA, and Brodie, J: Boric acid preservation of urine samples. BMJ 2:353–355, 1969.
10. Reilly, PA, and Wians, FH: Evaluation of a urine transport kit on urine reagent strips. Laboratory Medicine 18(3):167–169, 1987.
11. Rockerbie, RA, and Campbell, DJ: Effect of specimen storage and preservation on toxicological analysis of urine. Clin Biochem 11(3): 77–81, 1978.
12. Rous, SN: The Prostate Book. Consumers Union, Mt. Vernon, NY, 1988.
13. Saint Joseph Hospital Toxicology Laboratory/Creighton Medical Laboratories, Urine Drug Screening Collection Procedure, Omaha, NE, 1996.
14. STA United, Inc. and the Nebraska Department of Roads Federal Transit Administration Compliance 101 Seminar Workbook. Omaha, NE, 1996.

STUDY QUESTIONS

1. State two characteristics of urine that make it an ideal laboratory specimen.
2. What is the primary constituent of normal urine?

3. Name the primary organic constituent of normal urine.

4. An unidentified fluid is received in the laboratory with a request to determine if the fluid is urine or another body fluid. Using routine laboratory tests, how could you determine that the fluid is most probably urine?

5. Place the following terms in order from lowest to highest urine volume: oliguria, polyuria, and anuria.

6. A patient presenting with polyuria, nocturia, polydipsia, and a high urine specific gravity is exhibiting symptoms of what disorder?

7. Why are disposable containers with a capacity of 50 mL recommended for the collection of specimens for routine urinalysis?

8. What error in specimen labeling could cause the improper reporting of two urine specimens?

9. List five reasons why a laboratory could consider a urine specimen unacceptable.

10. State two parameters of the routine urinalysis that are falsely increased if the specimen is not tested within 2 hours.

11. Describe three changes that will affect the results of the microscopic examination of urine that is not tested within 2 hours.

12. What is the primary cause of the changes that take place in unpreserved urine?

13. Name two chemical parameters not affected by the answer to Study Question #12?

14. Why is refrigeration the method of choice for preservation of routine urinalysis samples?

15. What chemical preservative can be used to preserve a specimen for a culture and a routine urinalysis? What urinalysis parameter is affected?

16. A properly labeled urine specimen for routine urinalysis is delivered to the laboratory in a gray-top blood collection tube. Is this specimen acceptable? Explain your answer.

17. What is the specimen of choice for routine urinalysis? Why?

18. Will failure to begin a 24-hour urine collection with an empty bladder cause the results to be falsely elevated or decreased?

19. Name three types of urine specimens that would be acceptable for culture to diagnose a bladder infection.

20. Why is the COC form an essential part of urine collections for drug analysis?

CASE STUDIES AND CLINICAL SITUATIONS

1. A 24-hour urine collection received in the laboratory for creatinine analysis has a volume of 500 mL.
   a. Should this specimen be rejected and a new specimen requested? Why or why not?
   b. State a possible source of error, if the creatinine concentration per 24 hours is abnormally low.

2. Mary Johnson brings a urine specimen to the laboratory for a glucose analysis. The test result is negative. The physician questions the result because the patient has a family history of diabetes mellitus and is experiencing mild clinical symptoms.
   a. What two sources of error related to the urine specimen could account for the negative test result?
   b. How could a specimen be collected that would more accurately reflect Mary's glucose metabolism?

3. A three-glass specimen for determination of possible prostatic infection is sent to the laboratory. Specimens #1 and #3 contain increased white blood cell levels.
   a. If all three specimens have positive bacterial cultures, does the patient have a prostatic infection? Explain your answer.
   b. Why is the presence of white blood cells in specimen #2 not part of the examination?
   c. If the amount of bacteria and white blood cells in specimen #1 is significantly lower than in specimen #3, what is the significance?

4. A worker suspects that he or she will be requested to collect an unwitnessed urine specimen for drug analysis. He or she carries a substitute specimen in his or her pocket for 2 days before being told to collect the specimen. Shortly after the worker delivers the specimen, he or she is instructed to collect another specimen.
   a. What test was performed on the specimen to determine possible specimen manipulation?
   b. How was the specimen in this situation affected?
   c. If a specimen for drug analysis tests positive, state a possible defense related to specimen collection and handling that an attorney might employ.
   d. How can this defense be avoided?

CHAPTER 4

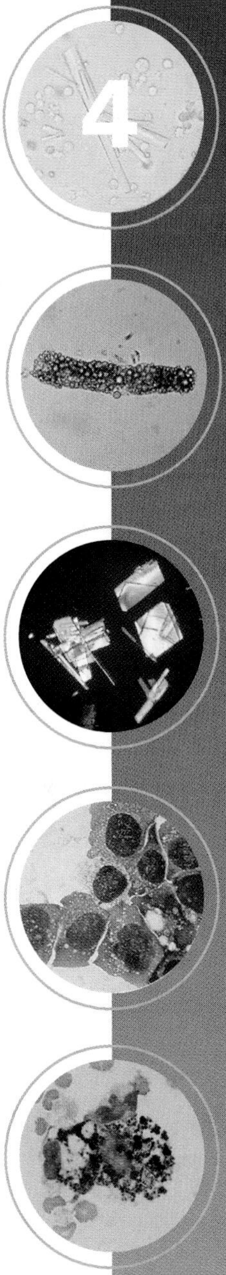

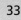

Physical Examination of Urine

LEARNING OBJECTIVES

Upon completion of this chapter, the reader will be able to:

1 List the common terminology used to report normal urine color.
2 Discuss the relationship of urochrome to normal urine color.
3 State how the presence of bilirubin in a specimen may be suspected.
4 Discuss the significance of cloudy red urine and clear red urine.
5 Name two pathologic causes of black or brown urine.
6 Discuss the significance of phenazopyridine in a specimen.
7 State the clinical significance of urine clarity.
8 List the common terminology used to report clarity.
9 Describe the appearance and discuss the significance of amorphous phosphates and amorphous urates in freshly voided urine.
10 List three pathologic and four nonpathologic causes of cloudy urine.
11 Define specific gravity, and tell why this measurement can be significant in the routine analysis.
12 Describe the principles of the urinometer, refractometer, and harmonic oscillation densitometry methods for determining specific gravity.
13 State two advantages of performing specific gravity by refractometer rather than by urinometer.
14 Given the concentration of glucose and protein in a specimen, calculate the correction needed to compensate for these high-molecular-weight substances in the refractometer specific gravity reading.
15 Name two nonpathogenic causes of abnormally high specific gravity readings using a refractometer.

KEY TERMS

clarity
harmonic oscillation densitometry
hypersthenuric
hyposthenuric
isosthenuric
refractometry
specific gravity
urinometry

The physical examination of urine includes the determination of the urine color, ***clarity***, and ***specific gravity***. As mentioned in Chapter 3, early physicians based many medical decisions on the color and clarity of urine. Today, observation of these characteristics provides preliminary information concerning disorders such as glomerular bleeding, liver disease, inborn errors of metabolism, and urinary tract infection. Measurement of specific gravity aids in the evaluation of renal tubular function. The results of the physical portion of the urinalysis also can be used to confirm or to explain findings in the chemical and microscopic areas of urinalysis.

Color

The color of urine varies from almost colorless to black. These variations may be due to normal metabolic functions, physical activity, ingested materials, or pathologic conditions. A noticeable change in urine color is often the reason a patient seeks medical advice; it then becomes the responsibility of the laboratory to determine whether this color change is normal or pathologic. The more common normal and pathologic correlations of urine colors are summarized in Table 4–1.

NORMAL URINE COLOR

Terminology used to describe the color of normal urine may differ slightly among laboratories but should be consistent within each laboratory. Common descriptions include light yellow, yellow, dark yellow, and amber. Care should be taken to examine the specimen under a good light source, looking down through the container against a white background. The yellow color of urine is caused by the presence of a pigment, which Thudichum named **urochrome** in 1864. Urochrome is a product of endogenous metabolism, and under normal conditions the body produces it at a constant rate. The actual amount of urochrome produced is dependent on the body's metabolic state, with increased amounts produced in thyroid conditions and fasting states.[4] Urochrome also increases in urine that stands at room temperature.[9]

Because urochrome is excreted at a constant rate, the intensity of the yellow color in a fresh urine specimen can give a rough estimate of urine concentration. A dilute urine will be pale yellow and a concentrated specimen will be dark yellow. Remember that, owing to variations in the body's state of hydration, these differences in the yellow color of urine can be normal.

Two additional pigments, **uroerythrin** and **urobilin**, are also present in the urine in much smaller quantities and contribute little to the color of normal, fresh urine. The presence of uroerythyrin, a pink pigment, is most evident in specimens that have been refrigerated, resulting in the precipitation of amorphous urates. Uroerythrin attaches to the urates, producing a pink color to the sediment. *Urobilin*, an oxidation product of the normal urinary constituent, urobilinogen, imparts an orange-brown color to urine that is not fresh.

ABNORMAL URINE COLOR

As can be seen in Table 4–1, abnormal urine colors are as numerous as their causes. Certain colors, however, are seen more frequently and have a greater clinical significance than others.

Dark Yellow/Amber/Orange

Dark yellow or amber urine may not always signify a normal concentrated urine but can be caused by the presence of the abnormal pigment bilirubin. If bilirubin is present, it will be detected during the chemical examination; however, its presence is suspected if a yellow foam appears when the specimen is shaken. Normal urine produces only a small amount of rapidly disappearing foam when shaken, and a large amount of white foam indicates an increased concentration of protein. A urine specimen that contains bilirubin may also contain hepatitis virus, reinforcing the need to follow Standard Precautions. The photo-oxidation of large amounts of excreted urobilinogen to urobilin will also produce a yellow-orange urine; however, yellow foam does not appear when the specimen is shaken. Photo-oxidation of bilirubin imparts a yellow-green color to the urine.

Also frequently encountered in the urinalysis laboratory is the yellow-orange specimen caused by the administration of phenazopyridine (Pyridium) or azo-gantrisin compounds to persons with urinary tract infections. This thick, orange pigment not only obscures the natural color of the specimen but also interferes with chemical tests based on color reactions. Recognition of the presence of phenazopyridine in a specimen is important so that laboratories can use alternate testing procedures. Specimens containing phenazopyridine will produce a yellow foam when shaken, which could be mistaken for bilirubin.

Red/Pink/Brown

One of the most common causes of abnormal urine color is the presence of blood. Red is the usual color that blood produces in urine, but the color may range from pink to brown, depending on the amount of blood, the pH of the urine, and the length of contact. Red blood cells (**RBCs**) remaining in an acidic urine for several hours will produce a brown urine due to the oxidation of hemoglobin to methemoglobin. A fresh brown urine containing blood may also indicate glomerular bleeding.[1]

Besides RBCs, two other substances, hemoglobin and myoglobin, produce a red urine and result in a positive chemical test result for blood (Figure 4–1). When RBCs are present, the urine will be red and cloudy; however, if hemoglobin or myoglobin is present, the specimen will be red and clear. Distinguishing between hemoglobinuria and myoglobinuria may be possible by examining the patient's plasma. Hemoglobinuria resulting from the in vivo breakdown of RBCs is accompanied by red plasma. Breakdown of skeletal muscle produces myoglobin. Myoglobin is more rapidly cleared from the plasma than is hemoglobin and, therefore, does not affect the color of the plasma. Fresh

TABLE 4–1 **Laboratory Correlation of Urine Color[6]**

Color	Cause	Clinical/Laboratory Correlations
Colorless	Recent fluid consumption	Commonly observed with random specimens
Pale yellow	Polyuria or diabetes insipidus	Increased 24-hour volume
	Diabetes mellitus	Elevated specific gravity and positive glucose test result
Dark yellow	Concentrated specimen	May be normal after strenuous exercise or in first morning specimen
Amber		Dehydration from fever or burns
Orange	Bilirubin	Yellow foam when shaken and positive chemical test results for bilirubin
	Acriflavine	Negative bile test results and possible green fluorescence
	Phenazopyridine (Pyridium)	Drug commonly administered for urinary tract infections May have orange foam and thick orange pigment that can obscure or interfere with reagent strip readings
	Nitrofurantoin	Antibiotic administered for urinary tract infections
	Phenindione	Anticoagulant, orange in alkaline urine, colorless in acid urine
Yellow-green Yellow-brown	Bilirubin oxidized to biliverdin	Colored foam in acidic urine and false-negative chemical test results for bilirubin
Green	*Pseudomonas* infection	Positive urine culture
Blue-green	Amitriptyline	Antidepressant
	Methocarbamol (Robaxin)	Muscle relaxant, may be green-brown
	Clorets	None
	Indican	Bacterial infections
	Methylene blue	Fistulas
	Phenol	When oxidized
Pink Red	RBCs	Cloudy urine with positive chemical test results for blood and RBCs visible microscopically
	Hemoglobin	Clear urine with positive chemical test results for blood; intravascular hemolysis
	Myoglobin	Clear urine with positive chemical test results for blood; muscle damage
	Porphyrins	Negative chemical test results for blood Detect with Watson-Schwartz screening test or fluorescence under ultraviolet light
	Beets	Alkaline urine of genetically susceptible persons
	Rifampin	Tuberculosis medication
	Menstrual contamination	Cloudy specimen with RBCs, mucus, and clots
Brown Black	RBCs oxidized to methemoglobin	Seen in acidic urine after standing; positive chemical test result for blood
	Methemoglobin	Denatured hemoglobin
	Homogentisic acid (alkaptonuria)	Seen in alkaline urine after standing; specific tests are available
	Melanin or melanogen	Urine darkens on standing and reacts with nitroprusside and ferric chloride
	Phenol derivatives	Interferes with copper reduction tests
	Argyrol (antiseptic)	Color disappears with ferric chloride
	Methyldopa or levodopa	Antihypertensive
	Metronidazole (Flagyl)	Darkens on standing

urine containing myoglobin frequently exhibits a more reddish-brown color than that of hemoglobin. The possibility of hemoglobinuria being produced from the in vitro lysis of RBCs also must be considered. Chemical tests to distinguish between hemoglobin and myoglobin are available (see Chap. 5).

Urine specimens containing porphyrins also may appear red resulting from the oxidation of **porphobilinogen** to **porphyrins**. They are often referred to as having the color of port wine.

Nonpathogenic causes of red urine include menstrual contamination, ingestion of highly pigmented foods, and

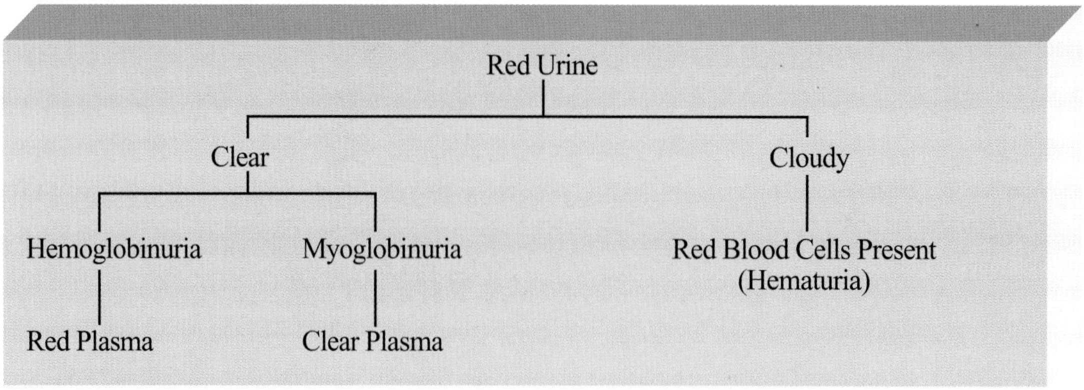

FIGURE 4–1 Differentiation of red urine testing chemically positive for blood.

medications. In genetically susceptible persons, eating fresh beets will cause a red color in alkaline urine.[10] Ingestion of blackberries can produce a red color in acidic urine. Many medications, including rifampin, phenolphthalein, phenindione, and phenothiazines, produce red urine.

Brown/Black

Additional testing is recommended for urine specimens that turn brown or black on standing and have negative chemical test results for blood, inasmuch as they may contain melanin or homogentisic acid. Melanin is an oxidation product of the colorless pigment, melanogen, produced in excess when a malignant **melanoma** is present. Homogentisic acid, a metabolite of phenylalanine, imparts a black color to alkaline urine from persons with the inborn-error of metabolism, called alkaptonuria. These conditions are discussed in Chapter 9. Medications producing brown/black urines include levodopa, methyldopa, phenol derivatives, and metronidazole (Flagyl).

Blue/Green

Pathogenic causes of blue/green urine color are limited to bacterial infections, including urinary tract infection by *Pseudomonas* species and intestinal tract infections resulting in increased urinary indican. Ingestion of breath deodorizers (Clorets) can result in a green urine color.[5] The medications methocarbamol (Robaxin), methylene blue, and amitriptyline (Elavil) may cause blue urine.

PROCEDURE

Color and Clarity Procedure

- Use a well-mixed specimen.
- View through a clear container.
- View against a white background.
- Maintain adequate room lighting.
- Evaluate a consistent volume of specimen.
- Determine color and clarity.

Observation of specimen collection bags from hospitalized patients frequently detects abnormally colored urine. This may signify a pathologic condition that requires the urine to stand for a period of time before color development or the presence of medications. Phenol derivatives found in certain intravenous medications will produce green urine on oxidation.[2] A purple staining may occur in catheter bags and is caused by the presence of indican in the urine or a bacterial infection frequently caused by *Klebsiella* or *Providencia* species.[3]

Clarity

Clarity is a general term that refers to the transparency/turbidity of a urine specimen. In routine urinalysis, clarity is determined in the same manner that ancient physicians used; that is, by visually examining the mixed specimen while holding it in front of a light source. The specimen should, of course, be in a clear container. Color and clarity are routinely determined at the same time. Common terminology used to report clarity includes clear, hazy, cloudy, turbid, and milky. As discussed under the section on urine color, terminology should be consistent within a laboratory. A description of urine clarity reporting is presented in Table 4–2.

NORMAL CLARITY

Freshly voided normal urine is usually clear, particularly if it is a midstream clean-catch specimen. Precipitation of amorphous phosphates and carbonates may cause a white cloudiness.

TABLE 4–2 **Urine Clarity**

Clarity	Term
Clear	No visible particulates, transparent.
Hazy	Few particulates, print easily seen through urine.
Cloudy	Many particulates, print blurred through urine.
Turbid	Print cannot be seen through urine.
Milky	May precipitate or be clotted.

TABLE 4–3 **Nonpathologic Causes of Urine Turbidity**

Squamous epithelial cells
Mucus
Amorphous phosphates, carbonates, urates
Semen, spermatozoa
Fecal contamination
Radiographic contrast media
Talcum powder
Vaginal creams

NONPATHOLOGIC TURBIDITY

The presence of squamous epithelial cells and mucus, particularly in specimens from women, can result in a hazy but normal urine.

Specimens that are allowed to stand or are refrigerated also may develop turbidity that is nonpathologic. As discussed in Chapter 3, improper preservation of a specimen results in bacterial growth and this will increase specimen turbidity but is not representative of the actual specimen.

Refrigerated specimens frequently develop a thick turbidity caused by the precipitation of amorphous phosphates, carbonates, and urates. Amorphous phosphates and carbonates produce a white precipitate in urine with an alkaline pH, whereas amorphous urates produce a precipitate in acidic urine that resembles pink brick dust due to the presence of uroerythyrin.

Additional nonpathologic causes of urine turbidity include semen, fecal contamination, radiographic contrast media, talcum powder, and vaginal creams (Table 4–3).

PATHOLOGIC TURBIDITY

The most commonly encountered pathologic causes of turbidity in a fresh specimen are RBCs, white blood cells (**WBCs**), and bacteria. Other less frequently encountered causes of pathologic turbidity include abnormal amounts of nonsquamous epithelial cells, yeast, abnormal crystals, lymph fluid, and lipids (Table 4–4).

The clarity of a urine specimen certainly provides a key to the microscopic examination results, because the degree of turbidity should correspond with the amount of material observed under the microscope. Questionable causes of urine turbidity can be confirmed by chemical tests shown in Table 4–5.

A clear urine is not always normal. However, with the increased sensitivity of the routine chemical tests, most abnormalities in clear urine will be detected prior to the microscopic analysis. Current criteria used to determine the necessity of performing a microscopic examination on all urine specimens include both clarity and chemical tests for RBCs, WBCs, bacteria, and protein.

TABLE 4–4 **Pathologic Causes of Urine Turbidity**

Red blood cells
White blood cells
Bacteria
Yeast
Nonsquamous epithelial cells
Abnormal crystals
Lymph fluid
Lipids

TABLE 4–5 **Laboratory Correlations in Urine Turbidity[6]**

Acidic Urine
Amorphous urates
Radiographic contrast media
Alkaline Urine
Amorphous phosphates, carbonates
Soluble with Heat
Amorphous urates, uric acid crystals
Soluble in Dilute Acetic Acid
Red blood cells
Amorphous phosphates, carbonates
Insoluble in Dilute Acetic Acid
White blood cells
Bacteria, yeast
Spermatozoa
Soluble in Ether
Lipids
Lymphatic fluid, chyle

Specific Gravity

The ability of the kidneys to selectively reabsorb essential chemicals and water from the glomerular filtrate is one of the body's most important functions. The intricate process of reabsorption is often the first renal function to become impaired; therefore, an assessment of the kidney's ability to reabsorb is a necessary component of the routine urinalysis. This evaluation can be performed by measuring the specific gravity of the specimen. Specific gravity also will detect possible dehydration or abnormalities in antidiuretic hormone and can be used to determine whether specimen concentration is adequate to ensure the accuracy of chemical tests.

Specific gravity is defined as the **density** of a solution compared with the density of a similar volume of distilled water at a similar temperature. Because urine is actually water that contains dissolved chemicals, the specific gravity of urine is a measure of the density of the dissolved chemicals in the specimen. As a measure of specimen density, specific gravity is influenced not only by the number of particles present but also by their size. Large urea molecules contribute more to the reading than do the small sodium and chloride molecules. Therefore, because urea is of less value than sodium and chloride in the evaluation of renal concentrating ability, it also may be necessary to test the specimen's osmolarity. This procedure is discussed in Chapter 2. For purposes of routine urinalysis, however, the specific gravity provides valuable preliminary information and can be easily performed using a urinometer (hydrometer), a refractometer, a reagent strip, or an automated instrument. This chapter will discuss the physical methods for determining specific gravity. The chemical reagent strip method is covered in Chapter 5.

URINOMETER

The urinometer consists of a weighted float attached to a scale that has been calibrated in terms of urine specific gravity. The weighted float displaces a volume of liquid equal to its weight and has been designed to sink to a level of 1.000 in distilled water. The additional mass provided by the dissolved substances in urine causes the float to displace a volume of urine smaller than that of distilled water. The level to which the urinometer sinks, as shown in Figure 4–2, represents the specimen's mass or specific gravity.

Urinometry is less accurate than the other methods currently available and is not recommended by the National Committee for Clinical Laboratory Standards (NCCLS).[8] A major disadvantage of using a urinometer to measure specific gravity is that it requires a large volume (10 to 15 mL) of specimen. The container in which the urinometer is floated must be wide enough to allow it to float without touching the sides and from resting on the bottom. When using the urinometer, an adequate amount of urine is first poured into a proper-size container, and the urinometer is added with a spinning motion. The scale reading is then taken at the bottom of the urine meniscus.

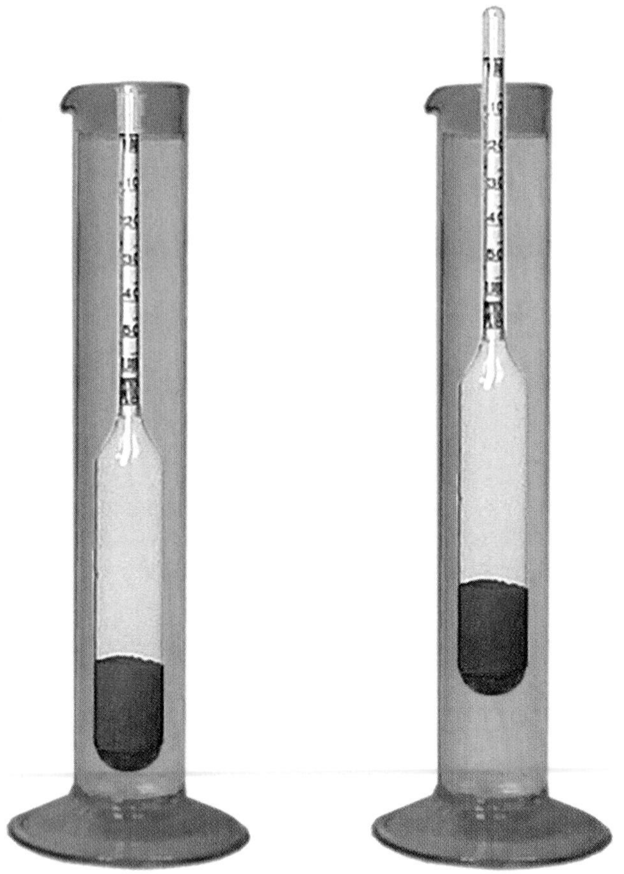

FIGURE 4–2 Urinometers representing various specific gravity readings.

The urinometer reading may also need to be corrected for temperature, inasmuch as urinometers are calibrated to read 1.000 in distilled water at a particular temperature. The calibration temperature is printed on the instrument and is usually about 20°C. If the specimen is cold, 0.001 must be subtracted from the reading for every 3°C that the specimen temperature is below the urinometer calibration temperature. Conversely, 0.001 must be added to the reading for every 3°C that the specimen measures above the calibration temperature.

A correction also must be calculated when using either the urinometer or the refractometer if large amounts of glucose or protein are present. Both glucose and protein are high-molecular-weight substances that have no relationship to renal concentrating ability but will increase specimen density. Therefore, their contribution to the specific gravity is subtracted to give a more accurate report of the kidney's concentrating ability. A gram of protein per deciliter of urine will raise the urine specific gravity by 0.003, and 1 g glucose/dL will add 0.004 to the reading. Consequently, for each gram of protein present, 0.003 must be subtracted from the specific gravity reading, and 0.004 must be subtracted for each gram of glucose present.

EXAMPLE

A specimen containing 1 g/dL of protein and 1 g/dL of glucose has a specific gravity reading of 1.030. Calculate the corrected reading.

1.030 − 0.003 (protein) = 1.027 − 0.004 (glucose)
= 1.023 corrected specific gravity

REFRACTOMETER

Refractometry, like urinometry, determines the concentration of dissolved particles in a specimen. It does this by measuring refractive index. Refractive index is a comparison of the velocity of light in air with the velocity of light in a solution. The concentration of dissolved particles present in the solution determines the velocity and angle at which light passes through a solution. Clinical refractometers make use of these principles of light by using a prism to direct a specific (monochromatic) wavelength of daylight against a manufacturer-calibrated specific gravity scale. The concentration of the specimen determines the angle at which the light beam enters the prism. Therefore, the specific gravity scale is calibrated in terms of the angles at which light passes through the specimen.

The refractometer provides the distinct advantage of determining specific gravity using a small volume of specimen (one or two drops). Temperature corrections are not necessary because the light beam passes through a temperature-

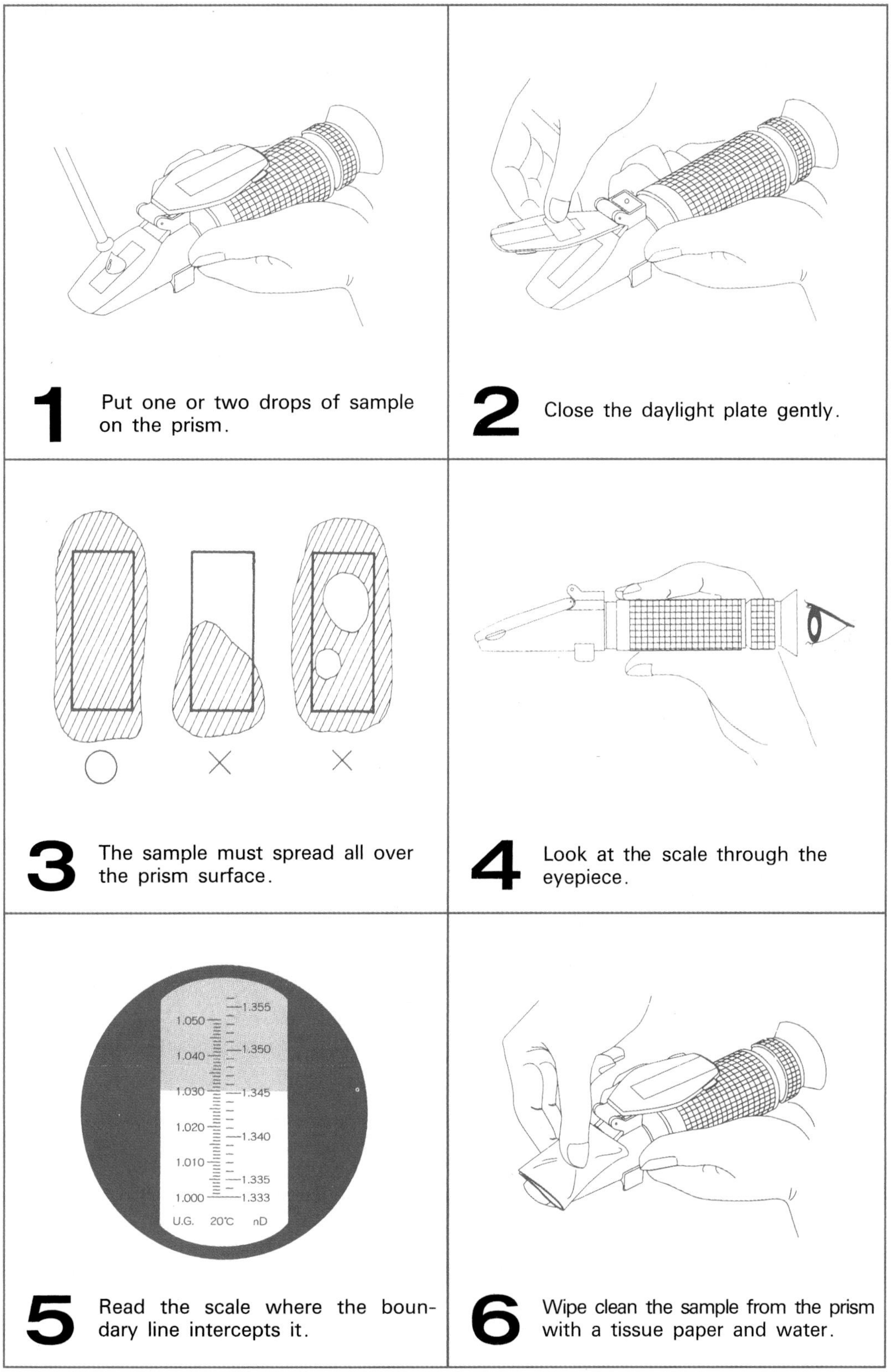
1 Put one or two drops of sample on the prism.
2 Close the daylight plate gently.
3 The sample must spread all over the prism surface.
4 Look at the scale through the eyepiece.
1.050
1.040
1.030
1.020
1.010
1.000
1.355
1.350
1.345
1.340
1.335
1.333
U.G. 20℃ nD
5 Read the scale where the boundary line intercepts it.
6 Wipe clean the sample from the prism with a tissue paper and water.

FIGURE 4–3 Steps in the use of the urine specific gravity refractometer. (Courtesy of NSG Precision Cells, Inc., 195G Central Ave., Farmingdale, NY, 11735, 516-249-7474.)

compensating liquid prior to being directed at the specific gravity scale. Temperature is compensated between 15°C and 38°C. Corrections for glucose and protein are still calculated, although refractometer readings are less affected by particle density than are urinometer readings.

When using the refractometer, a drop of urine is placed on the prism, the instrument is focused at a good light source, and the reading is taken directly from the specific gravity scale. The prism and its cover should be cleaned after each specimen is tested. Figure 4–3 illustrates the use of the refractometer.

Calibration of the refractometer is performed using distilled water that should read 1.000. If necessary, the instrument contains a zero set screw to adjust the distilled water reading (Figure 4–4). The calibration is further checked using 5 percent NaCl, which as shown in the refractometer conversion tables should read 1.022 ± 0.001, or 9 percent sucrose that should read 1.034 ± 0.001. Urine control samples representing low, medium, and high concentrations should also be run at the beginning of each shift. Calibration and control results are always recorded in the appropriate quality control records.

HARMONIC OSCILLATION DENSITOMETRY

Harmonic oscillation densitometry is based on the principle that the frequency of a sound wave entering a solution will change in proportion to the density of the solution. The Yellow Iris (International Remote Imaging Systems, Chatsworth, CA) automated urinalysis workstations discussed in more detail in Appendix A use this method to determine specific gravity. A portion of the urine sample enters a U-shaped tube. A sound wave of specific frequency is generated at one end of the tube, and as the sound wave passes (oscillates) through the urine its frequency is altered by the density of the specimen. A microprocessor at the other end of the tube measures the change in sound wave frequency, compensates for temperature variations, and converts the reading to specific gravity (Figure 4–5).

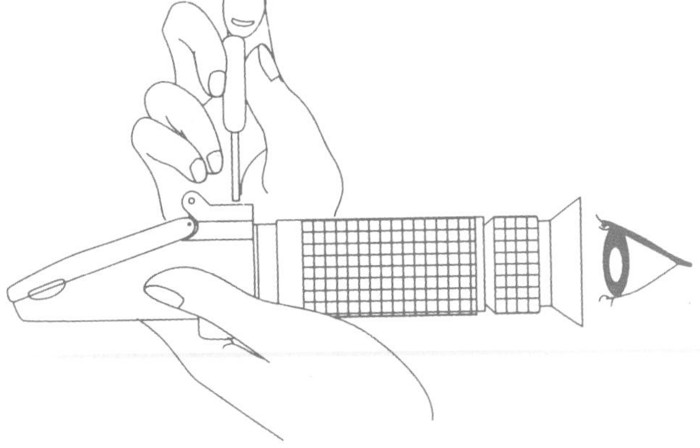

FIGURE 4–4 Calibration of the urine specific gravity refractometer. (Courtesy of NSG Precision Cells, Inc., 195G Central Ave., Farmingdale, NY, 11735, 516-249-7474.)

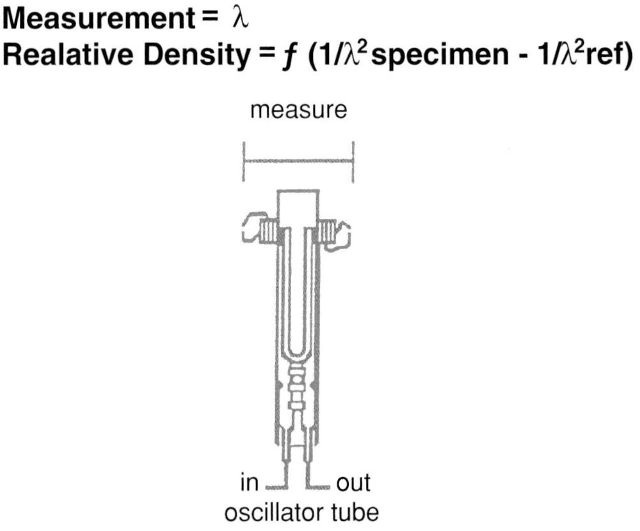

FIGURE 4–5 Mass gravity meter used to perform specific gravity measurement by harmonic oscillation. (Courtesy of International Remote Imaging Systems, Chatsworth, CA.)

Clinical Correlations

The specific gravity of the plasma filtrate entering the glomerulus is 1.010. The term ***isosthenuric*** is used to describe urine with a specific gravity of 1.010. Specimens below 1.010 are ***hyposthenuric***, and those above 1.010 are ***hypersthenuric***. One would expect urine that has been concentrated by the kidney to be hypersthenuric; however, this is not always true. Normal random specimens may range from 1.003 to 1.035, depending on the patient's degree of hydration. Specimens measuring lower than 1.003 probably are not urine. Most random specimens fall between 1.015 and 1.025, and any random specimen with a specific gravity of 1.023 or higher is generally considered normal. If a patient exhibits consistently low results, specimens may be collected under controlled conditions as discussed in Chapter 2.

Abnormally high results—over 1.035—are seen in patients who have recently undergone an intravenous pyelogram. This is caused by the excretion of the injected radiographic contrast media. Patients who are receiving dextran or other high-molecular-weight intravenous fluids (plasma expanders) will also produce urine with an abnormally

Summary of Urine Specific Gravity Measurements

Method	Principle
Urinometry	Density
Refractometry	Refractive index
Harmonic oscillation densitometry	Density
Reagent strip	pK_a changes of a polyelectrolyte

TABLE 4–6 **Common Causes of Urine Odor**[6]

Odor	Cause
Aromatic	Normal
Foul, ammonia-like	Bacterial decomposition, urinary tract infection
Fruity, sweet	Ketones (diabetes mellitus, starvation, vomiting)
Maple syrup	Maple syrup urine disease
Mousy	Phenylketonuria
Rancid	Tyrosinemia
Sweaty feet	Isovaleric acidemia
Cabbage	Methionine malabsorption
Bleach	Contamination

high specific gravity. Once the foreign substance has been cleared from the body, the specific gravity will return to normal. In these circumstances, urine concentration can be measured using the reagent strip chemical test or osmometry because they are not affected by these high-molecular-weight substances.[11] When the presence of glucose or protein is the cause of high results, this will be detected in the routine chemical examination. As discussed previously, this can be corrected for mathematically.

Specimens with specific gravity readings greater than the refractometer or urinometer scale can be diluted and retested. If this is necessary, only the decimal portion of the observed specific gravity is multiplied by the dilution factor. For example, a specimen diluted 1:2 with a reading of 1.025 would have an actual specific gravity of a 1.050.

Odor

Although it is seldom of clinical significance and is not a part of the routine urinalysis, urine odor is a noticeable physical property. Freshly voided urine has a faint aromatic odor. As the specimen stands, the odor of ammonia becomes more prominent. The breakdown of urea is responsible for the characteristic ammonia odor. Causes of unusual odors include bacterial infections, which cause a strong, unpleasant odor, and diabetic ketones, which produce a sweet or fruity odor. A serious metabolic defect results in urine with a strong odor of maple syrup and is appropriately called maple syrup urine disease. This and other metabolic disorders with characteristic urine odors are discussed in Chapter 9. Ingestion of certain foods, including onions, garlic, and asparagus, can cause an unusual or pungent urine odor. Studies have shown that although everyone who eats asparagus produces an odor, only certain genetically predisposed people can smell the odor.[7] Common causes of urine odors are summarized in Table 4–6.

REFERENCES

1. Berman, L: When urine is red. JAMA 237:2753–2754, 1977.
2. Bowling, P, Belliveau, RR, and Butler, TJ: Intravenous medications and green urine. JAMA 246(3):216, 1981.
3. Dealler, SF, et al: Purple urine bags. J Urol 142(3):769–770, 1989.
4. Drabkin, DL: The normal pigment of urine: The relationship of urinary pigment output to diet and metabolism. J Biol Chem 75: 443–479, 1927.
5. Evans, B: The greening of urine: Still another "Cloret sign." N Engl J Med 300(4):202, 1979.
6. Henry, JB, Lauzon, RB, and Schumann, GB: Basic examination of urine. In Henry, JB (ed): Clinical Diagnosis and Management by Laboratory Methods. WB Saunders, Philadelphia, 1996.
7. Mitchell, SC, et al: Odorous urine following asparagus ingestion in man. Experimenta 43(4):382–383, 1987.
8. National Committee for Clinical Laboratory Standards Approved Guideline GP16-A: Urinalysis and Collection, Transportation, and Preservation of Urine Specimens. NCCLS, Villanova, PA, 1995.
9. Ostow, M, and Philo, S: The chief urinary pigment: The relationship between the rate of excretion of the yellow pigment and the metabolic rate. Am J Med Sci 207:507–512, 1944.
10. Reimann, HA: Re: Red urine. JAMA 241(22):2380, 1979.
11. Smith, C, Arbogast, C, and Phillips, R: Effect of x-ray contrast media on results for relative density of urine. Clin Chem 19(4):730–731, 1983.

STUDY QUESTIONS

1. Why is it possible to estimate the concentration of a normal urine specimen by its color?
2. State a pathologic cause of yellow urine foam and of white urine foam.
3. How does the presence of phenazopyridine affect routine urinalysis testing?
4. What is the significance of a cloudy, red urine?
5. Why is there a difference in the color of the serum from persons with hemoglobinuria and myoglobinuria?
6. Under what conditions will a port-wine urine color be observed in a urine specimen?
7. Why might a brown/black urine have a positive chemical test result for blood?
8. State the conditions required for urines containing melanin or homogentisic acid to appear brown/black.
9. Name a pathologic cause and a nonpathologic cause of blue/green urine.
10. Differentiate between the appearance of amorphous phosphates and urates in a refrigerated urine specimen. What chemical test is critical to the differentiation?
11. In what circumstance might a sediment be slightly warmed prior to microscopic examination?
12. How will collection of a urine specimen using the midstream clean-catch method affect urine clarity?
13. When should a microscopic examination be performed on a clear urine specimen?
14. For what part of the routine urinalysis does specimen clarity serve as a method of quality control?
15. Define specific gravity.

16. Can a cloudy urine specimen have a low specific gravity? Why or why not?

17. How can specific gravity be used to determine the quality of a specimen for urinalysis?

18. Why is specific gravity of less value than osmolarity in evaluating renal concentration ability?

19. State three disadvantages of the urinometer not encountered with the refractometer.

20. Describe the calibration of the refractometer.

21. What conclusion can be drawn from a specimen with a specific gravity of 1.001?

22. The specific gravity of a first morning specimen containing 2 g of protein and 2 g of glucose is 1.023 measured by refractometer. Does this indicate normal concentrating ability? Why or why not?

23. Describe two methods by which a specific gravity that is higher than the refractometer scale can be measured.

24. Why might a urine specimen from a patient who has just returned from radiology have an abnormally high specific gravity? Why might a urine specimen from a patient who has recently experienced a severe hemorrhage have an abnormally high specific gravity?

25. State a pathologic and nonpathologic reason why a urine specimen would have a strong odor of ammonia.

CASE STUDIES AND CLINICAL SITUATIONS

1. A concerned male athlete brings a clear, red urine specimen to the physician's office.
   a. Would you expect to see RBCs in the microscopic examination? Why or why not?
   b. Name two pathologic causes of a clear, red urine. Under what conditions do these substances appear in the urine?
   c. The patient reported that the urine appeared cloudy when he collected it the previous evening, but it was clear in the morning. Is this possible? Explain your answer.
   d. If the urine is chemically negative for blood, what questions should the physician ask the patient?

2. Upon arriving at work, a technologist notices that a urine specimen left beside the sink by personnel on the nightshift has a black color. The initial report describes the specimen as yellow.
   a. Should the technologist be concerned about this specimen? Explain your answer.
   b. If the specimen had an initial pH of 6.0 and now has a pH of 8.0, what is the most probable cause of the black color?
   c. If the specimen has a pH of 6.0 and was sitting uncapped, what is the most probable cause of the black color?
   d. If the original specimen was reported to be red and to contain RBCs, what is a possible cause of the black color?

3. While performing a routine urinalysis on a specimen collected from a patient in the urology clinic, the technician finds a specific gravity reading that exceeds the 1.035 scale on the refractometer.
   a. If the urinalysis report has a 1+ protein and a negative glucose, what is the most probable cause of this finding?
   b. The technician makes a 1:4 dilution of the specimen, repeats the specific gravity, and gets a reading of 1.015. What is the actual specific gravity?
   c. Using 1 mL of urine, how would the technician make the above dilution?
   d. How could a specific gravity be obtained from this specimen without diluting it?

4. Mrs. Smith frequently shops at the farmer's market near her home. She notices her urine has a red color and brings a sample to her physician. The specimen tests negative for blood.
   a. What is a probable cause of Mrs. Smith's red urine?
   b. Mrs. Smith collects a specimen at the physician's office. The color is yellow and the pH is 5.5. Is this consistent with the previous answer? Why or why not?

5. A urinalysis supervisor requests a new specimen in each of the following situations. Support or disagree with the decisions.
   a. A green-yellow specimen with negative test results for glucose and bilirubin
   b. A dark yellow specimen that produces a large amount of white foam
   c. A cloudy urine with a strong odor of ammonia
   d. A hazy specimen with a specific gravity greater than 1.035 by refractometer

CHAPTER 5

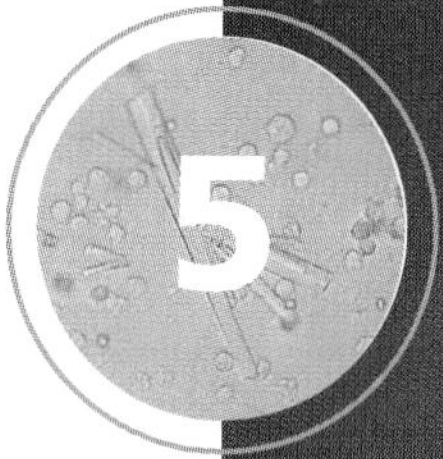

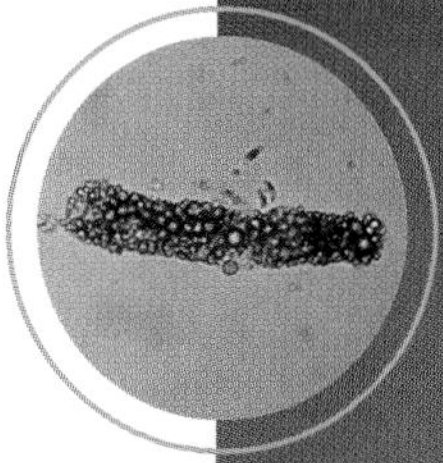

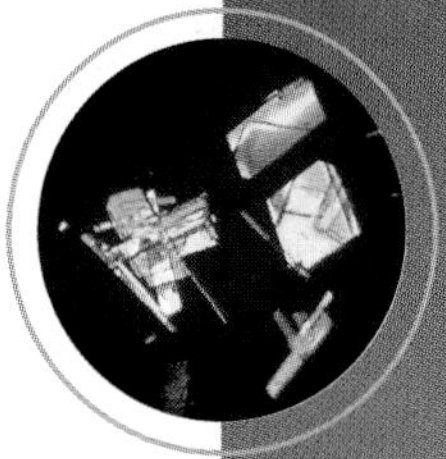

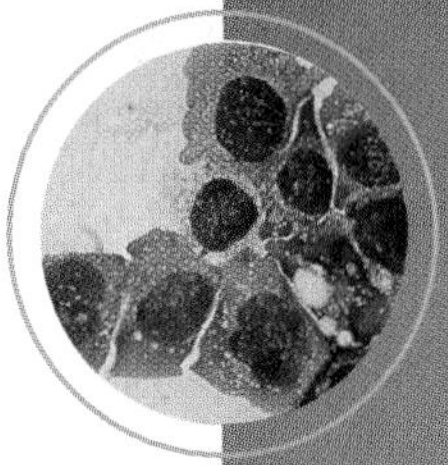

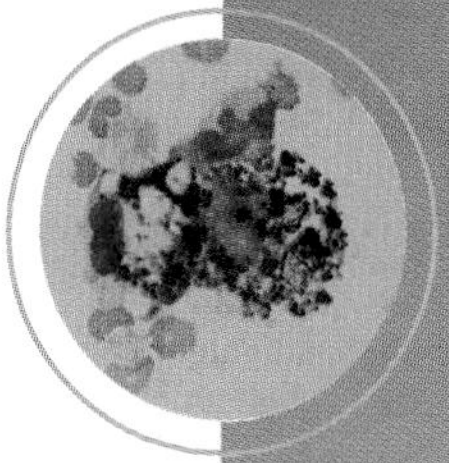

Chemical Examination of Urine

LEARNING OBJECTIVES

Upon completion of this chapter, the reader will be able to:

1. Describe the proper technique for performing reagent strip testing.
2. List four causes of premature deterioration of reagent strips, and tell how to avoid them.
3. List five quality-control procedures routinely performed with reagent strip testing.
4. Name two reasons for measuring urinary pH, and discuss their clinical applications.
5. Discuss the principle of pH testing by reagent strip.
6. Differentiate between prerenal, renal, and postrenal proteinuria, and give clinical examples of each.
7. Explain the "protein error of indicators," and list any sources of interference that may occur with this method of protein testing.
8. Discuss the sulfosalicylic acid (SSA) test for urine protein, including interpretation and sources of interference.
9. Describe the unique solubility characteristics of Bence Jones protein, and tell how they can be used to perform a screening test for the presence of this protein.
10. Explain why glucose that is normally reabsorbed in the proximal convoluted tubule may appear in the urine, and state the renal threshold levels for glucose.
11. Describe the principle of the glucose oxidase method of reagent strip testing for glucose, and name possible causes of interference with this method.
12. Describe the copper reduction method for detection of urinary reducing substances, and list possible causes of interference.
13. Interpret matching and nonmatching results between the glucose oxidase and the copper reduction tests for glucose.
14. Name the three "ketone bodies" appearing in urine and three causes of ketonuria.
15. Discuss the principle of the sodium nitroprusside reaction, including sensitivity and possible causes of interference.
16. Differentiate between hematuria, hemoglobinuria, and myoglobinuria with regard to the appearance of urine and serum and clinical significance.
17. Describe the chemical principle of the reagent strip method for blood testing, and list possible causes of interference.
18. Discuss methods used to differentiate between hemoglobinuria and myoglobinuria.
19. Outline the steps in the degradation of hemoglobin to bilirubin, urobilinogen, and finally urobilin.

20 Describe the relationship of urinary bilirubin and urobilinogen to the diagnosis of bile duct obstruction, liver disease, and hemolytic disorders.
21 Discuss the principle of the reagent strip test for urinary bilirubin, including possible sources of error.
22 Discuss the advantages and disadvantages of performing an Ictotest for detection of urine bilirubin.
23 State two reasons for increased urine urobilinogen and one reason for a decreased urine urobilinogen.
24 Describe the Watson-Schwartz test used to differentiate among urobilinogen, porphobilinogen, Ehrlich reactive compounds, and the Hoesch screening test for porphobilinogen.
25 Discuss the principle of the nitrite-reagent-strip test for bacteriuria.
26 List five possible causes of a false-negative results in the reagent-strip test for nitrite.
27 State the principle of the reagent strip test for leukocytes.
28 Discuss the advantages and sources of error of the reagent strip test for leukocytes.
29 Explain the principle of the chemical test for specific gravity.
30 Compare reagent strip testing for urine specific gravity with urinometer and refractometer testing.
31 Correlate physical and chemical urinalysis results.

KEY TERMS

bacteriuria
bilirubin
glycosuria
hematuria
hemoglobinuria
ketonuria
leukocyturia
microalbuminuria
myoglobinuria
orthostatic proteinuria
postrenal proteinuria
prerenal proteinuria
protein error of indicators
proteinuria
renal proteinuria
urobilinogen

Reagent Strips

Routine chemical examination of the urine has changed dramatically since the early days of urine testing, owing to the development of the reagent strip method for chemical analysis. Reagent strips currently provide a simple, rapid means for performing medically significant chemical analysis, including pH, protein, glucose, ketones, blood, ***bilirubin***, ***urobilinogen***, nitrite, leukocytes, and specific gravity. The two major types of reagent strips are manufactured under the tradenames Multistix (Bayer Corporation, Elkhart, IN) and Chemstrip (Roche-Boehringer Mannheim Diagnostics, Indianapolis, IN). These products are available with single- or multiple-testing areas, and the brand and number of tests used are a matter of laboratory preference. Certain variations relating to chemical reactions, sensitivity, specificity, and interfering substances occur among the products and are discussed in the following sections. Reagent strip brands are also specified by instrumentation manufacturers.

Reagent strips consist of chemical-impregnated absorbent pads attached to a plastic strip. A color-producing chemical reaction takes place when the absorbent pad comes in contact with urine. Color reactions are interpreted by comparing the color produced on the pad with a chart supplied by the manufacturer. Several colors or intensities of a color for each substance being tested appear on the chart. By careful comparison of the colors on the chart and the strip, a semiquantitative value of trace, 1+, 2+, 3+, or 4+ can be reported. An estimate of the milligrams per deciliter present is available for appropriate testing areas. Automated reagent strip readers also provide Système International units.

REAGENT STRIP TECHNIQUE

Testing methodology includes dipping the reagent strip completely, but briefly, into a well-mixed specimen; removing excess urine from the strip when withdrawing it from the specimen; waiting the specified length of time for reac-

PROCEDURE

Reagent Strip Technique

- Dip the reagent strip briefly into a well-mixed uncentrifuged urine specimen at room temperature.
- Remove excess urine by touching the edge of the strip to the container as the strip is withdrawn. Blot the edge of the strip.
- Wait the specified amount of time for the reaction to occur.
- Compare the color reaction of the strip pads to the manufacturer's color chart in good lighting.

tions to take place; and comparing the colored reactions against the manufacturer's chart using a good light source.

Improper technique can result in errors. Formed elements such as red and white blood cells sink to the bottom of the specimen and will be undetected in an unmixed specimen. Allowing the strip to remain in the urine for an extended period may cause leaching of reagents from the pads. Likewise, excess urine remaining on the strip after its removal from the specimen can produce a runover between chemicals on adjacent pads, producing distortion of the colors. To ensure against runover, blotting the edge of the strip on absorbent paper and holding the strip horizontally while comparing it with the color chart is recommended. The amount of time needed for reactions to take place varies between tests and manufacturers and ranges from an immediate reaction for pH to 120 seconds for leukocytes. For the best semiquantitative results, the manufacturer's stated time should be followed; however, when precise timing cannot be adhered to, manufacturers recommend that reactions be read between 60 and 120 seconds, with the leukocyte reaction read at 120 seconds. A good light source is, of course, essential for accurate interpretation of color reactions. The strip must be held close to the color chart without actually placing it on the chart. Reagent strips and color charts from different manufacturers are not interchangeable. Specimens that have been refrigerated must be allowed to return to room temperature prior to reagent strip testing, as the enzymatic reactions on the strips are temperature dependent.

HANDLING AND STORAGE OF REAGENT STRIPS

In addition to the use of correct testing technique, reagent strips must be protected from deterioration caused by moisture, volatile chemicals, heat, and light. Reagent strips are packaged in opaque containers with a desiccant to protect them from light and moisture. Strips are removed just prior to testing, and the bottle is tightly resealed immediately. Bottles should not be opened in the presence of volatile fumes. Manufacturers recommend that reagent strips be stored at room temperature below 30°C. All bottles are stamped with an expiration date that represents the functional life expectancy of the chemical pads. Reagent strips must not be used past the expiration date. Care must be taken not to touch the chemical pads when removing the strips.

QUALITY CONTROL OF REAGENT STRIPS

Reagent strips must be checked with both positive and negative controls a minimum of once every 24 hours. Many laboratories perform this check at the beginning of each shift.[12] Testing is also performed when a new bottle of reagent strips is opened, questionable results are obtained, or there is concern about the integrity of the strips. All quality control results must be recorded following laboratory protocol. Several companies manufacture both positive and negative controls, and many methods of preparing and preserving in-house controls have been published.[8] Distilled water is not recommended as a negative control because reagent strip chemical reactions are designed to perform at ionic concentrations similar to urine.[18] All readings of the negative control must be negative, and positive control readings should agree with the published value by ± one color block.[12] Results that do not agree with the published values must be resolved through the testing of additional strips and controls (see Chap. 7).

Summary of Reagent Strip Testing

Care of Reagent Strips

1. Store with desiccant in an opaque, tightly closed container.
2. Store below 30°C; do not freeze.
3. Do not expose to volatile fumes.
4. Do not use past the expiration date.
5. Do not use if chemical pads become discolored.
6. Remove strips immediately prior to use.

Technique

1. Mix specimen well.
2. Dip the strip completely, but briefly, into specimen.
3. Remove excess urine by withdrawing the strip against the rim of the container and by blotting the edge of the strip.
4. Compare reaction colors with the manufacturer's chart under a good light source at the specified time.
5. Perform backup tests when indicated.
6. Be alert for the presence of interfering substances.
7. Understand the principles and significance of the test.
8. Relate chemical findings to each other and to the physical and microscopic urinalysis results.

Quality Control

1. Test open bottles of reagent strips with known positive and negative controls every 24 h.
2. Resolve control results that are out of range by further testing.
3. Test reagents used in backup tests with positive and negative controls.
4. Perform positive and negative controls on new reagents and newly opened bottles of reagent strips.
5. Record all control results and reagent lot numbers.

Demonstration of chemically acceptable reagent strips does not entirely rule out the possibility of inaccurate results. Interfering substances in the urine, technical carelessness, and color blindness also will produce errors. Reagent strip manufacturers have published information concerning the limitations of their chemical reactions, and laboratory personnel should be aware of these conditions. As mentioned in Chapter 4, a primary example of reagent strip interference is the masking of color reactions by the orange pigment present in the urine of persons taking phenazopyridine compounds. If laboratory personnel do not recognize the presence of this pigment or other pigments, they will report many erroneous results.

Nonreagent strip testing procedures using tablets and liquid chemicals are available when questionable results are obtained or highly pigmented specimens are encountered. In the past, many of these procedures were used routinely to confirm positive results. Increased specificity and sensitivity of reagent strips and the use of automated strip readers have reduced the need for routine use of these procedures.[14] The chemical reliability of these procedures also must be checked using positive and negative controls. Specific backup tests are discussed in this chapter under the sections devoted to the chemical parameters for which they are used.

TABLE 5–1 **Causes of Acid and Alkaline Urine**

Acid Urine	Alkaline Urine
Emphysema	Hyperventilation
Diabetes mellitus	Vomiting
Starvation	Renal tubular acidosis
Dehydration	Presence of urease-producing bacteria
Diarrhea	Vegetarian diet
Presence of acid-producing bacteria (*Escherichia coli*)	Old specimens
High-protein diet	
Cranberry juice	
Medications (methenamine mandelate [Mandelamine], fosfomycin tromethamine)	

pH

Along with the lungs, the kidneys are the major regulators of the acid-base content in the body. They do this through the secretion of hydrogen in the form of ammonium ions, hydrogen phosphate, and weak organic acids, and by the reabsorption of bicarbonate from the filtrate in the convoluted tubules (see Chap. 2). A healthy individual will usually produce a first morning specimen with a slightly acidic pH of 5.0 to 6.0; a more alkaline pH is found following meals (alkaline tide). The pH of normal random samples can range from 4.5 to 8.0. Consequently, no normal values are assigned to urinary pH, and it must be considered in conjunction with other patient information, such as the acid-base content of the blood, the patient's renal function, the presence of a urinary tract infection, the patient's dietary intake, and the age of the specimen (Table 5–1).

CLINICAL SIGNIFICANCE

The importance of urinary pH is primarily as an aid in determining the existence of systemic acid-base disorders of metabolic or respiratory origin and in the management of urinary conditions that require the urine to be maintained at a specific pH. In respiratory or metabolic acidosis not related to renal function disorders, the urine will be acidic; conversely, if respiratory or metabolic alkalosis is present, the urine will be alkaline. Therefore, a urinary pH that does not conform to this pattern may be used to rule out the suspected condition, or, as discussed in Chapter 2, it may indicate a disorder resulting from the kidneys' inability to secrete or to reabsorb acid or base.

The precipitation of inorganic chemicals dissolved in the urine forms urinary crystals and renal calculi. This precipitation depends on urinary pH and can be controlled by maintaining the urine at a pH that is incompatible with the precipitation of the particular chemicals causing the calculi formation. For example, calcium oxalate, a frequent constituent of renal calculi, precipitates primarily in acidic and not alkaline urine. Therefore, maintaining urine at an alkaline pH will discourage formation of the calculi. Knowledge of urinary pH is important in the identification of crystals observed during microscopic examination of the urine sediment. This will be discussed in detail in Chapter 6.

The maintenance of an acidic urine can be of value in the treatment of urinary tract infections caused by urea-splitting organisms because they do not multiply as readily in an acidic medium. These same organisms are also responsible for the highly alkaline pH found in specimens that have been allowed to sit unpreserved for extended periods. Urinary pH is controlled primarily by dietary regulation, although medications also may be used. Persons on high-protein and high-meat diets tend to produce acidic urine, whereas urine from vegetarians is more alkaline, owing to the formation of bicarbonate following digestion of many fruits and vegetables.[13] An exception to the rule is cranberry juice, which produces an acidic urine and has long been used as a home remedy for minor bladder infections. Medications prescribed for urinary tract infections, such as methenamine mandelate (Mandelamine) and fos-

Summary of Clinical Significance of Urine pH

1. Respiratory or metabolic acidosis/ketosis
2. Respiratory or metabolic alkalosis
3. Defects in renal tubular secretion and reabsorption of acids and bases—renal tubular acidosis
4. Renal calculi formation
5. Treatment of urinary tract infections
6. Precipitation/identification of crystals
7. Determination of unsatisfactory specimens

pH Reagent Strip Summary

Reagents	Methyl red, bromthymol blue
Sensitivity	5–9
Sources of error/interference	No known interfering substances Runover from adjacent pads Old specimens
Correlations with other tests	Nitrite Leukocytes Microscopic

fomycin tromethamine, are metabolized to produce an acidic urine.

The pH of freshly excreted urine does not reach 9 in normal or abnormal conditions. A pH of 9 is associated with an improperly preserved specimen and indicates that a fresh specimen should be obtained to ensure the validity of the analysis.

REAGENT STRIP REACTIONS

The Multistix and Chemstrip brands of reagent strips measure urine pH in 0.5- or 1-unit increments between pH 5 and 9. To provide differentiation of pH units throughout this wide range, both manufacturers use a double-indicator system of methyl red and bromthymol blue. Methyl red produces a color change from red to yellow in the pH range 4 to 6, and bromthymol blue turns from yellow to blue in the range of 6 to 9. Therefore, in the pH range 5 to 9 measured by the reagent strips, one will see colors progressing from orange at pH 5 through yellow and green to a final deep blue at pH 9.

$$\text{Methyl red} + H^+ \rightarrow \text{Bromthymol blue} - H^+$$
$$(\text{Red} \rightarrow \text{Yellow}) \qquad (\text{Yellow} \rightarrow \text{Blue})$$

No known substances interfere with urinary pH measurements performed by reagent strips. Care must be taken, however, to prevent runover between the pH testing area and the adjacent, highly acidic protein testing area on Multistix, as this may produce a falsely acidic reading in an alkaline urine.

Protein

Of the routine chemical tests performed on urine, the most indicative of renal disease is the protein determination. The presence of ***proteinuria*** is often associated with early renal disease, making the urinary protein test an important part of any physical examination. Normal urine contains very little protein: usually, less than 10 mg/dL or 100 mg per 24 hours is excreted. This protein consists primarily of low-molecular-weight serum proteins that have been filtered by the glomerulus and proteins produced in the genitourinary tract. Owing to its low molecular weight, albumin is the major serum protein found in normal urine. Even though it is present in high concentrations in the plasma, the normal urinary albumin content is low because the majority of the albumin presented to the glomerulus is not filtered, and much of the filtered albumin is reabsorbed by the tubules. Other proteins include small amounts of serum and tubular microglobulins, Tamm-Horsfall protein produced by the tubules, and proteins from prostatic, seminal, and vaginal secretions.

CLINICAL SIGNIFICANCE

Demonstration of proteinuria in a routine analysis does not always signify renal disease; however, its presence does require additional testing to determine whether the protein represents a normal or a pathologic condition. The causes of proteinuria are varied and can be grouped into three major categories: ***prerenal***, ***renal***, and ***postrenal***, based on the origin of the protein.

PRERENAL PROTEINURIA

As the name implies, prerenal proteinuria is caused by conditions affecting the plasma prior to its reaching the kidney and, therefore, is not indicative of actual renal disease. This condition is frequently transient, caused by increased levels of low-molecular-weight plasma proteins such as hemoglobin, myoglobin, and the **acute phase reactants** associated with infection and inflammation. The increased filtration of these proteins exceeds the normal reabsorptive capacity of the renal tubules resulting in an overflow of the proteins into the urine. Because reagent strips detect primarily albumin, prerenal proteinuria is usually not discovered in a routine urinalysis.

Bence Jones Protein

A primary example of proteinuria due to increased serum protein levels is the excretion of Bence Jones protein by persons with multiple myeloma. In multiple myeloma, a proliferative disorder of the immunoglobulin-producing plasma cells, the serum contains markedly elevated levels of monoclonal immunoglobulin light chains (Bence Jones protein). This low-molecular-weight protein is filtered in quantities exceeding the tubular reabsorption capacity and is excreted in the urine.

When Bence Jones protein is suspected, a screening test that uses the unique solubility characteristics of the protein can be performed. Unlike other proteins, which coagulate and remain coagulated when exposed to heat, Bence Jones protein coagulates at temperatures between 40°C and 60°C and dissolves when the temperature reaches 100°C. Therefore, a specimen that appears turbid between 40°C and 60°C and clear at 100°C can be suspected of containing Bence Jones protein. Interference due to other precipitated proteins can be removed by filtering the specimen at 100°C and observing the specimen for turbidity as it cools to between 40°C and 60°C. Not all persons with multiple myeloma excrete detectable levels of Bence Jones protein. Suspected cases of multiple myeloma must be diagnosed by performing serum electrophoresis.

RENAL PROTEINURIA

Proteinuria associated with true renal disease may be the result of either glomerular or tubular damage. When the glomerular membrane is damaged, selective filtration is impaired, and increased amounts of serum albumin and eventually red and white blood cells pass through the membrane and are excreted in the urine. Conditions that present the glomerular membrane with abnormal substances (e.g., **amyloid material**, toxic substances, and the immune complexes found in lupus erythematosus and streptococcal glomerulonephritis) are the major causes of proteinuria due to glomerular damage.

Increased pressure from the blood entering the glomerulus may override the selective filtration of the glomerulus, causing increased albumin to enter the filtrate. This condition may be reversible, such as occurs during strenuous exercise and dehydration or associated with hypertension. Proteinuria that occurs during the latter months of pregnancy may indicate a pre-eclamptic state and should be considered in conjunction with other clinical symptoms, such as hypertension, to determine if this condition exists.

Increased albumin is also present in disorders affecting tubular reabsorption because the normally filtered albumin can no longer be reabsorbed. Other low-molecular-weight proteins that are usually reabsorbed also will be present. Causes of tubular dysfunction include exposure to toxic substances and heavy metals, severe viral infections, and **Fanconi's syndrome**. The amount of protein that appears in the urine following glomerular damage will range from slightly above normal to 4 g/day, whereas markedly elevated protein levels are seldom seen in tubular disorders.

The discovery of protein, particularly in a random sample, is not always of pathologic significance, because several benign causes of renal proteinuria exist. Benign proteinuria is usually transient and can be produced by conditions such as exposure to cold, strenuous exercise, high fever, and dehydration.

Orthostatic (Postural) Proteinuria

A persistent benign proteinuria occurs frequently in young adults and is termed ***orthostatic***, or postural, proteinuria. It occurs following periods spent in a vertical posture and disappears when a horizontal position is assumed. Increased pressure on the renal vein when in the vertical position is believed to account for this condition. Patients suspected of orthostatic proteinuria are requested to empty their bladder before going to bed, collect a specimen immediately upon arising in the morning, and collect a second specimen after remaining in a vertical position for several hours. Both specimens are tested for protein, and, if orthostatic proteinuria is present, a negative reading will be seen on the first morning specimen and a positive result will be found on the second specimen.

Microalbuminuria

The development of diabetic nephropathy leading to reduced glomerular filtration and eventual renal failure is a common occurrence in persons with both type 1 and type 2 diabetes mellitus. Onset of renal complications can first be predicted by detection of ***microalbuminuria***, and the progression of renal disease can be prevented through better stabilization of blood glucose levels and controlling of hypertension.[19] The presence of microalbuminuria is also associated with an increased risk of cardiovascular disease.[3]

The term microalbuminuria is used to denote proteinuria that cannot be detected by routinely used reagent strips. Values are reported as the albumin excretion rate (**AER**) in µg/min, mg/24 h, and the albumin:creatinine ratio, depending on the testing methodology in use. Microalbuminuria is considered to be significant when the AER is 20 to 200 µg/min, 30 to 300 mg of albumin are excreted in 24 hours, or the albumin:creatinine ratio is greater than 3.4 mg/mmol.

Determination of AER and 24-hour albumin excretion requires collection of timed specimens. The albumin:creatinine ratio and the semiquantitative Micral-Test (BMC, Indianapolis, IN) can be performed on random specimens. To avoid the presence of orthostatic protein, overnight timed specimens and first morning specimens are recommended for testing. The Clinitek 50 or Clinitek 100 microalbumin reagent strips (Bayer Diagnostics, Elkhart, IN) provide an automated calculation of the albumin:creatinine ratio using semiquantitative results for albumin and creatinine obtained by reactions on the chemical pads (Appendix A). The Micral-Test is a reagent strip test employing an antibody-enzyme conjugate to bind human albumin. The resulting conjugate reacts with substrate to produce a colored reaction that can be compared to a color chart calibrated between 0 to 10 mg/dL. Development of rapid testing methods is increasing the routine testing of patients with diabetes for the presence of microalbuminuria.

Summary of Clinical Significance of Urine Protein

Prerenal	***Tubular Disorders***
Intravascular hemolysis Muscle injury Severe infection and inflammation Multiple myeloma	Fanconi's syndrome Toxic agents/heavy metals Severe viral infections
Renal	***Postrenal***
Glomerular disorders Immune complex disorders Amyloidosis Toxic agents Diabetic nephropathy Strenuous exercise Dehydration Hypertension Pre-eclampsia Orthostatic or postural proteinuria	Lower urinary tract infections/inflammation Injury/trauma Menstrual contamination Prostatic fluid/spermatozoa Vaginal secretions

POSTRENAL PROTEINURIA

Protein can be added to a urine specimen as it passes through the structures of the lower urinary tract (ureters, bladder, urethra, prostate, and vagina). Bacterial and fungal infections and inflammations produce exudates containing protein from the interstitial fluid. The presence of blood as the result of injury or menstrual contamination contributes protein, as does the presence of prostatic fluid and large amounts of spermatozoa.

REAGENT STRIP REACTIONS

Reagent strip testing for protein uses the principle of the ***protein error of indicators*** to produce a visible colorimetric reaction. Contrary to the general belief that indicators produce specific colors in response to particular pH levels, certain indicators change color in the presence of protein even though the pH of the medium remains constant. This is because protein (primarily albumin) accepts ions from the indicator. Depending on the manufacturer, the protein area of the strip contains either tetrabromphenol blue or 3′, 3″, 5′, 5″-tetrachlorophenol-3, 4, 5, 6-tetrabromosulfonphthalein and an acid buffer to maintain the pH at a constant level. At a pH level of 3, both indicators will appear yellow in the absence of protein; however, as the protein concentration increases, the color will progress through various shades of green and finally to blue. Readings are usually reported in terms of negative, trace, 1+, 2+, 3+, and 4+; however, the manufacturers also supply a semiquantitative value in milligrams per deciliter corresponding to each color change. Interpretation of trace readings can be difficult. The specific gravity of the specimen should be considered because a trace protein in a dilute specimen is more significant than in a concentrated specimen.

$$\underset{\text{(Yellow)}}{\text{Indicator}} + \text{Protein} \xrightarrow{\text{pH 3.0}} \text{Protein} + H^+ \quad \underset{\text{(Blue-green)}}{\text{Indicator} - H^+}$$

REACTION INTERFERENCE

The major source of error with reagent strips occurs with highly buffered alkaline urine that overrides the acid buffer system, producing a rise in pH and a color change unrelated to protein concentration. Likewise, a technical error of allowing the reagent pad to remain in contact with the urine for a prolonged period may remove the buffer. False-positive readings will be obtained when the reaction does not take place under acidic conditions. Highly pigmented urine and contamination of the container with quaternary ammonium compounds, detergents, and antiseptics will also cause false-positive readings. When using Multistix, a false-positive trace reading may occur in specimens with a high specific gravity. The fact that reagent strips detect primarily albumin can result in a false-negative reading in the presence of proteins other than albumin.

Traditionally most laboratories chose to confirm all positive protein results using the sulfosalicyclic acid **(SSA)** precipitation test. Currently this practice is being replaced by more selective criteria to determine the need for additional testing. For example, some laboratories perform SSA testing only on highly alkaline urines, and others acidify the specimen and retest using a reagent strip. Also, a laboratory with an automated strip reader can opt not to record trace readings.

Protein Reagent Strip Summary

Reagents	Multistix: Tetrabromphenol blue Chemstrip: 3′, 3″, 5′, 5″ tetrachlorophenol 3, 4, 5, 6-tetrabromosulfophthalein
Sensitivity	Multistix: 15–30 mg/dL albumin Chemstrip: 6 mg/dL albumin
Sources of error/interference	False-positive: Highly buffered alkaline urine Pigmented specimens, phenazopyridine Quaternary ammonium compounds (detergents) Antiseptics, chlorhexidine Loss of buffer from prolonged exposure of the reagent strip to the specimen High specific gravity False-negative: Proteins other than albumin
Correlations with other tests	Blood Nitrite Leukocytes Microscopic

SULFOSALICYLIC ACID PRECIPITATION TEST

The SSA test is a cold precipitation test that reacts equally with all forms of protein (Table 5–2). Various concentrations and amounts of SSA can be used to precipitate protein, and methods vary greatly among laboratories. All

TABLE 5–2 **Reporting SSA Turbidity**

Grade	Turbidity	Protein Range (mg/dL)
Negative	No increase in turbidity	<6
Trace	Noticeable turbidity	6–30
1+	Distinct turbidity with no granulation	30–100
2+	Turbidity with granulation with no flocculation	100–200
3+	Turbidity with granulation and flocculation	200–400
4+	Clumps of protein	>400

PROCEDURE

Sulfosalicylic Acid (SSA) Precipitation Test

- Add 3 mL of 3% SSA reagent to 3 mL of centrifuged urine.
- Mix by inversion and observe for cloudiness.
- Grade the degree of turbidity (see Table 5–2).

precipitation tests must be performed on centrifuged specimens to remove any extraneous contamination.

Any substance precipitated by acid will, of course, produce false turbidity in the SSA test. The most frequently encountered substances are radiographic dyes, tolbutamide metabolites, cephalosporins, penicillins, and sulfonamides.[1] The presence of radiographic material can be suspected when a markedly elevated specific gravity is obtained. In the presence of radiographic dye, the turbidity will also increase on standing due to the precipitation of crystals rather than protein. The patient's history will provide the necessary information on tolbutamide and antibiotic ingestion. In contrast to the reagent strip test, a highly alkaline urine will produce false-negative readings in precipitation tests as the higher pH interferes with precipitation. Use of a more concentrated solution of SSA may overcome the effect of a highly buffered, alkaline urine.

Glucose

Because of its value in the detection and monitoring of diabetes mellitus, the glucose test is the most frequent chemical analysis performed on urine. Owing to the nonspecific symptoms associated with the onset of diabetes, it is estimated that more than half of the cases in the world are undiagnosed. Therefore, blood and urine glucose tests are included in all physical examinations and are often the focus of mass health screening programs. Early diagnosis of diabetes mellitus through blood and urine glucose tests provides a greatly improved prognosis. Using currently available reagent strip methods for both blood and urine glucose testing, patients can monitor themselves at home and can detect regulatory problems prior to the development of serious complications.

CLINICAL SIGNIFICANCE

Under normal circumstances, almost all the glucose filtered by the glomerulus is reabsorbed in the proximal convoluted tubule; therefore, urine contains only minute amounts of glucose. Tubular reabsorption of glucose is by active transport in response to the body's need to maintain an adequate concentration of glucose. Should the blood level of glucose become elevated (**hyperglycemia**), as occurs in diabetes mellitus, the tubular transport of glucose ceases, and glucose appears in the urine. The blood level at which tubular reabsorption stops (renal threshold) for glucose is approximately 160 to 180 mg/dL. Blood glucose levels will fluctuate, and a normal person may have ***glycosuria*** following a meal with a high glucose content. Therefore, the most informative glucose results are obtained from specimens collected under controlled conditions. Fasting prior to the collection of samples for screening tests is recommended. For purposes of diabetes monitoring, specimens are usually tested 2 hours after meals. A first morning specimen does not always represent a fasting specimen because glucose from an evening meal may remain in the bladder overnight, and patients should be advised to empty the bladder and collect the second specimen.[5] Urine for glucose testing also may be collected in conjunction with the blood samples drawn during the course of a glucose tolerance test, which is used to confirm the diagnosis of diabetes mellitus or hypoglycemia.

Hyperglycemia that occurs during pregnancy and disappears after delivery is called gestational diabetes. The onset of the hyperglycemia and glycosuria is normally around the sixth month of pregnancy. Hormones secreted by the placenta are believed to block the action of insulin, resulting in hyperglycemia. Detection of gestational diabetes is important to the welfare of the baby, because glucose will cross the placenta whereas insulin does not. Women who have gestational diabetes are prone to developing type 2 diabetes mellitus in later years.

Hyperglycemia of nondiabetic origin is seen in a variety of disorders and also will produce glycosuria. Many of these disorders are associated with hormonal function and include pancreatitis, pancreatic cancer, acromegaly, Cushing's syndrome, hyperthyroidism, and pheochromocytoma. The hormones glucagon, epinephrine, cortisol, thyroxine, and growth hormone, which are increased in these disorders, work in opposition to insulin, thereby producing hyperglycemia and glucosuria. Whereas a primary function of insulin is to convert glucose to glycogen for storage (**glycogenesis**), these opposing hormones cause the breakdown of

Summary of Clinical Significance of Urine Glucose

Hyperglycemia Associated

Diabetes mellitus
Pancreatitis
Pancreatic cancer
Acromegaly
Cushing's syndrome
Hyperthyroidism
Pheochromocytoma
Central nervous system damage
Stress
Gestational diabetes

Renal Associated

Fanconi's syndrome
Advanced renal disease
Osteomalacia
Pregnancy

glycogen to glucose (**glycogenolysis**), resulting in increased levels of circulating glucose. Epinephrine is also a strong inhibitor of insulin secretion and is increased when the body is subjected to severe stress, which accounts for the glucosuria seen in conjunction with cerebrovascular trauma and myocardial infarction.

Glycosuria will occur in the absence of hyperglycemia when the reabsorption of glucose by the renal tubules is compromised. This is frequently referred to as "renal glycosuria" and is seen in end-stage renal disease, osteomalacia, and Fanconi's syndrome. Glycosuria not associated with gestational diabetes is occasionally seen as a result of a temporary lowering of the renal threshold for glucose during pregnancy.

REAGENT STRIP (GLUCOSE OXIDASE) REACTIONS

Two very different tests have been used by laboratories to measure urinary glucose. The glucose oxidase procedure provides a specific test for glucose, and the copper reduction test is a general test for glucose and other reducing substances. Reagent strips employ the glucose oxidase testing method by impregnating the testing area with a mixture of glucose oxidase, peroxidase, chromogen, and buffer to produce a double sequential enzyme reaction. In the first step, glucose oxidase catalyzes a reaction between glucose and room air to produce gluconic acid and peroxide. In the second step, peroxidase catalyzes the reaction between peroxide and chromogen to form an oxidized colored compound that represents the presence of glucose.

$$1.\ \text{Glucose} + O_2\ (\text{air}) \xrightarrow[\text{oxidase}]{\text{glucose}} \text{gluconic acid} + H_2O_2$$

$$2.\ H_2O_2 + \text{chromogen} \xrightarrow{\text{peroxidase}} \text{oxidized colored chromogen} + H_2O$$

Reagent strip manufacturers use several different chromogens, including potassium iodide (green to brown) and tetramethylbenzidine (yellow to green). Urine glucose may be reported in terms of negative, trace, 1+, 2+, 3+, and 4+; however, the color charts also provide quantitative measurements ranging from 100 mg/dL to 2 g/dL, or 0.1 percent to 2 percent. The American Diabetes Association recommends quantitative reporting.

REACTION INTERFERENCE

Because the glucose oxidase method is specific for glucose, false-positive reactions will not be obtained from other urinary constituents, including other sugars that may be present. False-positive reactions may occur, however, if containers become contaminated with peroxide or strong oxidizing detergents.

Substances that interfere with the enzymatic reaction or reducing agents, such as ascorbic acid, that prevent oxidation of the chromogen may produce false-negative results. To minimize interference from ascorbic acid, reagent strip manufacturers are incorporating additional chemicals such as iodate, which oxidizes ascorbic acid into the test pads. Product literature should be carefully reviewed for current information regarding all interfering substances. High levels of ketones also affect glucose oxidase tests at low glucose concentrations; however, because ketones are usually accompanied by marked glycosuria, this seldom presents a problem. High specific gravity and low temperature may decrease the sensitivity of the test. By far the greatest source of false-negative glucose results is the technical error of allowing specimens to remain unpreserved at room temperature for extended periods. False-negative results will be obtained with both the glucose oxidase and the copper reduction methods owing to the rapid glycolysis of glucose.

Glucose Reagent Strip Summary

Reagents	Multistix: Glucose oxidase Peroxidase Potassium iodide Chemstrip: Glucose oxidase Peroxidase Tetramethylbenzidine
Sensitivity	Multistix: 75–125 mg/dL Chemstrip: 40 mg/dL
Interference	False-positive: Contamination by oxidizing agents and detergents False-negative: High levels of ascorbic acid High levels of ketones High specific gravity Low temperatures Improperly preserved specimens
Correlations with other tests	Ketones

COPPER REDUCTION TEST

Measurement of glucose by the copper reduction method was one of the earliest chemical tests performed on urine. The test relies on the ability of glucose and other substances to reduce copper sulfate to cuprous oxide in the presence of alkali and heat. A color change progressing from a negative blue ($CuSO_4$) through green, yellow, and orange/red (Cu_2O) occurs when the reaction takes place.

$$CuSO_4\ (\text{cupric ions}) + \text{reducing substance} \xrightarrow[\text{alkali}]{\text{heat}}$$

$$Cu_2O\ (\text{cuprous ions}) + \text{oxidized substance} \rightarrow \text{color}\ (\text{blue/green} \rightarrow \text{orange/red})$$

The classic Benedict's solution was developed in 1908 and contained copper sulfate, sodium carbonate, and sodium citrate buffer.[2] Urine was then added to the solution, heat was applied, and the resulting precipitate was observed for color. A more convenient method that employs Benedict's principle is the Clinitest tablet (Bayer Diagnostics, Elkhart, IN). The tablets contain copper sulfate, sodium carbonate, sodium citrate, and sodium hydroxide. Upon addition of the tablet to water and urine, heat is produced by the hydrolysis of sodium hydroxide and its reaction with sodium citrate, and carbon dioxide is released from the sodium carbonate to prevent room air from interfering with the reduction reaction. Tubes should be placed in a rack and not held in the hand because the reaction heat could cause a burn. At the conclusion of the effervescent reaction, the tube is gently shaken, and the color ranging from blue to orange/red can be compared with the manufacturer's color chart to determine the approximate amount of reducing substance.

Care must be taken to observe the reaction closely as it is taking place, because at high glucose levels, a phenomenon known as "pass through" may occur. When this happens, the color produced passes through the orange/red stage and returns to a blue or blue-green color, and if not observed, a high glucose level may be reported as negative. The manufacturers of Clinitest have suggested a method using two drops instead of five drops of urine to minimize the occurrence of "pass through." A separate color chart must be used to interpret the reaction.

The sensitivity of Clinitest to glucose is reduced to a minimum of 200 mg/dL. As a nonspecific test for reducing substances, Clinitest is subject to interference from other reducing sugars, including galactose, lactose, fructose, maltose, and pentoses, ascorbic acid, certain drug metabolites, and antibiotics such as the cephalosporins. Therefore, Clinitest does not provide a confirmatory test for glucose.

Clinitest tablets are very hygroscopic and should be stored in their tightly closed packages. A strong blue color in the unused tablets suggests deterioration due to moisture accumulation, as does vigorous tablet fizzing.

PROCEDURE

Clinitest Procedure

- Place five drops of urine into a glass test tube.
- Add 10 drops of distilled water to the urine in the test tube.
- Drop one Clinitest tablet into the test tube and observe the reaction until completion (cessation of boiling).

  CAUTION: The reaction mixture gets very hot. Do not touch the bottom area of the test tube. Use glass test tube only.
- Wait 15 seconds after boiling has stopped and gently shake the contents of the tube.
- Compare the color of the mixture to the Clinitest color chart and record the result (negative, trace, 1+, 2+, 3+, 4+).
- Observe for the possibility of the "pass-through" phenomenon.

Summary of Glucose Oxidase and Clinitest Reactions

Glucose Oxidase	Clinitest	Interpretation
1+ positive	Negative	Small amount of glucose present
4+ positive	Negative	Possible oxidizing agent interference on reagent strip
Negative	Positive	Nonglucose reducing substance present Possible interfering substance for reagent strip

COMPARISON OF GLUCOSE OXIDASE AND CLINITEST

Several reasons exist to explain the finding of conflicting results between the two glucose tests. As stated previously, the Clinitest is not as sensitive as the glucose oxidase test, so the finding of a 1+ reagent strip reading and a negative Clinitest should not be surprising. A strongly positive reagent strip and a negative Clinitest, however, should cause concern about the possible contamination by strong oxidizing agents. The most significant discrepancy is the negative reagent strip with a positive Clinitest. Although interfering substances affecting either test may cause this problem, the most frequent cause is the presence of other reducing sugars in the urine. Commonly found reducing sugars include galactose, fructose, pentose, and lactose, of which galactose is the most clinically significant. Galactose in the urine of a newborn represents an "inborn error of metabolism" in which lack of the enzyme galactose-1-phosphate uridyl transferase prevents breakdown of ingested galactose and results in failure to thrive and other complications, including death. All newborns should be screened for galactosuria because early detection followed by dietary restriction will control the condition. Depending on the laboratory population, Clinitest is routinely performed on pediatric specimens from patients up to at least the age of 2 years. The appearance of other reducing sugars is usually of minimal clinical significance, and lactose is frequently found in the urine of nursing mothers. Keep in mind that table sugar is sucrose, a nonreducing sugar, and will not react with Clinitest or glucose oxidase strips.

Ketones

The term ketones represents three intermediate products of fat metabolism, namely, acetone, acetoacetic acid, and beta-hydroxybutyric acid. Normally, measurable amounts of ketones do not appear in the urine, because all the metabolized fat is completely broken down into carbon dioxide and water. However, when the use of available carbohydrate as the major source of energy becomes compromised and body stores of fat must be metabolized to supply energy, ketones will be detected in urine.

Summary of Clinical Significance of Urine Ketones

1. Diabetic acidosis
2. Insulin dosage monitoring
3. Starvation
4. Malabsorption/pancreatic disorders
5. Strenuous exercise
6. Vomiting
7. Inborn errors of amino acid metabolism (see Chap. 9)

CLINICAL SIGNIFICANCE

Clinical reasons for increased fat metabolism include the inability to metabolize carbohydrate, as occurs in diabetes mellitus; increased loss of carbohydrate from vomiting; and inadequate intake of carbohydrate associated with starvation and malabsorption.

Testing for urinary ketones is most valuable in the management and monitoring of insulin-dependent (type 1) diabetes mellitus. ***Ketonuria*** shows a deficiency in insulin, indicating the need to regulate dosage. It is often an early indicator of insufficient insulin dosage in type 1 diabetes and in patients with diabetes experiencing medical problems in addition to their diabetes. Increased accumulation of ketones in the blood leads to electrolyte imbalance, dehydration, and, if not corrected, acidosis and eventual diabetic coma. To aid in the monitoring of diabetes, ketone tests not only are included in all multiple-test strips but also are combined with glucose on strips used primarily for at-home testing by diagnosed patients with diabetes.

The use of multiple-test strips in hospital laboratories will often produce positive ketone tests unrelated to diabetes because the patient's illness is either preventing adequate intake or absorption of carbohydrates or is producing an accelerated loss, as in the case of vomiting. Obesity clinics can use a practical application of ketonuria produced by starvation to determine whether patients on high-protein or fasting diets have been cheating. Frequent strenuous exercise can cause overuse of available carbohydrates and produce ketonuria.

REAGENT STRIP REACTIONS

The three ketone compounds are not present in equal amounts in urine. Both acetone and beta-hydroxybutyric acid are produced from acetoacetic acid, and the proportions of 78 percent beta-hydroxybutyric acid, 20 percent acetoacetic acid, and 2 percent acetone are relatively constant in all specimens.

PROCEDURE

Acetest Procedure

- Remove the Acetest tablet from the bottle and place on a clean dry piece of white paper.
- Place one drop of urine on top of the tablet.
- Wait 30 seconds.
- Compare the tablet color with the manufacturer-supplied color chart.
- Report as negative, small, moderate, or large.

Reagent strip tests use the sodium nitroprusside (nitroferricyanide) reaction to measure ketones. In this reaction, acetoacetic acid in an alkaline medium will react with sodium nitroprusside to produce a purple color. The test does not measure beta-hydroxybutyric acid and is only slightly sensitive to acetone when glycine is also present; however, inasmuch as these compounds are derived from acetoacetic acid, their presence can be assumed, and it is not necessary to perform individual tests. Results are reported qualitatively as negative, small, moderate, or large, or as negative, 1+, 2+, or 3+.

In cases of severe ketosis, it may be necessary to perform tests on serial dilutions to provide more information as to the degree of ketosis.

$$\text{acetoacetate (and acetone)} + \text{sodium nitroprusside} + \text{(glycine)} \xrightarrow{\text{alkaline}} \text{purple color}$$

Acetest (Bayer Diagnostics, Elkhart, IN) provides sodium nitroprusside, glycine, disodium phosphate, and lactose in tablet form. The addition of lactose gives better color differentiation; however, the primary advantage of the Acetest tablets is that they can be used for serum and other body fluid testing. Acetest tablets are hygroscopic, and, if the specimen is not completely absorbed within 30 seconds, a new tablet should be used.

REACTION INTERFERENCE

Specimens obtained following diagnostic procedures using the dyes phenolsulfonphthalein and bromsulphalein may produce an interfering red color in the alkaline test medium, as will highly pigmented red urine. Large amounts of levodopa and medications containing sulfhydryl groups, including mercaptoethane sulfonate sodium (MESNA) and captopril, may produce atypical color reactions. Reactions

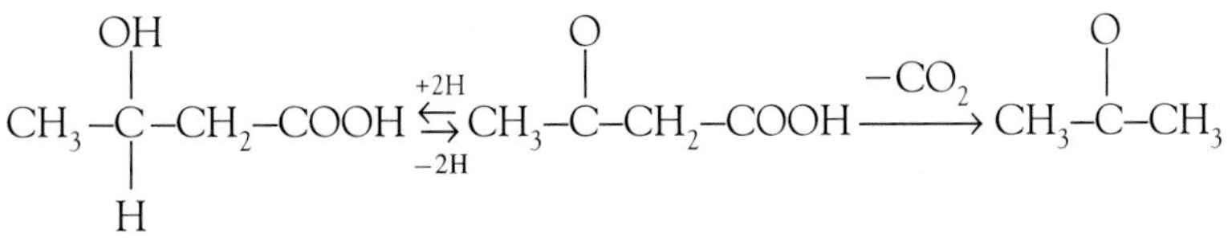

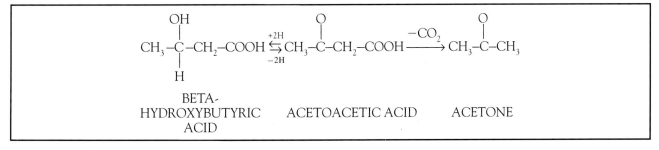

BETA-HYDROXYBUTYRIC ACID   ACETOACETIC ACID   ACETONE

Ketone Reagent Strip Summary

Reagents	Sodium nitroprusside Glycine (Chemstrip)
Sensitivity	Multistix: 5–10 mg/dL acetoacetic acid Chemstrip: 9 mg/dL acetoacetic acid 70 mg/dL acetone
Interference	False-positive: Phthalein dyes Highly pigmented red urine Levodopa Medications containing free sulfhydryl groups False-negative: Improperly preserved specimens
Correlations with other tests	Glucose

with interfering substances frequently fade on standing, whereas color development from acetoacetic acid increases, resulting in false-positive results from improperly timed readings. Falsely decreased values due to the volatilization of acetone and the breakdown of acetoacetic acid by bacteria will be seen in improperly preserved specimens.

Blood

Blood may be present in the urine either in the form of intact red blood cells (***hematuria***) or as the product of red blood cell destruction, hemoglobin (***hemoglobinuria***). As discussed in Chapter 4, blood present in large quantities can be detected visually; hematuria produces a cloudy red urine, and hemoglobinuria appears as a clear red specimen. Because any amount of blood greater than five cells per microliter of urine is considered clinically significant, visual examination cannot be relied on to detect the presence of blood. Microscopic examination of the urinary sediment will show intact red blood cells, but free hemoglobin produced either by hemolytic disorders or lysis of red blood cells will not be detected. Therefore, chemical tests for hemoglobin provide the most accurate means for determining the presence of blood. Once blood has been detected, the microscopic examination can be used to differentiate between hematuria and hemoglobinuria.

CLINICAL SIGNIFICANCE

The finding of a positive reagent strip test result for blood indicates the presence of red blood cells, hemoglobin, or myoglobin. Each of these has a different clinical significance.

HEMATURIA

Hematuria is most closely related to disorders of renal or genitourinary origin in which bleeding is the result of trauma or damage to the organs of these systems. Major causes of hematuria include renal calculi, glomerular diseases, tumors, trauma, pyelonephritis, exposure to toxic chemicals, and anticoagulant therapy. The laboratory is frequently requested to perform a urinalysis when patients presenting with severe back and abdominal pain are suspected of having renal calculi. In such cases, hematuria is usually of a small to moderate degree, but its presence can be essential to the diagnosis. Hematuria of nonpathologic significance is observed following strenuous exercise and during menstruation.

HEMOGLOBINURIA

Hemoglobinuria may result from the lysis of red blood cells produced in the urinary tract, particularly in dilute, alkaline urine. It also may result from intravascular hemolysis and the subsequent filtering of hemoglobin through the glomerulus. Lysis of red blood cells in the urine will usually show a mixture of hemoglobinuria and hematuria, whereas no red blood cells will be seen in cases of intravascular hemolysis. Under normal conditions, the formation of large hemoglobin-haptoglobin complexes in the circulation prevents the glomerular filtration of hemoglobin. When the amount of free hemoglobin present exceeds the haptoglobin content—as occurs in hemolytic anemias, transfusion reactions, severe burns, infections, and strenuous exercise—hemoglobin is available for glomerular filtration. Reabsorption of filtered hemoglobin also will result in the appearance of large yellow-brown granules of denatured **ferritin** called **hemosiderin** in the renal tubular epithelial cells and in the urine sediment.

Summary of Clinical Significance of a Positive Reaction for Blood

Hematuria

1. Renal calculi
2. Glomerulonephritis
3. Pyelonephritis
4. Tumors
5. Trauma
6. Exposure to toxic chemicals
7. Anticoagulants
8. Strenuous exercise

Hemoglobinuria

1. Transfusion reactions
2. Hemolytic anemias
3. Severe burns
4. Infections/malaria
5. Strenuous exercise/red blood cell trauma

Myoglobinuria

1. Muscular trauma/crush syndromes
2. Prolonged coma
3. Convulsions
4. Muscle-wasting diseases
5. Alcoholism/overdose
6. Drug abuse
7. Extensive exertion

MYOGLOBINURIA

Myoglobin, a heme-containing protein found in muscle tissue, not only reacts positively with the reagent strip test for blood but also produces a clear red-brown urine. The presence of myoglobin rather than hemoglobin should be suspected in patients with conditions associated with muscle destruction (**rhabdomyolysis**). Examples of these conditions include trauma, crush syndromes, prolonged coma, convulsions, muscle-wasting diseases, alcoholism, heroin abuse, and extensive exertion. The heme portion of myoglobin is toxic to the renal tubules, and high concentrations can cause acute renal failure. The massive hemoglobinuria seen in hemolytic transfusion reactions also is associated with acute renal failure.

HEMOGLOBINURIA VERSUS MYOGLOBINURIA

Occasionally the laboratory may be requested to differentiate between the presence of hemoglobin and myoglobin in a urine specimen. The diagnosis of ***myoglobinuria*** usually is based on the patient's history and elevated serum levels of the enzymes creatinine kinase and lactic dehydrogenase. The appearance of the patient's plasma also can aid in the differentiation. The kidneys rapidly clear myoglobin from the plasma, leaving a normal appearing plasma, whereas hemoglobin bound to haptoglobin remains in the plasma and imparts a red color.

The concentration of myoglobin in the urine must be at least 25 mg/dL before the red pigmentation can be visualized. At this concentration, a precipitation test can be used to screen for the presence of myoglobin; 2.8 g of ammonium sulfate are added to 5 mL of centrifuged urine. After mixing and allowing the specimen to sit for 5 minutes, the urine is filtered or centrifuged, and the supernatant is tested for a reaction for blood with a reagent strip. The principle of this screening test is based on the fact that the larger hemoglobin molecules will be precipitated by the ammonium sulfate, and myoglobin will remain in the supernatant. Therefore, when myoglobin is present, the supernatant will retain the red color and give a positive reagent strip test for blood. Conversely, hemoglobin will produce a red precipitate and a supernatant that tests negative for blood. Myoglobin is not stable in acid urine and, if denatured, may precipitate with the ammonium sulfate. Specimens that cannot be tested immediately should be neutralized and frozen.

REAGENT STRIP REACTIONS

Chemical tests for blood use the pseudoperoxidase activity of hemoglobin to catalyze a reaction between hydrogen peroxide and the chromogen tetramethylbenzidine to produce an oxidized chromogen, which has a green-blue color.

$$H_2O_2 + \text{chromogen} \xrightarrow[\text{peroxidase}]{\text{hemoglobin}} \text{oxidized chromogen} + H_2O$$

Reagent strip manufacturers incorporate peroxide, tetramethylbenzidine, and buffer into the blood testing area. Two color charts are provided that correspond to the reactions that occur with hemoglobinuria and myoglobinuria and hematuria. In the presence of free hemoglobin/myoglobin, uniform color ranging from a negative yellow through green to a strongly positive green-blue will appear on the pad. In contrast, intact red blood cells are lysed when they come in contact with the pad, and the liberated hemoglobin produces an isolated reaction that results in a speckled pattern on the pad. The degree of hematuria can then be estimated by the intensity of the speckled pattern. Reagent strip tests can detect concentrations as low as five red blood cells per microliter; however, care must be taken when comparing these figures with the actual microscopic values, because the absorbent nature of the pad will attract more than 1 μL of urine. The value of the test lies primarily in its ability to differentiate between hemoglobinuria/myoglobinuria and hematuria, not in the quantitation. The terms trace, small, moderate, and large or trace, 1+, 2+ and 3+ are used for reporting.

REACTION INTERFERENCE

False-positive reactions owing to menstrual contamination may be seen. They also will occur if strong oxidizing detergents are present in the specimen container. Vegetable peroxidase and bacterial enzymes, including an *Escherichia coli* peroxidase, also may cause false-positive reactions. Therefore, sediments containing bacteria should be checked closely for the presence of red blood cells.[21]

Traditionally ascorbic acid has been associated with false-negative reagent strip reactions for blood. Both Mul-

Blood Reagent Strip Summary

Reagents	Multistix: Diisopropylbenzene dehydroperoxide tetramethylbenzidine Chemstrip: 2,5-dimethyl-2,5-dihydroperoxide tetramethylbenzidine
Sensitivity	Multistix: 5–20 RBCs/μL, 0.015–0.062 mg/dL hemoglobin Chemstrip: 5 RBCs/μL, hemoglobin corresponding to 10 RBCs/μL
Interference	False-positive: Strong oxidizing agents Bacterial peroxidases Menstrual contamination False-negative: High specific gravity/crenated cells Formalin Captopril High concentrations of nitrite Ascorbic acid >25 mg/dL Unmixed specimens
Correlations with other tests	Protein Microscopic

tistix and Chemstrip have modified their reagent strips to reduce this interference to very high levels (25 mg/dL) of ascorbic acid. Multistix uses a peroxide that is less subject to reduction by ascorbic acid, and Chemstrip overlays the reagent pad with an iodate-impregnated mesh that oxidizes the ascorbic acid prior to its reaching the reaction pad. False-negative reactions can result when urine with a high specific gravity contains crenated red blood cells that do not lyse when they come in contact with the reagent pad. Decreased reactivity also may be seen when formalin is used as a preservative or when the hypertension medication, captopril, or high concentrations of nitrite (greater than 10 mg/dL) are present. Red blood cells settle to the bottom of the specimen container, and failure to mix the specimen prior to testing will cause a falsely decreased reading.

Bilirubin

The appearance of bilirubin in the urine can provide an early indication of liver disease. It is often detected long before the development of **jaundice**.

PRODUCTION OF BILIRUBIN

Bilirubin, a highly pigmented yellow compound, is a degradation product of hemoglobin. Under normal conditions, the life span of red blood cells is approximately 120 days, at which time they are destroyed in the spleen and liver by the phagocytic cells of the reticuloendothelial system. The liberated hemoglobin is broken down into its component parts: iron, protein, and protoporphyrin. The body reuses the iron and protein, and the cells of the reticuloendothelial system convert the remaining protoporphyrin to bilirubin. The bilirubin is then released into the circulation, where it binds with albumin and is transported to the liver. At this point, the kidneys cannot excrete the circulating bilirubin because not only is it bound to albumin but also it is water insoluble. In the liver, bilirubin is conjugated with glucuronic acid by the action of glucuronyl transferase to form water-soluble bilirubin diglucuronide (conjugated bilirubin). Usually, this conjugated bilirubin will not appear in the urine because it is passed directly from the liver into the bile duct and on to the intestine. In the intestine, intestinal bacteria reduce bilirubin to urobilinogen, which is then oxidized and excreted in the feces in the form of urobilin. In Figure 5–1, bilirubin metabolism is illustrated for reference with this section and the subsequent discussion of urobilinogen.

CLINICAL SIGNIFICANCE

Conjugated bilirubin will appear in the urine when the normal degradation cycle is disrupted by obstruction of the bile duct (e.g., gallstones or cancer) or when the integrity of the liver is damaged, allowing leakage of conjugated bilirubin into the circulation. Hepatitis and cirrhosis are common examples of conditions that produce liver damage resulting in bilirubinuria. Not only does the detection of urinary bilirubin provide an early indication of liver disease, but also its presence or absence can be used in determining the cause of clinical jaundice. As shown in Table 5–3, this determination can be even more significant when bilirubin results are combined with urinary urobilinogen. Jaundice due to increased destruction of red blood cells does not produce bilirubinuria. This is because the serum bilirubin is present in the unconjugated form and the kidneys cannot excrete it.

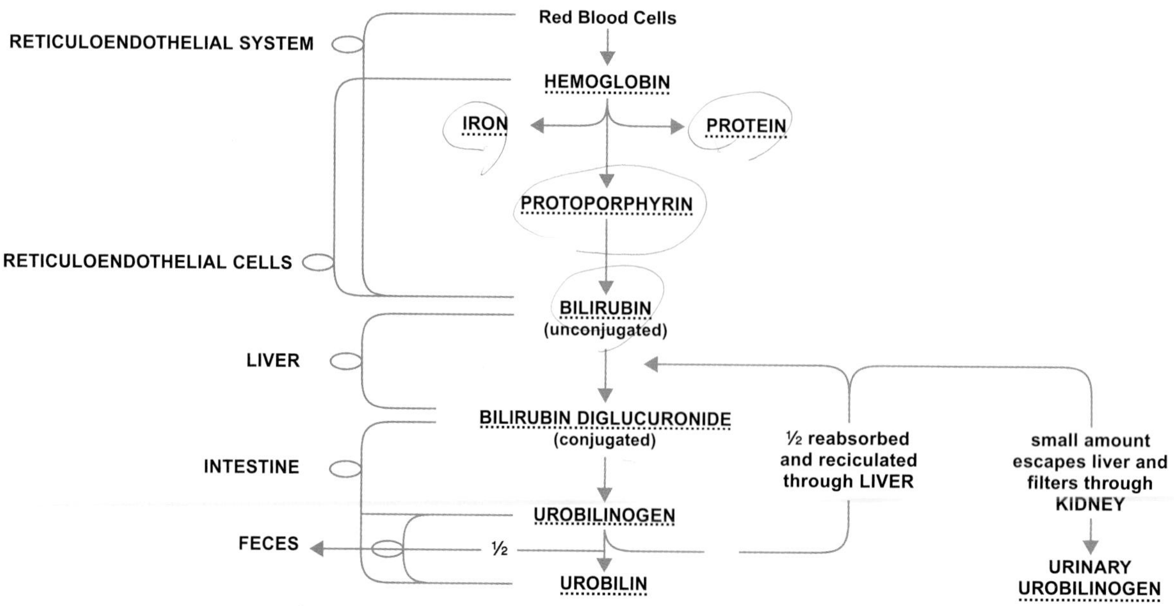

FIGURE 5–1 Hemoglobin degradation.

Specific gravity — assessment of the kidney's ability to reabsorb

Normal 1.003 ~ 1.035

< 1.010 hyposthenuric

> 1.010 hypersthenuric

Odor bacterial inf — strong unpl

diabetic ketones — sweet / fruity odor

metabolic defect — maple syrup odor

P46 pH along w/ the lungs, the kidneys are the major regulators of acid-base content in the body.

protein albumin is the major serum protein in urine

— clinical sig-

① prerenal proteinuria — usually not discovered in a routine urinalysis

Bence Jones protein — persons w/ multiple myeloma

↑ monoclonal Ig light chain (= Bence Jones protein)

coagulate at 40–60°C, dissolves at 100°C

② renal proteinuria

glomerular membrane damaged — ↑ serum albumin

WBC. RBC in urine

a) orthostatic (postural) proteinuria ··· pos on second specimen

neg on the 1st morning specimen

b) microalbuminuria = ↓ levels of urine protein not detected by reagent strips

③ postrenal proteinuria — bacteria and fungal infection & inflammation

Reaction interference

highly buffered alkaline urine that overrides the acid buffer system

glucose

hyperglycemia (↑ glucose in blood) — diabetes mellitus

glycosuria w/ absence of hyperglycemia — end-stage renal disease

(1) pediatric specimen

(2) drug specimen collection

COC (chain of custody) = process that provides this documentation of proper sample ID from collection to the results

Physical Exam

1) color

- Dark yellow / Amber / Orange … can be presence of bilirubin
  Yellow foam appears when the specimen is shake
  Medications … administration of phenazopyridine (Pyridium) or azo-gantrisin compounds ⇒ alternate resu
- Red / Pink / Brown … possible of RBCs, hemoglobin and myoglobin
  (Red/cloudy) (Red/clear)
  porphyrins (port wine color) – neg for blood
  Medications … rifampin, phenolphthalein, phenindione, phenothiazine
- Brown / Black … possible of melanoma, alkaptonuria
  Medications … levodopa, methyldopa, phenol derivatives, and metronidazole (Flagyl)
- Blue / Green … bacterial infection ex) UT inf by Pseudomonas
  Medications – methocarbomol (Robaxin), methylene blue, amitriptyline (Elavil)

Clarity

- Nonpathogenic turbidity … presence of squamous epithelial cells, mucus
  refrigerated specimen – amorphous phosphates (alkaline pH), carbonates, urates (acid)
- Pathologic turbidity … RBCs, WBCs, and bacteria, also abnormal amount of nonsquamous epithelial cells, yeast, abnormal crystals, lymph fluid and lipids

false negative glucose — when specimens to remain unpreserved at RT

Ketones - 3 intermediate products of fat metabolism

↑ fat metabolism — diabetes mellitus, vomitting, starvation

Type I diabetes mellitus (insulin-dependent) → Ketonuria
(deficiency in insulin)

(cloudy red)
blood hematuria - intact red blood cells in the urine
(clear red)
hemoglobinuria - destructed RBC " , as hemoglobin

* differentiate above 2 by microscopic exam

clinical sig

a) hematuria ··· disorders of renal or genitourinary origin
severe back & abdominal pain
ex) renal calculi, glomerular diseases, tumors, trauma,
therapy
pyelonephritis, exposure to toxic chem, anticoag

b) hemoglobinuria ··· lysis of RBC in urinary tract
through glomerulus
intravascular hemolysis, subsequent filtering

c) myoglobinuria ··· heme-containing protein
→ rhabdomydysis [=muscle destruction]

* false-positive rxn due to menstrual contamination may be seen

Bilirubin liver disease indication, often long before jaundice.

bilirubin = degradation product of hemoglobulin

TABLE 5–3 **Urine Bilirubin and Urobilinogen in Jaundice**

	Urine Bilirubin	Urine Urobilinogen
Bile duct obstruction	+ + +	Normal
Liver damage	+ or –	+ +
Hemolytic disease	Negative	+ + +

REAGENT STRIP (DIAZO) REACTIONS

Routine testing for urinary bilirubin by reagent strip uses the diazo reaction. Bilirubin combines with 2,4-dichloroaniline diazonium salt or 2,6-dichlorobenzene-diazonium-tetrafluoroborate in an acid medium to produce an azodye, with colors ranging from increasing degrees of tan or pink to violet, respectively. Qualitative results are reported as negative, small, moderate, or large, or as negative, 1+, 2+, or 3+. Reagent strip color reactions for bilirubin are more difficult to interpret than other reagent strip reactions and are easily influenced by other pigments present in the urine. Atypical color reactions are frequently noted on visual examination and are measured by automated readers. Further testing should be performed on any questionable results.[15]

$$\text{bilirubin glucuronide} + \text{diazonium salt} \xrightarrow{\text{acid}} \text{azodye}$$

Questionable results can be repeated using the Ictotest (Bayer Diagnostics, Elkhart, IN). The Ictotest is less subject to interference and is sensitive to 0.05 to 0.10 mg/dL of bilirubin, whereas the reagent strips have a lower sensitivity level of 0.40 mg/dL. Ictotest kits consist of testing mats and tablets containing *p*-nitrobenzene-diazonium-*p*-toluenesulfonate, SSA, sodium carbonate, and boric acid. Ten drops of urine are added to the mat, which has special absorbent properties that cause bilirubin to remain on the surface as the urine absorbs into the mat. Following the chemical reaction, a blue-to-purple color will appear on the mat when bilirubin is present. Colors other than blue or purple appearing on the mat are considered to be a negative result. If interference in the Ictotest is suspected, it can usually be removed by adding water directly to the mat after the urine has been added. Interfering substances will be washed into the mat, and only bilirubin will remain on the surface. An Ictotest may be requested when early cases of liver disorders, such as hepatitis, are suspected.

Summary of Clinical Significance of Urine Bilirubin

1. Hepatitis
2. Cirrhosis
3. Other liver disorders
4. Biliary obstruction (gallstones, carcinoma)

PROCEDURE

Ictotest Procedure

- Place 10 drops of urine onto one square of the absorbent test mat.
- Using forceps, remove one Ictotest reagent tablet, recap the bottle promptly, and place the tablet in the center of the moistened area.
- Place one drop of water onto the tablet and wait 5 seconds.
- Place a second drop of water onto the tablet so that the water runs off the tablet onto the mat.
- Observe the color of the mat around the tablet at the end of 60 seconds. The presence of a blue-to-purple color on the mat indicates that bilirubin is present. A slight pink or red color should be ignored. Report as positive or negative.

REACTION INTERFERENCE

As discussed previously, false-positive reactions are primarily due to urine pigments. Of particular concern are the yellow-orange urines from persons taking phenazopyridine compounds, because the thick pigment produced may be mistaken for bilirubin on initial examination. The presence of indican and metabolites of the medication Lodine may cause false-positive readings.

The false-negative results caused by the testing of specimens that are not fresh are the most frequent errors associated with bilirubin testing. Bilirubin is an unstable com-

Bilirubin Reagent Strip Summary

Reagents	Multistix: 2,4-dichloroaniline diazonium salt Chemstrip: 2,6-dichlorobenzene-diazonium-tetrafluoroborate
Sensitivity	Multistix: 0.4–0.8 mg/dL bilirubin Chemstrip: 0.5 mg/dL bilirubin
Interference	False-positive: Highly pigmented urines, phenazopyridine Indican, (intestinal disorders) Metabolites of Lodine False-negative: Specimen exposure to light Ascorbic acid >25 mg/dL High concentrations of nitrite
Correlations with other tests	Urobilinogen

pound that is rapidly photo-oxidized to biliverdin when exposed to light. Biliverdin does not react with diazo tests. False-negative results also will occur when hydrolysis of bilirubin diglucuronide produces free bilirubin, because this is less reactive in the reagent strip tests.[4] High concentrations of ascorbic acid (greater than 25 mg/dL) and nitrite may lower the sensitivity of the test, because they combine with the diazonium salt and prevent its reaction with bilirubin.

Urobilinogen

Like bilirubin, urobilinogen is a bile pigment that results from the degradation of hemoglobin. As shown in Figure 5–1, it is produced in the intestine from the reduction of bilirubin by the intestinal bacteria. Approximately half of the urobilinogen is reabsorbed from the intestine into the blood, recirculates to the liver, and is excreted back into the intestine through the bile duct. The urobilinogen remaining in the intestine is excreted in the feces, where it is oxidized to urobilin, the pigment responsible for the characteristic brown color of the feces. Urobilinogen appears in the urine because, as it circulates in the blood en route to the liver, it passes through the kidney and is filtered by the glomerulus. Therefore, a small amount of urobilinogen—less than 1 mg/dL or Ehrlich unit—is normally found in the urine.

CLINICAL SIGNIFICANCE

Increased urine urobilinogen (greater than 1 mg/dL) is seen in liver disease and hemolytic disorders. Measurement of urine urobilinogen can be valuable in the detection of early liver disease; however, studies have shown that when urobilinogen tests are routinely performed, 1 percent of the nonhospitalized population and 9 percent of a hospitalized population exhibit elevated results.[6] This is frequently caused by constipation.

Impairment of liver function decreases the ability of the liver to process the urobilinogen recirculated from the intestine. The excess urobilinogen remaining in the blood is filtered by the kidneys and appears in the urine.

The clinical jaundice associated with hemolytic disorders results from the increased amount of circulating unconjugated bilirubin. This unconjugated bilirubin is presented to the liver for conjugation, resulting in a markedly increased amount of conjugated bilirubin entering the intestines. As a result, increased urobilinogen is produced, and increased amounts of urobilinogen are reabsorbed into the blood and circulated through the kidneys where filtration takes place. In addition, the overworked liver does not process the reabsorbed urobilinogen as efficiently, and additional urobilinogen is presented for urinary excretion.

Although it cannot be determined by reagent strip, the absence of urobilinogen in the urine and feces also is diagnostically significant and represents an obstruction of the bile duct that prevents the normal passage of bilirubin into the intestine. See Table 5–3 for an outline of the relationship of urine urobilinogen and bilirubin to the pathologic conditions associated with them.

Summary of Clinical Significance of Urine Urobilinogen

1. Early detection of liver disease
2. Liver disorders, hepatitis, cirrhosis, carcinoma
3. Hemolytic disorders

REAGENT STRIP REACTIONS AND INTERFERENCE

The reagent strip reactions for urobilinogen differ between Multistix and Chemstrip much more significantly than with other reagent strip parameters. Multistix uses Ehrlich's aldehyde reaction, in which urobilinogen reacts with *p*-diethylaminobenzaldehyde (Ehrlich's reagent) to produce colors ranging from light to dark pink. Results are reported as Ehrlich units (**EU**), which are equal to mg/dL, ranging from normal readings of 0.2 and 1 through abnormal readings of 2, 4, and 8. Chemstrip incorporates an azo-coupling (diazo) reaction using 4-methoxybenzene-diazonium-tetrafluoroborate to react with urobilinogen, producing colors ranging from white to pink. The reaction is much more specific for urobilinogen than the Ehrlich reaction. Results are reported in mg/dL. Both tests will detect urobilinogen present in normal quantities, and color comparisons are provided for the upper limits of normal as well as abnormal concentrations. Reagent strip tests cannot determine the absence of urobilinogen, which is significant in biliary obstruction.

MULTISTIX:

$$\underset{\text{(Ehrlich's reactive substances)}}{\text{urobilinogen}} + \underset{\text{(Ehrlich's reagent)}}{p\text{-diethylaminobenzaldehyde}} \xrightarrow{\text{acid}} \text{red color}$$

CHEMSTRIP:

$$\text{urobilinogen} + \text{diazonium salt} \xrightarrow{\text{acid}} \text{red azodye}$$

REACTION INTERFERENCE

The Ehrlich reaction on Multistix is subject to a variety of interferences, referred to as Ehrlich-reactive compounds, that will produce false-positive reactions. These include porphobilinogen, indican, *p*-aminosalicylic acid, sulfonamides, methyldopa, procaine, and chlorpromazine compounds. The presence of porphobilinogen is clinically significant; however, the reagent strip test is not considered a reliable method to screen for its presence. Porphobilinogen is discussed later in this section and in Chapter 9.

The sensitivity of the Ehrlich reaction increases with temperature, and testing should be performed at room temperature. Highly pigmented urines will cause atypical readings with both brands of reagent strips.

Urobilinogen Reagent Strip Summary

Reagents	Multistix: *p*-diethylaminobenzaldehyde Chemstrip: 4-methoxybenzene-diazonium-tetrafluroborate
Sensitivity	Multistix: 0.2 mg/dL urobilinogen Chemstrip: 0.4 mg/dL urobilinogen
Interference	Multistix: False-positive: Porphobilinogen, Indican, *p*-aminosalicylic acid, Sulfonamides, Methyldopa, Procaine, Chlorpromazine, Highly pigmented urine False-negative: Old specimens, Preservation in formalin Chemstrip: False-positive: Highly pigmented urine False-negative: Old specimens, Preservation in formalin, High concentrations of nitrate
Correlations with other tests	Bilirubin

False-negative results occur most frequently when specimens are improperly preserved, allowing urobilinogen to be photo-oxidized to urobilin. High concentrations of nitrite will interfere with the azo-coupling reaction on Chemstrip. False-negative readings also are obtained with both strips when formalin is used as a preservative.

EHRLICH'S TUBE TEST

Until development of reagent strip methods, tests for urobilinogen were not performed routinely because the available procedures were time consuming and nonspecific. The tube test described here was used when clinically necessary and serves as the basis for the Watson-Schwartz and Hoesch screening tests for porphobilinogen. The reagent used in both tests is *p*-diethylaminobenzaldehyde (Ehrlich's reagent). Addition of Ehrlich's reagent to urine containing urobilinogen produces a cherry-red color, as do the Ehrlich-reactive compounds. To produce a semiquantitative measurement, the original method of adding one part Ehrlich's reagent to 10 parts urine and observing against a white background for the presence of a red color was modified to test serial dilutions of urine. Positive results in dilutions greater than 1 to 20 were considered significant. To avoid missing the presence of a faint pink color in higher dilutions, tubes should be examined by looking down through the top while holding the bottom against a white background. Sodium acetate can be added to enhance the reaction. Results are reported in Ehrlich units, which are essentially equivalent to 1 mg/mL of urobilinogen. Whereas reagent strip testing for urobilinogen is usually performed on random or first morning specimens, the recommended specimen for quantitative testing is one col-

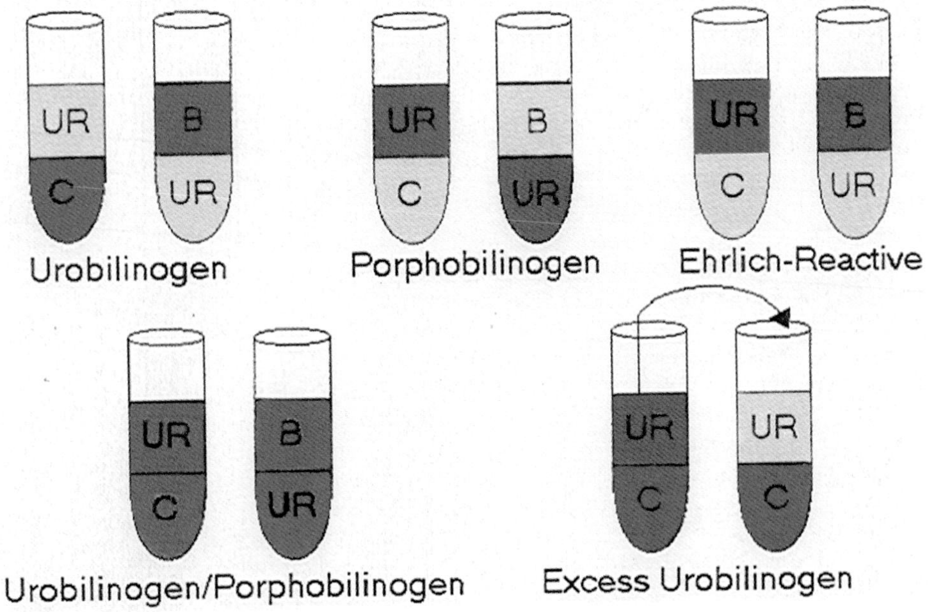

FIGURE 5–2 Typical Ehrlich reactions. (Adapted from Henry, Lauzon, and Schumann,[7] p. 434.)

lected after the noon meal, between 2 PM and 4 PM. This is the time of greatest urobilinogen excretion. As mentioned previously, the Ehrlich reaction is not specific for urobilinogen, and a red color also will be seen in the presence of porphobilinogen and other Ehrlich-reactive compounds. A positive reaction may require additional testing to determine which compound is present.

WATSON-SCHWARTZ DIFFERENTIATION TEST

The classic test for differentiating between urobilinogen and porphobilinogen is the Watson-Schwartz test.[20] After production of the cherry-red color using sodium acetate and Ehrlich's reagent, the specimen is divided into two tubes. The addition of chloroform to one tube will result in the extraction of urobilinogen into the chloroform (bottom) layer, producing a colorless urine (top) layer, and a red chloroform layer on the bottom. Neither porphobilinogen nor other Ehrlich-reactive compounds are soluble in chloroform. Porphobilinogen is also not soluble in butanol; however, urobilinogen and other Ehrlich reactive compounds will be extracted into butanol. Therefore, the addition of butanol to the second tube will produce a red (upper) butanol layer if urobilinogen or Ehrlich reactive compounds are present and a colorless butanol layer if porphobilinogen is present. As shown in Figure 5–2 and Table 5–4, urobilinogen is soluble in both chloroform and butanol, and porphobilinogen is soluble in neither. If both urobilinogen and porphobilinogen are present, both layers will appear red. Before reporting the test as positive for both substances, an additional chloroform extraction should be performed on the red urine layer to ensure that the red color is not due to excess urobilinogen.

HOESCH SCREENING TEST FOR PORPHOBILINOGEN

The Hoesch test is used for rapid screening or monitoring of urinary porphobilinogen. Two drops of urine are added to approximately 2 mL of Hoesch reagent (Ehrlich's reagent dissolved in 6 M HCl), and the top of the solution is immediately observed for the appearance of a red color, which indicates the presence of porphobilinogen. When the tube is shaken, the red color is seen throughout the solution. The test will detect approximately 2 mg/dL of porphobilinogen, and urobilinogen is inhibited by the highly acidic pH. High concentrations of methyldopa and indican and highly pigmented urines may produce false-positive results.

Nitrite

CLINICAL SIGNIFICANCE

The reagent strip test for nitrite provides a rapid screening test for the presence of urinary tract infection (**UTI**). The test is designed to detect those cases in which the need for a culture may not be apparent and is not intended to replace the urine culture as the primary test for diagnosing and monitoring bacterial infection. Most UTIs are believed to start in the bladder as a result of external contamination and, if untreated, to progress upward through the ureters to the tubules, renal pelvis, and kidney. The nitrite test is valuable for detecting initial bladder infection (cystitis), because patients are often asymptomatic or have vague symptoms that would not lead the physician to order a urine culture. Pyelonephritis, an inflammatory process of the kidney and adjacent renal pelvis, is a frequent complication of untreated cystitis and can lead to renal tissue damage, impairment of renal function, hypertension, and even septicemia. Therefore, detection of ***bacteriuria*** through the use of the nitrite screening test and subsequent antibiotic therapy can prevent these serious complications. The nitrite test also can be used to evaluate the success of antibiotic therapy and to periodically screen persons with recurrent infections, patients with diabetes, and pregnant women, all of whom are considered to be at high risk for UTI.[10] As discussed in the following section, many laboratories use the nitrite test in combination with the leukocyte esterase test to determine the necessity of performing urine cultures.

TABLE 5–4 **Watson-Schwartz Test Interpretation**

	Urobilinogen	Other Ehrlich-Reactive Substances	Porphobilinogen
Chloroform Extraction			
Urine (Top Layer)	Colorless	Red	Red
Chloroform (Bottom Layer)	Red	Colorless	Colorless
Butanol Extraction			
Butanol (Top Layer)	Red	Red	Colorless
Urine (Bottom Layer)	Colorless	Colorless	Red

Summary of Clinical Significance of Urine Nitrite

1. Cystitis
2. Pyelonephritis
3. Evaluation of antibiotic therapy
4. Monitoring of patients at high risk for urinary tract infection
5. Screening of urine culture specimens

REAGENT STRIP REACTIONS

The chemical basis of the nitrite test is the ability of certain bacteria to reduce nitrate, a normal constituent of urine, to nitrite, which does nor normally appear in the urine. Nitrite is detected by the Greiss reaction, in which nitrite at an acidic pH reacts with an aromatic amine (para-arsanilic acid or sulfanilamide) to form a diazonium compound that then reacts with tetrahydrobenzoquinolin compounds to produce a pink-colored azodye. To prevent false-positive reactions in externally contaminated specimens, the sensitivity of the test is standardized to correspond with a quantitative bacterial culture criterion of 100,000 organisms per milliliter. Although different shades of pink may be produced, the test does not measure the degree of bacteriuria, and any shade of pink is considered to represent a clinically significant amount of bacteria. Results are reported only as negative or positive.

$$\text{para-arsanilic acid or sulfanilamide} + \underset{\text{(nitrite)}}{NO_2} \xrightarrow{\text{acid}} \text{diazonium salt}$$

$$\text{diazonium salt} + \text{tetrahydrobenzoquinolin} \xrightarrow{\text{acid}} \text{pink azodye}$$

REACTION INTERFERENCE

Several major factors can influence the reliability of the nitrite test, and tests with negative results in the presence of even vaguely suspicious clinical symptoms should always be repeated or followed by a urine culture.

1. Bacteria that lack the enzyme reductase do not possess the ability to reduce nitrate to nitrite. Reductase is found in the gram-negative bacteria (*Enterobacteriaceae*) that most frequently cause UTIs. Non-nitrate-reducing gram-positive bacteria and yeasts, however, cause a significant number of infections, and the nitrite test will not detect the presence of these organisms.
2. Bacteria capable of reducing nitrate must remain in contact with the urinary nitrate long enough to produce nitrite. Therefore, all nitrite tests should be performed on first morning specimens because urine will have been held in the bladder for several hours. The correlation between positive cultures and positive nitrite test results is significantly lower when testing is performed on random samples.[11]

Nitrite Reagent Strip Summary

Reagents	Multistix:	*p*-arsanilic acid Tetrahydrobenzo(h)-quinolin-3-ol
	Chemstrip:	Sulfanilamide 3-hydroxy-1,2,3,4-tetrahydro-7,8 benzoquinoline
Sensitivity	Multistix:	0.06–0.1 mg/dL nitrite ion
	Chemstrip:	0.05 mg/dL nitrite ion
Interference	False-negative:	Nonreductase-containing bacteria Insufficient contact time between bacteria and urinary nitrate Lack of urinary nitrate Large quantities of bacteria converting nitrite to nitrogen Presence of antibiotics High concentrations of ascorbic acid High specific gravity
	False-positive:	Improperly preserved specimens Highly pigmented urine
Correlations with other tests	Protein Leukocytes Microscopic	

3. The reliability of the test depends on the presence of adequate amounts of nitrate in the urine. This is seldom a problem in patients on a normal diet that contains green vegetables; however, because diet usually is not controlled prior to testing, the possibility of a false-negative result owing to lack of dietary nitrate does exist.
4. Further reduction of nitrite to nitrogen may occur when large numbers of bacteria are present and cause a false-negative reaction.
5. Other causes of false-negative results include inhibition of bacterial metabolism by the presence of antibiotics, large quantities of ascorbic acid interfering with the diazo reaction, and decreased sensitivity in specimens with a high specific gravity.

False-positive results will be obtained if nitrite testing is not performed on fresh samples, because multiplication of contaminant bacteria will soon produce measurable amounts of nitrite. When fresh urine is used, false-positive results will not be obtained, even if a nonsterile container is used. Pink discoloration or spotting on the edges of the reagent pad should not be considered a positive reaction. Highly pigmented urines will produce atypical color reactions. Visual examination of the strip will determine that the characteristic pink color is not present. Automated strip readers will report any color change as positive, and strips should be visually examined when discrepancies are observed.

Leukocyte Esterase

Prior to development of the reagent strip leukocyte esterase (**LE**) test, detection of increased urinary leukocytes required microscopic examination of the urine sediment. This can be subject to variation depending on the method used to prepare the sediment and the technical personnel examining the sediment. Therefore, the chemical test for leukocytes offers a more standardized means for the detection of leukocytes. The test is not designed to measure the concentration of leukocytes, and the manufacturers recommend that quantitation be done by microscopic examination. An additional advantage to the chemical LE test is that it will detect the presence of leukocytes that have been lysed, particularly in dilute alkaline urine, and would not appear in the microscopic examination.

CLINICAL SIGNIFICANCE

Normal values for leukocytes are based on the microscopic sediment examination and vary from 0 to 2 to 0 to 5 per high power field. Women tend to have higher numbers than men as a result of vaginal contamination. Increased urinary leukocytes are indicators of UTI. The LE test detects the presence of esterase in the granulocytic white blood cells (neutrophils, eosinophils, basophils, and monocytes). Neutrophils are the leukocytes most frequently associated with bacterial infections. Esterases also are present in *Trichomonas* and histiocytes. Lymphocytes, erythrocytes, bacteria, and renal tissue cells do not contain esterases. A positive LE test result is most frequently accompanied by the presence of bacteria, which, as discussed previously, may or may not produce a positive nitrite reaction. Infections caused by *Trichomonas*, *Chlamydia*, yeast, and inflammation of renal tissues (i.e., interstitial nephritis) produce ***leukocyturia*** without bacteriuria.

Screening urine specimens using the LE and nitrite chemical reactions to determine the necessity of performing urine cultures can be a cost-effective measure.[22] The LE test contributes significantly more to the reliability of this practice than does the nitrite test.

REAGENT STRIP REACTION

The reagent strip reaction uses the action of LE to catalyze the hydrolysis of an acid ester imbedded on the reagent pad to produce an aromatic compound and acid. The aromatic compound then combines with a diazonium salt present on the pad to produce a purple azodye.

Summary of Clinical Significance of Urine Leukocytes

1. Bacterial and nonbacterial urinary tract infection
2. Inflammation of the urinary tract
3. Screening of urine culture specimens

Leukocyte Esterase Reagent Strip Summary

Reagents	Multistix: Derivatized pyerole amino acid ester Diazonium salt Chemstrip: Indoxylcarbonic acid ester Diazonium salt
Sensitivity	Multistix: 5–15 WBC/hpf Chemstrip: 10–25 WBC/hpf
Interference	False-positive: Strong oxidizing agents Formalin Highly pigmented urine, nitrofurantoin False-negative: High concentrations of protein, glucose, oxalic acid, ascorbic acid, gentamicin, cephalosporins, tetracyclines
Correlations with other tests	Protein Nitrite Microscopic

$$\text{indoxylcarbonic acid ester} \xrightarrow[\text{esterases}]{\text{leukocyte}} \text{indoxyl} + \text{acid indoxyl}$$

$$+ \text{ diazonium salt} \xrightarrow{\text{acid}} \text{purple azodye}$$

The LE reaction requires the longest time of all the reagent strip reactions (2 minutes). Reactions are reported as trace, small, moderate, and large or trace, 1+, 2+, and 3+. Trace readings may not be significant and should be repeated on a fresh specimen.

REACTION INTERFERENCE

The presence of strong oxidizing agents or formalin in the collection container will cause false-positive reactions. Highly pigmented urines and the presence of nitrofurantoin will obscure the color reaction.

False-negative results may occur in the presence of high concentrations of protein (greater than 500 mg/dL), glucose (greater than 3 g/dL), oxalic acid, and ascorbic acid. Crenation of leukocytes preventing release of esterases may occur in urines with a high specific gravity.[17] The presence of the antibiotics gentamicin, cephalexin, cephalothin, and tetracycline decreases the sensitivity of the reaction.

Specific Gravity

The addition of a specific gravity testing area to reagent strips has eliminated a time-consuming step in routine urinalysis and has provided a convenient method for routine screening. Replacing osmometry or refractometry for criti-

Summary of Clinical Significance of Urine Specific Gravity

1. Monitoring patient hydration and dehydration
2. Loss of renal tubular concentrating ability
3. Diabetes insipidus
4. Determination of unsatisfactory specimens due to low concentration

cal fluid monitoring is not recommended.[16] The clinical significance of the specific gravity test is discussed in Chapter 4.

REAGENT STRIP REACTION

The reagent strip reaction is based on the change in pK_a (dissociation constant) of a polyelectrolyte in an alkaline medium. The polyelectrolyte ionizes releasing hydrogen ions in proportion to the number of ions in the solution. The higher the concentration of urine, the more hydrogen ions are released, thereby lowering the pH. Incorporation of the indicator bromthymol blue on the reagent pad measures the change in pH. As the specific gravity increases, the indicator changes from blue (1.000 [alkaline]), through shades of green, to yellow (1.030 [acid]). Readings can be made in 0.005 intervals by careful comparison with the color chart. The specific gravity reaction is diagramed in Figure 5–3.

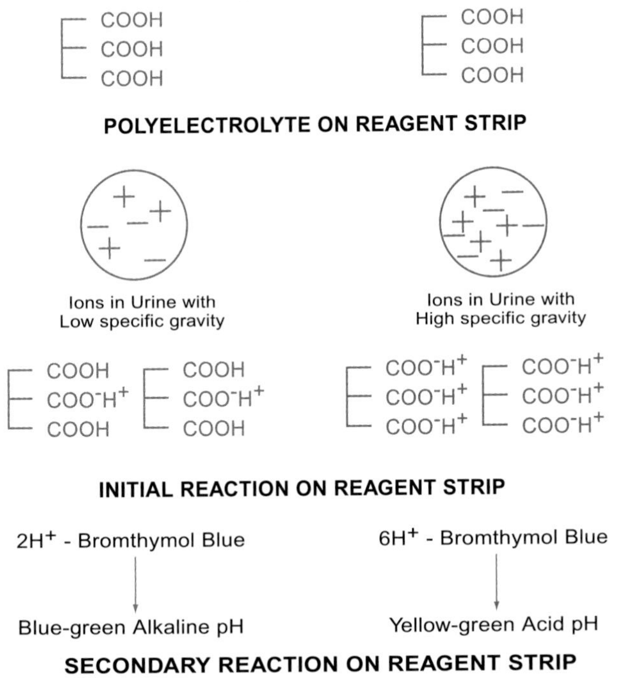

FIGURE 5–3 Diagram of reagent strip specific gravity reaction.

Urine Specific Gravity Reagent Strip Summary

Reagents	Multistix: Poly (methyl vinyl ether/maleic anhydride) bromthymol blue Chemstrip: Ethyleneglycol-Bis (aminoethylether) bromthymol blue
Sensitivity	1.000–1.030
Interference	False-positive: High concentrations of protein False-negative: Highly alkaline urines (>6.5)

REACTION INTERFERENCE

The reagent strip specific gravity measures only ionic solutes, thereby eliminating the interference by the large organic molecules, such as urea and glucose, and by radiographic contrast media and plasma expanders that are included in physical measurements of specific gravity.[9] This difference must be considered when comparing specific gravity results obtained by a different method. Elevated concentrations of protein will slightly increase the readings as a result of protein anions.

Specimens with a pH of 6.5 or higher will have decreased readings caused by interference with the bromthymol blue indicator (the blue-green readings associated with an alkaline pH correspond to a low specific gravity reading). Therefore, manufacturers recommend adding 0.005 to specific gravity readings when the pH is 6.5 or higher.

REFERENCES

1. Abuela, G: Proteinuria: Diagnostic principles and procedures. Ann Intern Med 98:1986–1991, 1983.
2. Benedict, SR: A reagent for the detection of reducing sugars. J Biol Chem 5:485–487, 1909.
3. Bianchi, S, et al: Microalbuminurea in essential hypertension. J Nephrol 10(4):216–219, 1997.
4. Free, AH, and Free, HM: Urodynamics: Concepts Relating to Routine Urine Chemistry. Ames Division, Miles Laboratories, Elkhart, IN, 1978.
5. Guthrie, D, Hinnen, D, and Guthrie, R: Single-voided vs. double-voided urine testing. Diabetes Care 2(3):269–271, 1979.
6. Hager, CB, and Free, AH: Urine urobilinogen as a component of routine urinalysis. Am J Med Technol 36(5):227–233, 1970.
7. Henry, JB, Lauzon, RB, and Schumann, BG: Basic examination of urine. In Henry, JB (ed): Clinical Diagnosis and Management by Laboratory Methods. WB Saunders, Philadelphia, 1996.
8. Hoeltge, GA, and Ersts, A: A quality control system for the general urinalysis laboratory. Am J Clin Pathol 73(3):404–408, 1980.
9. Kavelman, DA: A representative of Ames responds. Clin Chem 29(1):210–211, 1983.
10. Kunin, CM, and DeGroot, JE: Self-screening for significant bacteriuria. JAMA 231(13):1349–1353, 1975.
11. Monte-Verde, D, and Nosanchuk, JS: The sensitivity and specificity of nitrite testing for bacteriuria. Lab Med 12(2):755–757, 1981.
12. National Committee for Clinical Laboratory Standards Approved Guideline GP16-A: Urinalysis and Collection, Transportation, and Preservation of Urine Specimens. NCCLS, Villanova, PA, 1995.
13. Rauber, AP, and Maroncelli, RD: Effects of dietary changes on alkalinization of urine pH. Vet Hum Toxicol (Suppl) 23:46–47, 1981.

14. Renfrew, G: Confirmatory testing in urinalysis. Urinalysis News 10(3), 1994.
15. Riddhimat, R, Hiranras, S, and Petchclair, B: Retesting atypical reactions in urine bilirubin tests. Clin Lab Sci 5(5):310–312, 1992.
16. Romolo, D, et al: Refractometry, test strip and osmometery compared as measures of relative density of urine. Clin Chem 33(1):190, 1987.
17. Scheer, WD: The detection of leukocyte esterase activity in urine with a new reagent strip. Am J Clin Pathol 87(1):86–93, 1987.
18. TechniTips, Miles Diagnostics, Elkhart, IN. October, 1992.
19. Ward, KM: Microalbuminuria: Clinical aspects. Clin Lab Sci 2(4): 212–213, 1989.
20. Watson, CJ, and Schwartz, S: A simple test for urinary porphobilinogen. Proc Soc Exp Biol Med 47:393–394, 1941.
21. Weaver, MR, and Gibb, I: Urinalysis for blood: Questionable interpretation of reagent strip results. Clin Chem 29(2):401–402, 1983.
22. Wise, KA, Sagert, LA, and Grammens, GL: Urine leukocyte esterase and nitrite tests as an aid to predict urine culture results. Lab Med 15(3):186–187, 1984.

STUDY QUESTIONS

1. Describe how each of the following errors in reagent strip technique will affect test results:
   a. Leaving the reagent strip in the urine specimen while recording results of the previous specimen
   b. Failing to remove excess urine while withdrawing the strip from the specimen
   c. Recording all results immediately after withdrawing the strip from the specimen
   d. Using a Chemstrip color chart with a Multistix reagent strip
2. How will failure to allow a refrigerated specimen to warm to room temperature before testing affect reagent strip testing? Why?
3. How are reagent strips protected from deterioration caused by:
   a. moisture
   b. volatile chemicals
   c. light
   d. heat
4. What is the significance of the expiration date stamped on reagent strip containers?
5. List four times when positive and negative controls must be run on reagent strips.
6. Explain the relationship of urine pH to the formation of crystals and renal calculi.
7. What is the significance of a urine pH of 9?
8. Why do reagent strip pH reactions use both methyl red and bromthymol blue indicators?
9. Indicate the source of the following proteinurias by placing a 1 for prerenal, 2 for renal, or 3 for postrenal in front of the condition.
   a. _____ Microalbuminuria
   b. _____ Acute phase reactants
   c. _____ Pre-eclampsia
   d. _____ Vaginal inflammation
   e. _____ Multiple myeloma
   f. _____ Orthostatic proteinuria
   g. _____ Prostatitis
10. Describe the unique solubility characteristics of Bence Jones protein.
11. Differentiate between glomerular and tubular proteinuria.
12. How does detection of microalbuminuria affect patient treatment?
13. Briefly explain the principle of the protein error of indicators. How does a highly alkaline urine affect this?
14. State a pathologic reason that would cause a negative reagent strip protein reaction and a positive SSA test result.
15. Explain why glycosuria occurs in the presence of hyperglycemia.
16. Why do persons with hyperthyroidism exhibit hyperglycemia and glucosuria? Why do persons under extreme stress exhibit hyperglycemia and glucosuria?
17. How can glycosuria occur in the absence of hyperglycemia?
18. Explain the purpose of glucose oxidase and peroxidase in the reagent strip test for glucose.
19. What is the primary cause of a false-negative test result for glucosuria?
20. Does the Clinitest detect oxidizing or reducing substances? How does it do this?
21. How will failure to detect "pass through" affect results?
22. What is the primary reason that laboratories perform the Clinitest?
23. State two reasons for a positive reagent strip test result for glucose and a negative Clinitest result.
24. State the three basic reasons for the presence of ketonuria.
25. What is the primary substance detected by sodium nitroprusside? Why is glycine added to the reaction?
26. How do the reactions between ketones and interfering substances differ on reagent strips?
27. Name three pathologic substances detected by the reagent strip blood reaction. State a reason why each of these appears in the urine.

	Substance	Reason
a.	__________	______________
b.	__________	______________
c.	__________	______________

28. Why is hemoglobinuria associated with pink plasma and myoglobinuria with normal-colored plasma?
29. Why may yellow-brown granules appear in the urine sediment?
30. Following precipitation of a clear red urine with ammonium sulfate, what is the significance of a red supernatant?

31. What is the purpose of peroxide on the reagent strip pad for blood?

32. What is the significance of a speckled reaction on the blood pad?

33. Why are high levels of ascorbic acid of concern with both the glucose and blood reactions?

34. List in order the three products formed in the degradation of hemoglobin to urobilin.

35. Name two causes of jaundice that produce bilirubinuria and one cause that does not produce bilirubinuria.

36. State two advantages of the Ictotest over the reagent strip bilirubin test.

37. What is the major cause of false-negative test results for bilirubin?

38. Why is it normal to have 0.1 to 1 mg/dL of urobilinogen in the urine?

39. How does hemolytic anemia affect urine urobilinogen? Why? How does biliary obstruction affect urine urobilinogen? Why?

40. How do the reagent strip reactions for urobilinogen differ between Multistix and Chemstrip? What other pathologic substance does Multistix detect?

41. Describe the reactions obtained with urobilinogen, porphobilinogen, and Ehrlich-reactive compounds in the Watson-Schwartz test.

42. How would you perform a rapid screening test for the presence of porphobilinogen?

43. Describe the diagnostic value of the nitrite test.

44. Why might an automated nitrite reading of positive be changed to negative when the strip is visually examined?

45. State four reasons why a specimen with a large amount of bacteria could have a negative nitrite reaction.

46. Can a nitrite test be performed on a fresh specimen collected in an unsterile container? Why or why not?

47. Why is it possible to have a positive LE reaction and not see any leukocytes in the urine microscopic examination?

48. When is it possible to have a positive LE test in the absence of bacteria?

49. Why do large quantities of ascorbic acid cause false-negative reactions for bilirubin, urobilinogen by Chemstrip, nitrite, and LE?

50. Why does a urine specimen with a low specific gravity produce an alkaline reaction with bromthymol blue in the specific gravity test?

51. How do specific gravity readings differ between reagent strips and refractometers?

52. Explain the need to add 0.005 to the specific gravity readings in urines with a pH of 6.5 or higher.

CASE STUDIES AND CLINICAL SITUATIONS

1. Preadmission laboratory work on an obese patient scheduled for surgery shows a fasting blood glucose level of 230 mg/dL. Results of the routine urinalysis are as follows:

COLOR: Pale yellow	KETONES: Negative
CLARITY: Clear	BLOOD: Negative
SP. GRAVITY: 1.030	BILIRUBIN: Negative
pH: 5.0	UROBILINOGEN: Negative
PROTEIN: 1+	NITRITE: Negative
GLUCOSE: 100 mg/dL	LEUKOCYTES: Negative

   a. Explain the correlation between the patient's blood and urine glucose results. blood glucose level ↑ → glycosuria
   b. What is the most probable metabolic disorder associated with this patient? Diabetes millitus
   c. Considering the patient's condition, what is the significance of the patient's protein result? Diabetic nephropathy
   d. What could have been done to delay the onset of proteinuria in this patient? Stablize blood sugar level
   e. If the patient in this study had a normal blood glucose level, to what would the urinary glucose be attributed? Tubular dysfunction.

2. Results of a urinalysis performed on a patient scheduled for gallbladder surgery are as follows:

COLOR: Amber	KETONES: Negative
CLARITY: Hazy	BLOOD: Negative
SP. GRAVITY: 1.022	BILIRUBIN: Moderate
pH: 6.0	UROBILINOGEN: Normal
PROTEIN: Negative	NITRITE: Negative
GLUCOSE: Negative	LEUKOCYTES: Negative

   a. What would be observed if this specimen were shaken? Yellow foam
   b. What confirmatory test could be performed on this specimen? Icto Test
   c. Explain the correlation between the patient's scheduled surgery and the normal urobilinogen. biliary duct obstruct prevent bilirubin into intestine?
   d. If blood were drawn from this patient, how might the appearance of the serum be described? Icteric
   e. What special handling is needed for serum and urine specimens from this patient? Protect from light

3. Results of a urinalysis on a very anemic and jaundiced patient are as follows:

COLOR: Red	KETONES: Negative
CLARITY: Clear	BLOOD: Large
SP. GRAVITY: 1.020	BILIRUBIN: Negative
pH: 6.0	UROBILINOGEN: 12 EU
PROTEIN: Negative	NITRITE: Negative
GLUCOSE: Negative	LEUKOCYTES: Negative

   a. Would these results be indicative of hematuria or hemoglobinuria?
   b. Correlate the patient's condition with the urobilinogen result.

↑ Hgb present to liver → ↑ bilirubin in liver → ↑ bilirubin in intestine → ↑ urobilinogen conversion

c. Why is the urine bilirubin result negative in this jaundiced patient? circulating bilirubin is unconjugated
d. If interference by porphyrins was suspected in this specimen, how could this be resolved? State two methods.

4. A female patient arrives at the outpatient clinic with symptoms of lower back pain and urinary frequency with a burning sensation. She is a firm believer in the curative powers of vitamins. She has tripled her usual dosage of vitamins in an effort to alleviate her symptoms; however, the symptoms have persisted. She is given a sterile container and asked to collect a midstream clean-catch urine specimen. Results of this routine urinalysis are as follows:

COLOR: Dark yellow	KETONES: Negative
CLARITY: Hazy	BLOOD: Trace
SP. GRAVITY: 1.012	BILIRUBIN: Negative
pH: 7.0	UROBILINOGEN: Normal
PROTEIN: Trace	NITRITE: Negative
GLUCOSE: Negative	LEUKOCYTES: 2+

Microscopic

8 TO 12 RBC/HPF	Heavy bacteria
40 TO 50 WBC/HPF	Moderate squamous epithelial cells

a. What discrepancies between the chemical and microscopic test results are present?
State a possible reason for each discrepancy.
b. What additional chemical tests could be affected by the patient's vitamin dosage?
c. Discuss the urine color and specific gravity results with regard to correlation, and give a possible cause for any discrepancy.
d. State three additional reasons not previously given for a negative nitrite test in the presence of increased bacteria.

5. Results of a urinalysis collected following practice from a 20-year-old college athlete are as follows:

COLOR: Dark yellow	KETONES: Negative
CLARITY: Hazy	BLOOD: 1+
SP. GRAVITY: 1.029	BILIRUBIN: Negative
pH: 6.5	UROBILINOGEN: 1 EU
PROTEIN: 2+	NITRITE: Negative
GLUCOSE: Negative	LEUKOCYTES: Negative

The physician requests the athlete to collect another specimen in the morning prior to classes and practice.
a. What is the purpose of the second sample?
b. What changes would you expect in the second sample?
c. Is the proteinuria present in the first sample of prerenal, renal, or postrenal origin?

6. A construction worker is pinned under collapsed scaffolding for several hours prior to being taken to the emergency room. His abdomen and upper legs are severely bruised, but no fractures are detected. A specimen for urinalysis obtained by catheterization has the following results:

COLOR: Red-brown	KETONES: Negative
CLARITY: Clear	BLOOD: 4+
SP. GRAVITY: 1.017	BILIRUBIN: Negative
pH: 6.5	UROBILINOGEN: 0.4 EU
PROTEIN: Trace	NITRITE: Negative
GLUCOSE: Negative	LEUKOCYTES: Negative

a. Would hematuria be suspected in this specimen? Why or why not?
b. What is the most probable cause of the positive blood reaction?
c. What is the source of the substance causing the positive blood reaction and the name of the condition?
d. Would this patient be monitored for changes in renal function? Why or why not?

7. Considering the correct procedures for care, technique, and quality control for reagent strips, state a possible cause for each of the following scenarios.
a. The urinalysis supervisor notices that an unusually large number of reagent strips are becoming discolored before the expiration date has been reached.
b. A physician's office is consistently reporting positive nitrite test results with negative LE test results.
c. A student's results for reagent strip blood and LE are consistently lower than those of the laboratory staff.
d. A physician questions the significant number of reports indicating elevated automated reagent strip bilirubin results accompanied by negative Ictotest results.

CHAPTER 6

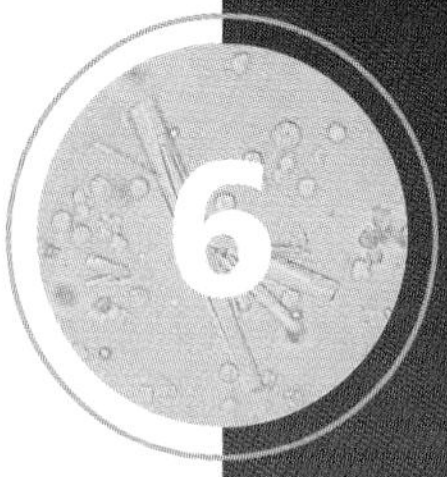

Microscopic Examination of the Urine

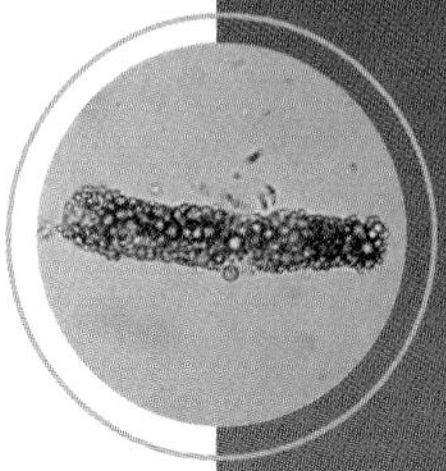

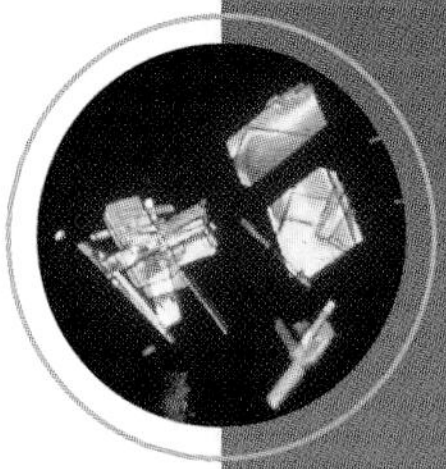

LEARNING OBJECTIVES

Upon completion of this chapter, the reader will be able to:

1. List the physical and chemical parameters included in macroscopic urine screening, and state their significance.
2. Discuss the advantages of commercial systems over the glass-slide method for sediment examination.
3. Describe the recommended methods for standardizing specimen preparation and volume, centrifugation, sediment preparation, volume and examination, and reporting of results.
4. State the purpose of Sternheimer-Malbin, acetic acid, toluidine blue, Sudan III, Gram, Hansel, and Prussian blue stains in the examination of the urine sediment.
5. Identify specimens that should be referred for cytodiagnostic testing.
6. Describe the basic principles of bright-field, phase-contrast, polarizing, and interference-contrast microscopy, and their relationship to sediment examination.
7. Differentiate between normal and abnormal sediment constituents.
8. Discuss the significance of red blood cells (RBCs) in the urinary sediment.
9. Discuss the significance of white blood cells (WBCs) in the urinary sediment.
10. Name, describe, and give the origin and significance of the three types of epithelial cells found in the urinary sediment.
11. Discuss the significance of oval fat bodies.
12. Describe the process of cast formation.
13. Describe and discuss the significance of hyaline, RBC, WBC, bacterial, epithelial cell, granular, waxy, fatty, and broad casts.
14. List and identify the normal crystals found in acidic urine.
15. List and identify the normal crystals found in alkaline urine.
16. Describe and state the significance of cystine, cholesterol, leucine, tyrosine, bilirubin, sulfonamide, radiographic dye, and ampicillin crystals.
17. Differentiate between actual sediment constituents and artifacts.
18. Correlate physical and chemical urinalysis results with microscopic observations and recognize discrepancies.

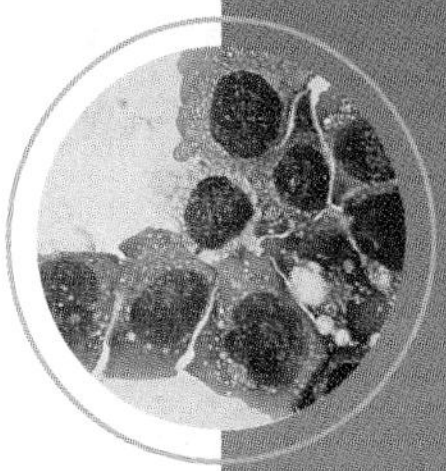

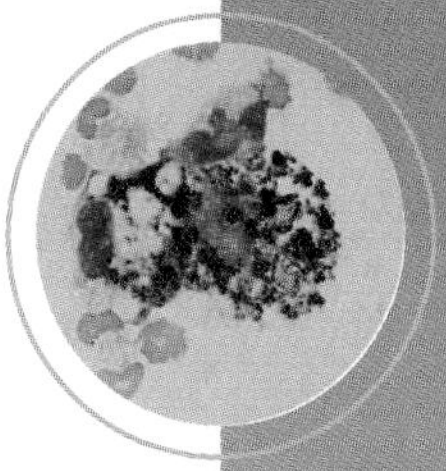

KEY TERMS

bright-field microscopy
casts
chemical sieving
cylindruria
interference-contrast microscopy
phase-contrast microscopy
polarizing microscopy
resolution
Tamm-Horsfall protein

The third part of the routine urinalysis is the microscopic examination of the urinary sediment. Its purpose is to detect and to identify insoluble materials present in the urine. The blood, kidney, lower genitourinary tract, and external contamination all contribute formed elements to the urine. These include RBCs, WBCs, epithelial cells, casts, bacteria, yeast, parasites, mucus, spermatozoa, crystals, and artifacts. Because some of these components are of no clinical significance and others are considered normal unless they are present in increased amounts, examination of the urinary sediment must include both identification and quantitation of the elements present. The urine microscopic examination is the least standardized and most time-consuming part of the routine urinalysis. Protocols have been developed to increase the standardization and cost-effectiveness of the microscopic urinalysis and are discussed in this chapter.

Macroscopic Screening

To enhance the cost-effectiveness of urinalysis, many laboratories have developed protocols, whereby microscopic examination of the urine sediment is performed only on specimens meeting specified criteria. Abnormalities in the physical and chemical portions of the urinalysis play a primary role in the decision to perform a microscopic analysis, thus the use of the term macroscopic screening, also referred to as ***chemical sieving***. Parameters considered significant vary among laboratories but usually include color, clarity, blood, protein, nitrite, leukocyte esterase, and possibly glucose.[5,15] Table 6–1 illustrates the significance of these parameters. Percentages of abnormal specimens that would go undetected using these parameters differ significantly among studies.[23,30,33] The patient population must also be considered when developing protocols for macroscopic screening.[12] Populations that have come under consideration include pregnant women as well as pediatric, geriatric, diabetic, immunocompromised, and renal patients. The National Committee for Clinical Laboratory Standards (NCCLS) recommends that microscopic examination be performed when requested by a physician, a laboratory-specified patient population is being tested, and any abnormal physical or chemical result is obtained.[24]

TABLE 6–1 **Macroscopic Screening Correlations**

Screening Test	Significance
Color	Blood
Clarity	Hematuria versus hemoglobinuria/myoglobinuria Confirm pathologic or nonpathologic cause of turbidity
Blood	RBCs/RBC casts
Protein	Casts/cells
Nitrite	Bacteria/WBCs
Leukocyte esterase	WBCs/WBC casts/bacteria
Glucose	Yeast

Preparation and Examination of the Urine Sediment

The microscopic analysis is subject to several procedural variations, including the methods by which the sediment is prepared, volume of sediment actually examined, methods and equipment used to obtain visualization, and manner in which the results are reported. The first procedure to standardize the quantitation of formed elements in the urine microscopic analysis was developed by Addis in 1926. The Addis count, as it is called, used a hemocytometer to count the number of RBCs, WBCs, casts, and epithelial cells present in a 12-hour specimen. Normal values have a wide range and are approximately 0 to 500,000 RBCs, 0 to 1,800,000 WBCs and epithelial cells, and 0 to 5000 hyaline casts.[1] The Addis count, which was used primarily to monitor the course of diagnosed cases of renal disease, has been replaced by various standardized commercial systems for the preparation, examination, and quantitation of formed elements in nontimed specimens.

COMMERCIAL SYSTEMS

The conventional method of placing a drop of centrifuged urine on a glass slide, adding a cover slip, and examining microscopically has been substantially improved through the use of commercial slide systems.[7,28] The NCCLS recommends their use together with standardization of all phases of the methodology, including the conventional method, as discussed in the following sections. Systems currently available include KOVA (ICL Scientific, Fountain Valley, CA), Urisystem (Fisher Scientific, Pittsburgh, PA), Count-10 (V-Tech, Inc., Palm Springs, CA), Quick-Read 10 (Globe Scientific, Paramus, NJ), Cen-Slide

(Davstar California, Newport Beach, CA), and R/S 2000 (DioSys, Waterbury, CA). The systems provide a variety of options including capped, calibrated centrifuge tubes; decanting pipettes to control sediment volume; and slides that control the amount of sediment examined, produce a consistent monolayer of sediment for examination, and provide calibrated grids for more consistent quantitation.

The Cen-Slide and R/S 2000 systems do not require manual loading of the centrifuged specimen onto a slide and are considered closed systems that minimize exposure to the specimen. Cen-Slide provides a specially designed tube that permits direct reading of the microscopic. The R/S 2000 system consists of a glass flow cell into which urine sediment is pumped, microscopically examined, and then flushed from the system.

SPECIMEN PREPARATION

Specimens should be examined while fresh or adequately preserved. Formed elements—primarily RBCs, WBCs, and hyaline casts—disintegrate rapidly, particularly in dilute alkaline urine. Refrigeration may cause precipitation of amorphous urates and phosphates and other nonpathologic crystals that can obscure other elements in the urine sediment. Warming the specimen to 37°C prior to centrifuging may dissolve some of these crystals.

The midstream clean-catch specimen minimizes external contamination of the sediment. As with the physical and chemical analyses, dilute random specimens may cause false-negative readings.

Care must be taken to thoroughly mix the specimen prior to decanting a portion into a centrifuge tube.

SPECIMEN VOLUME

A standard amount of urine, usually between 10 and 15 mL, is centrifuged in a conical tube. This will provide an adequate volume from which to obtain a representative sample of the elements present in the specimen. A 12-mL volume is frequently used because multiparameter reagent strips are easily immersed in this volume, and capped centrifuge tubes are often calibrated to this volume.

If obtaining a 12-mL specimen is not possible, as with pediatric patients, the volume of the specimen used should be noted on the report form. This allows the physician to correct the results, if indicated. Some laboratories choose to make this correction prior to reporting. For example, if 6 mL of urine is centrifuged the results are multiplied by 2.

CENTRIFUGATION

The speed of the centrifuge and the length of time the specimen is centrifuged should be consistent. Centrifugation for 5 minutes at a relative centrifugal force (**RCF**) of 400 will produce an optimum amount of sediment with the least chance of damaging the elements. To correct for differences in the diameter of centrifuge heads, the RCF rather than the revolutions per minute (**RPM**) is used. The RPM value shown on the centrifuge tachometer can be converted to RCF using nomograms available in many laboratory manuals or by using the formula:

$$\text{RCF} = 1.118 \times 10^{-5} \times \text{radius in centimeters} \times \text{RPM}^2$$

Centrifugation calibration should be routinely performed. Use of the braking mechanism to slow the centrifuge will cause disruption of the sediment prior to decantation and should not be used.

To prevent biohazardous aerosols, all specimens must be centrifuged in capped tubes.

SEDIMENT PREPARATION

A uniform amount of urine and sediment should remain in the tube after decantation. Volumes of 0.5 and 1.0 mL are frequently used. The volume of urine centrifuged divided by the sediment volume equals the concentration factor, which in the preceding examples is 24 and 12, respectively. The sediment concentration factor relates to the probability of detecting elements present in low quantities and is used when quantitating the number of elements present per milliliter.

To maintain a uniform sediment concentration factor, urine should be aspirated off rather than poured off, unless specified by the commercial system in use. Some systems provide pipettes for this purpose. The pipettes also are used for sediment resuspension and transfer of specimens to the slide.

The sediment must be thoroughly resuspended by gentle agitation. This can be performed using a commercial-system pipette or by repeatedly tapping the tip of the tube with the finger. Vigorous agitation should be avoided, as it may disrupt some cellular elements. Thorough resuspension is essential to provide equal distribution of elements in the microscopic examination fields.

VOLUME OF SEDIMENT EXAMINED

The volume of sediment placed on the microscope slide should be consistent for each specimen. When using the conventional glass-slide method, the recommended volume is 20 µL (0.02 mL) covered by a 22 × 22 mm glass cover slip. Allowing the specimen to flow outside of the cover slip may result in the loss of heavier elements such as casts.

Commercial systems control the volume of sediment examined by providing slides with chambers capable of containing a specified volume. Care must be taken to ensure the chambers are completely filled. Product literature supplies the chamber volume, size of the viewing area, and approximate number of low-power and high-power viewing areas, based on the area of the field of view using a standard microscope. This information, together with the sediment concentration factor, is necessary to quantitate cellular elements per milliliter of urine.

EXAMINATION OF THE SEDIMENT

The manner by which the microscopic examination is performed should be consistent and should include observation of a minimum of 10 fields under both low (10×) and high (40×) power. The slide is first examined under low power to detect casts and to ascertain the general composition of the sediment. When elements such as casts that require identification are encountered, the setting is changed to high power.

If the conventional glass-slide method is being used, casts have a tendency to locate near the edges of the cover slip; therefore, low-power scanning of the cover-slip perimeter is recommended. This does not occur when using standardized commercial systems.

When the sediment is examined unstained, many sediment constituents have a refractive index similar to urine. Therefore, it is essential that sediments be examined under reduced light when using ***bright-field microscopy***.

Initial focusing can be difficult with a fluid specimen, and care must be taken to ensure the examination is being performed in the correct plane. Often an epithelial cell will be present to provide a point of reference. Focusing on artifacts should be avoided, because they are often larger than the regular sediment elements and cause the microscopist to examine objects in the wrong plane. Continuous focusing with the fine adjustment aids in obtaining a complete representation of the sediment constituents.

REPORTING THE MICROSCOPIC EXAMINATION

The terminology and methods of reporting may differ slightly among laboratories but must be consistent with a particular laboratory system. Routinely, casts are reported as the average number per low-power field (**lpf**) following examination of 10 fields, and RBCs and WBCs, as the average number per 10 high-power fields (**hpfs**). Epithelial cells, crystals, and other elements are frequently reported in semiquantitative terms such as, rare, few, moderate, and many or as 1+, 2+, 3+, and 4+, following laboratory format as to lpf or hpf use. Laboratories must also determine their particular reference values based on the sediment concentration factor in use. For example, Urisystem, with a concentration factor of 30, states a reference value for WBCs of zero to eight per hpf, as opposed to the conventional value of zero to five per hpf used with a concentration factor of 12.

Conversion of the average number of elements per lpf or hpf to the number per milliliter will provide standardization among the various techniques in use. Steps include the following:

1. Calculation of the area of an lpf or hpf for the microscope in use using the manufacturer-supplied field of view diameter and the formula πr^2 = area.

EXAMPLE:
Diameter of hpf = 0.35 mm
$3.14 \times .175^2 = 0.096\ mm^2$

2. Calculation of the maximum number of lpfs or hpfs in the viewing area.

EXAMPLE:
Area under a 22 mm × 22 mm cover slip = 484 mm^2

$$\frac{484}{.096} = 5040 \text{ hpfs}$$

3. Calculation of the number of hpfs per milliliter of urine tested using the concentration factor and the volume of sediment examined.

EXAMPLE:

$$\frac{5040}{0.02 \text{ mL} \times 12} = \frac{5040}{.24} = 21{,}000 \text{ hpf/mL of urine}$$

4. Calculation of the number of formed elements per milliliter of urine by multiplying the number of hpfs per milliliter by the average number of formed elements per field.

EXAMPLE:
4 WBC/hpf × 21,000 = 84,000 WBC/mL

Provided the same microscope and volume of sediment examined are used, the number of lpfs and hpfs per milliliter of urine remains the same, thereby simplifying the calculation.

Laboratories should evaluate the advantages and disadvantages of adding an additional calculation step to the microscopic examination. The NCCLS states that all decisions with regard to reporting of the microscopic should be based on the needs of the individual laboratory. Procedures should be completely documented and followed by all personnel.

CORRELATION OF RESULTS

Microscopic results should be correlated with the physical and chemical findings to ensure the accuracy of the report. Specimens in which the results do not correlate must be rechecked for both technical and clerical errors. Table 6–2 shows some of the more common correlations in the urinalysis; however, the amount of formed elements or chemicals must also be considered, as must the possibility of interference with chemical tests and the age of the specimen.

Sediment Examination Techniques

Many factors can influence the appearance of the urinary sediment, including cells and casts in various stages of development and degeneration, distortion of cells and crystals by the chemical content of the specimen, the presence of inclusions in cells and casts, and contamination by artifacts. Therefore, identification can sometimes be difficult even for experienced laboratory personnel. Identification can be enhanced through the use of sediment stains (Table 6–3) and different types of microscopy.

SEDIMENT STAINS

Staining increases the overall visibility of sediment elements being examined using bright-field microscopy by changing their refractive index. As mentioned previously, elements such as hyaline casts have a refractive index very similar to that of urine. Staining also imparts identifying

TABLE 6–2 **Routine Urinalysis Correlations**

Microscopic Elements	Physical	Chemical	Exceptions
Red blood cells	Turbidity Red color	+ Blood	Number Hemolysis
White blood cells	Turbidity	+ Protein + Nitrite + Leukocytes	Number Lysis
Epithelial cells	Turbidity		Number
Casts		+ Protein	Number
Bacteria	Turbidity	pH + Nitrite + Leukocytes	Number and type
Crystals	Turbidity Color	pH	Number and type

characteristics to cellular structures, such as the nuclei, cytoplasm, and inclusions.

The most frequently used stain in urinalysis is the Sternheimer-Malbin stain, which consists of crystal violet and safranin O.[32] The stain is available commercially under a variety of names, including Sedi-Stain (Becton-Dickinson, Parsippany, NJ) and KOVA stain (ICL Scientific, Fountain Valley, CA). Commercial brands contain stabilizing chemicals to prevent the precipitation that occurred with the original stain. The dye is absorbed well by WBCs, epithelial cells, and casts, providing clearer delineation of structure and contrasting colors of the nucleus and cytoplasm. Table 6–4 provides an example of the staining reactions as shown in the product literature.

A 0.5 percent solution of toluidine blue, a metachromatic stain, provides enhancement of nuclear detail. It can be useful in the differentiation between WBCs and renal tubular epithelial cells and also is used in the examination of cells from other body fluids.

Nuclear detail is also enhanced by the addition of 2 percent acetic acid to the sediment. This method cannot be used for initial sediment analysis because RBCs will be lysed by the acetic acid.

Lipid Stains

The passage of lipids (triglycerides, neutral fats, and cholesterol) across the glomerular membrane results in the appearance of free fat droplets and lipid-containing cells and casts in the urinary sediment. The lipid stains, Oil Red O and Sudan III, and polarizing microscopy can be used to confirm the presence of these elements. Triglycerides and neutral fats stain orange-red in the presence of stain, whereas cholesterol does not stain but is capable of polarization. The three lipids are usually present concurrently in the sediment, thereby permitting use of either staining or polarization for their confirmation.

Gram Stain

The Gram stain is used primarily in the Microbiology section for the differentiation between gram-positive (blue)

TABLE 6–3 **Sediment Stain Characteristics**

Stain	Action	Function
Sternheimer-Malbin	Delineates structure and contrasting colors of the nucleus and cytoplasm	Identifies WBCs, epithelial cells, and casts
Toluidine blue	Enhances nuclear detail	Differentiates WBCs and renal tubular epithelial (RTE) cells
2% acetic acid	Lyses RBCs and enhances nuclei of WBCs	Distinguishes RBCs from WBCs, yeast, oil droplets, and crystals
Lipid Stains: Oil Red O and Sudan III	Stains triglycerides and neutral fats orange-red	Identifies free fat droplets and lipid-containing cells and casts
Gram stain	Differentiates gram-positive and gram-negative bacteria	Identifies bacterial casts
Hansel stain	Methylene blue and eosin Y stain eosinophilic granules	Identifies urinary eosinophils
Prussian blue stain	Stains structures containing iron	Identifies yellow-brown granules of hemosiderin in cells and casts

TABLE 6–4 **Expected Staining Reactions of Sediment Constituents**

Elements in Urinary Sediment	Usual Distinguishing Color of Stained Elements		Comments
Red blood cells	Neutral—pink to purple Acid—pink (unstained) Alkaline—purple		
	Nuclei	***Cytoplasm***	
White blood cells—dark-staining cells	Purple	Purple granules	
Glitter cells (Sternheimer-Malbin positive cells)	Colorless or light blue	Pale blue or gray	Some glitter cells exhibit brownian movement
Renal tubular epithelial cells	Dark shade of blue-purple	Light shade of blue-purple	
Bladder tubular epithelial cells	Blue-purple	Light purple	
Squamous epithelial cells	Dark shade of orange-purple	Light purple or blue	
	Inclusions and Matrix		
Hyaline casts	Pale pink or pale purple		Very uniform color; slightly darker than mucous threads
Coarse granular inclusion casts	Dark purple granules in purple matrix		
Finely granular inclusion casts	Fine dark purple granules in pale pink or pale purple matrix		
Waxy casts	Pale pink or pale purple		Darker than hyaline casts, but of a pale even color; distinct broken ends
Fat inclusion casts	Fat globules unstained in a pink matrix		Rare; presence is confirmed if examination under polarized light indicates double refraction
Red cell inclusion casts	Pink to orange-red		Intact cells can be seen in matrix
Blood (hemoglobin) casts	Orange-red		No intact cells
Bacteria	Motile: do not stain Nonmotile: stain purple		Motile organisms are not impaired
Trichomonas vaginalis	Light blue-green		Motility is unimpaired in fresh specimens when recommended volumes of stain are used; immobile organisms also identifiable
Mucus	Pale pink or pale blue		
Background	Pale pink or pale purple		

From Product Profile: Sedi-Stain,[26] with permission.

and gram-negative (red) bacteria. Its role in routine urinalysis is limited to the identification of bacterial casts, which can easily be confused with granular casts. To perform Gram staining, a dried, heat-fixed preparation of the urine sediment must be used.

Hansel Stain

Polynuclear WBCs seen in the urinary sediment are almost always neutrophils associated with microbial infection. However, in cases of a drug-induced allergic reaction producing inflammation of the renal interstitium, eosinophils are present in the sediment. The preferred stain for urinary eosinophils is Hansel stain, consisting of methylene blue and eosin Y (Lide Labs, Inc, Florissant, MO); however, Wright's stain can also be used. Staining is performed on a dried smear of the centrifuged specimen or a cytocentrifuged preparation of the sediment.

Prussian Blue Stain

As discussed in Chapter 5, following episodes of hemoglobinuria, yellow-brown granules may be seen in renal tubular epithelial cells and casts or free-floating in the urine sediment. To confirm that these granules are hemosiderin, the Prussian blue stain is used and stains the hemosiderin granules a blue color.

CYTODIAGNOSTIC URINE TESTING

Although it is not a part of the routine examination of the urine sediment, the preparation of permanent slides using cytocentrifugation followed by staining with Papanicolaou's stain provides an additional method for detecting and monitoring renal disease. Cytodiagnostic urine testing is frequently performed independently of the routine urinalysis for detection of malignancies of the lower urinary tract. A voided first morning specimen is recommended for testing, which is performed by cytologists and pathologists.[14] Cytodiagnostic urine testing also provides more definitive information about renal tubular changes associated with transplant rejection; viral, fungal, and parasitic infections; cellular inclusions; pathologic casts; and inflammatory conditions. The urinalysis laboratory should refer specimens with unusual cellular findings to the cytology laboratory for further examination.

MICROSCOPY

The microscopic examination of the urine is best performed when the laboratorian is knowledgeable about the types of microscopes available, their primary characteristics, and the proper use of these microscopes.

Bright-field microscopy is the most common type of microscopy performed in the urinalysis laboratory. Other types of microscopy that are useful for examining the urine sediment are phase contrast, polarizing, and interference contrast (Table 6–5). All microscopes are designed to magnify small objects to a degree at which the details of their structure can be analyzed. Basically they do this by employing a variety of lenses and light sources as described in the following section.

The Microscope

Essentially all types of microscopes contain a lens system, illumination system, and a body consisting of a base, body tube, and nosepiece (Figure 6–1). Primary components of the lens system are the oculars, the objectives, and the coarse and fine adjustment knobs. The illumination system contains the light source, condenser, and field and iris diaphragms. Objects to be examined are placed on a platform, referred to as the mechanical stage.

The oculars or eyepieces of the microscope are located at the top of the body tube. Clinical laboratory microscopes are binocular, allowing the examination to be performed using both eyes to provide more complete visualization. For optimal viewing conditions, the oculars can be adjusted horizontally to adapt to differences in interpupillary distance between operators. A diopter adjustment knob on the oculars can be rotated to compensate for variations in vision between the operators' eyes. The oculars contain two lenses designed to further magnify the object that has been enhanced by the objectives. Laboratory microscopes normally contain objectives capable of increasing the magnification 10 times (10×).

Objectives are contained in the revolving nosepiece located above the mechanical stage. Objectives perform the initial magnification of the object on the mechanical stage. The image then passes to the oculars for further ***resolution*** (ability to visualize fine details). Routinely used objectives in the clinical laboratory have magnifications of 10× (low power), 40× (high power), and 100× (oil immersion). The objectives used for examination of the urine sediment are 10× and 40×. The final magnification of an object is the product of the objective magnification times the ocular magnification. Using a 10× ocular and a 10× objective provides a total magnification of 100× and in urinalysis is the lpf observation. The 10× ocular and the 40× objective provide a magnification of 400× for hpf observations.

Objectives are inscribed with information that describes their characteristics and includes the type of objective (plan used for bright field, ph for phase contrast), magnification, numerical aperture, microscope tube length, and cover-slip thickness to be used. The numerical aperture number represents the refractive index of the material between the slide and the outer lens (air or oil) and the angle of the light passing through it. The higher the numerical aperture, the greater is the resolving power. The length of the objectives attached to the nosepiece varies with magnification (length increases from 10× to 100× magnification), thereby changing the distance between the lens and the slide when they are rotated. Most microscopes are designed to be parfocal, indicating that they require only minimum adjustment when switching among objectives.

The distance between the slide and the objective is controlled by the coarse and fine focusing knobs located on the body tube. Initial focusing is performed using the coarse knob that moves the mechanical stage noticeably up and down. This is followed by adjustment using the fine focusing knob. When using a parfocal microscope, use of only the fine knob should be necessary when changing magnifications.

Illumination for the modern microscope is provided by a light source located in the base of the microscope. The light source is equipped with a rheostat to regulate the intensity of the light. Filters may also be placed on the light source to vary the illumination and wavelengths of the emitted light. A field diaphragm contained in the light source controls the diameter of the light beam reaching the slide. A condenser located below the stage then focuses the

TABLE 6–5 **Urinalysis Microscopic Techniques**

Technique	Function
Bright-field microscopy	Used for routine urinalysis
Phase-contrast microscopy	Enhances visualization of elements with low refractive indices, such as hyaline casts, mixed cellular casts, mucous threads, and *Trichomonas*
Polarizing microscopy	Aids in identification of cholesterol in oval fat bodies, fatty casts, and crystals
Interference-contrast microscopy	Produces a three-dimensional image and layer-by-layer imaging of a specimen

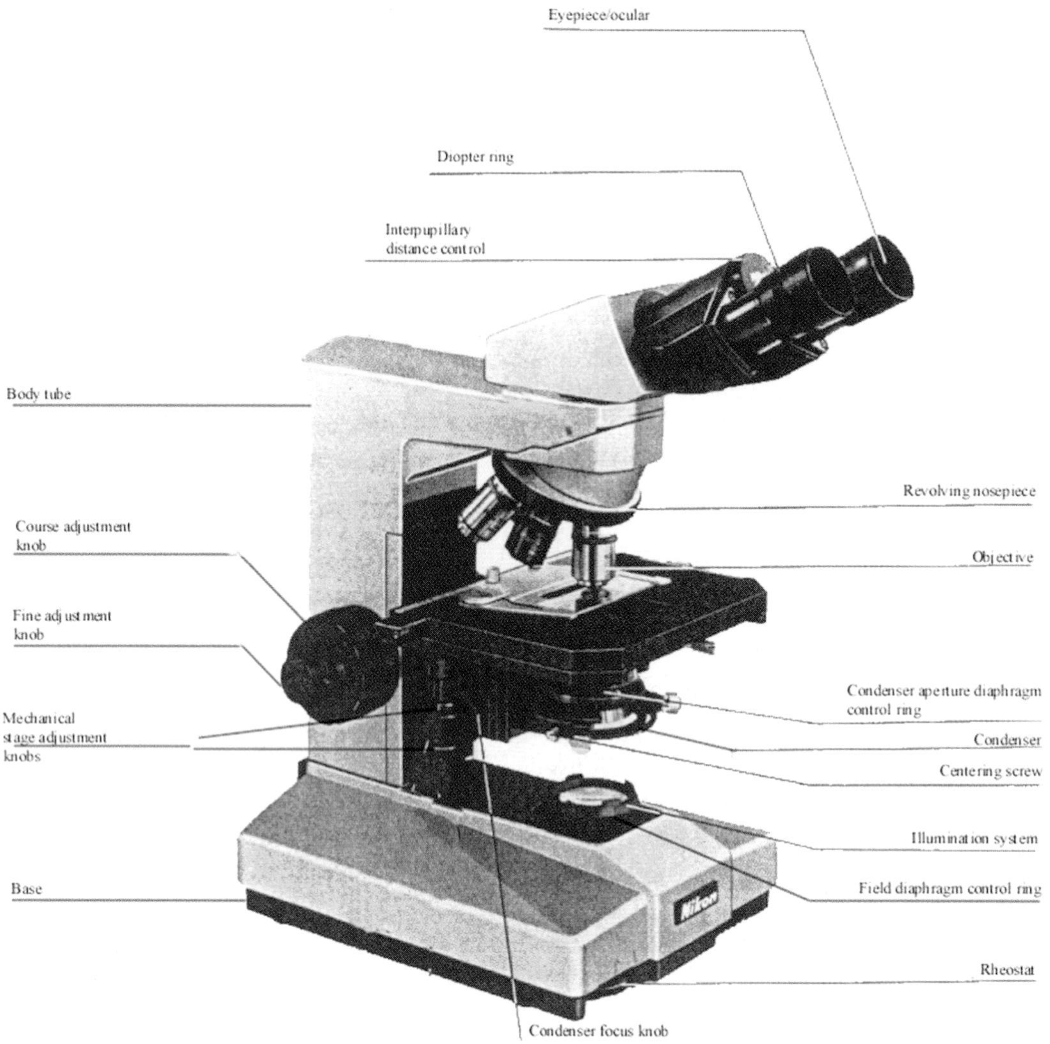

FIGURE 6–1 Parts of the binocular microscope. (Adapted from Nikon Labophot Instruction Manual.)

light on the specimen. The normal position of the condenser is almost completely up with the front lens of the condenser near the slide but not touching it. The condenser adjustment (focus) knob moves the condenser up and down to focus light on the object. An aperature diaphragm in the condenser controls the amount of light and the angle of light rays that will pass to the specimen and lens, which affects resolution, contrast, and depth of the field of image. The aperature diaphragm should not be used to reduce light intensity because it will decrease resolution. The microscope lamp rheostat is used for this adjustment.

Two adjustments to the condenser—centering and Köhler illumination—provide optimal viewing of the illuminated field. They should be performed whenever an objective is changed. To center the condenser and obtain Köhler illumination, the following steps should be taken:

- Place a slide on the stage and focus the object using the low-power objective with the condenser raised.
- Close the field diaphragm.

PROCEDURE

Care of the Microscope

1. Carry microscope with two hands, supporting the base with one hand.
2. Always hold the microscope in a vertical position.
3. Only clean optical surfaces with a good quality lens tissue and commercial lens cleaner.
4. Do not use the 10× and 40× objectives with oil.
5. Clean the oil immersion lens after use.
6. Always remove slides with the low-power objective raised.
7. Store the microscope with the low-power objective in position and the stage centered.

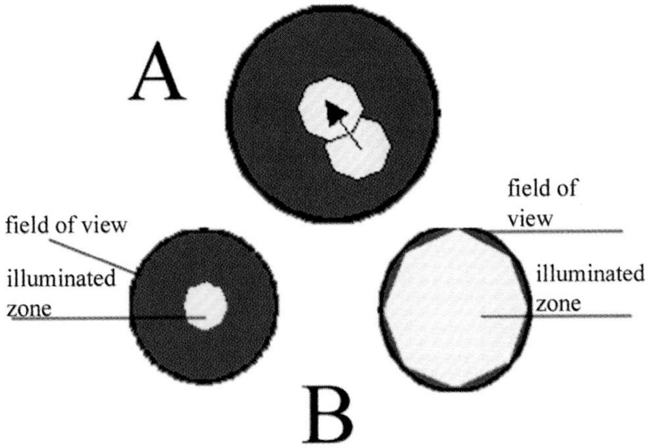

FIGURE 6–2 Centering the condenser and Köhler illumination.

- Lower the condenser until the edges of the field diaphragm are sharply focused.
- Center the image of the field diaphragm with the condenser centering screws as shown in Figure 6–2.
- Open the field diaphragm until its image is at the edge of the field.
- Remove an eyepiece and look down through the eyepiece tube.
- Adjust the aperature diaphragm until approximately 75 percent of the field is visible (see Fig. 6–2).
- Replace the eyepiece.

Additional focusing of the object should be performed using the adjustment knobs and the rheostat on the light source.

Bright-Field Microscopy

Bright-field microscopy, in which objects appear dark against a light background, is most frequently used in the clinical laboratory. This technique employs the basic microscope previously described with a light source emitting light in the visible wavelength range.

Use of bright-field microscopy for the examination of the urine sediment can present problems when the amount of light reaching the specimen is not properly controlled. Sediment constituents with a low refractive index will be overlooked when subjected to light of high intensity. Therefore, sediments must be examined using decreased light controlled by adjusting the rheostat on the light source, not by lowering the condenser. Staining of the sediment also will increase the visualization of these elements when using bright-field microscopy.

Phase-Contrast Microscopy

As light rays pass through an object, they are slowed in comparison to the rays passing through air (media), thereby decreasing the intensity of the light and producing contrast. This is called phase difference and is affected by the thickness of the object, refractive index, and other light-absorbance properties. The best contrast is obtained when the light that does not pass through the specimen is shifted one-quarter of a wavelength and compared with the phase difference of the specimen. ***Phase-contrast microscopy*** provides this contrast.

Phase-contrast microscopy is accomplished by adaptation of a bright-field microscope with a phase-contrast objective lens and a matching condenser. Two phase rings that appear as "targets" are placed in the condenser and the objective. One phase ring is placed in the condenser or below it permitting light to only pass through the central clear circular area. A second phase-shifting ring with a central circular area that retards the light by one-quarter wavelength is placed in the objective. Phase rings must match so it is important to check that both the objective and condenser mode is the same. The diameter of the rings varies with the magnification. The image has the best contrast when the background is darkest. Phase-contrast rings must be adjusted to have maximum contrast. The two rings are adjusted to make them concentric. Adjustment steps are as follows:[22]

- Focus the microscope in bright-field with a specimen slide.
- Select a low-power phase condenser ring.
- Select the corresponding ring objective.
- Remove an ocular, insert the adjustment telescope, and look through the telescope.
- Observe the dark and light rings (annuli).
- With the adjusting screw on the telescope, center the light annulus (condenser) over the dark annulus (objective) (Figure 6–3).
- Replace the ocular.

Light passes to the specimen through the clear circle in the phase ring in the condenser. The diffracted light then enters the central circle of the phase-shifting ring, and all other light is moved one-quarter of a wavelength out of phase. The variations of contrast in the specimen image due to the various refractive indexes in the object are observed as the light rays merge together, enhancing visualization and detail. Phase-contrast microscopy is particularly advantageous for identifying hyaline casts or mixed cellular casts, mucous threads, and *Trichomonas*.

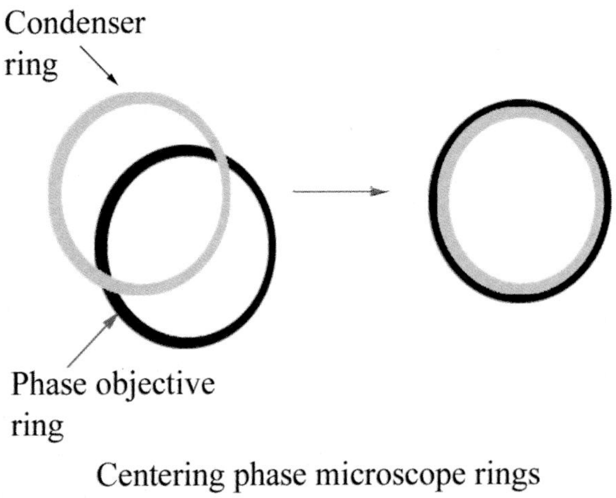

FIGURE 6–3 Phase-contrast ring adjustment.

Polarizing Microscopy

The use of polarized light aids in the identification of crystals and lipids. Both substances have the ability to rotate the path of the unidirectional polarized light beam to produce characteristic colors in crystals and Maltese cross formation in lipids. These elements seen under polarized light microscopy are birefringent, a property indicating that the element can refract light in two dimensions at 90 degrees to each other.

The halogen quartz lamp in the microscope produces light rays of many different waves. Each wave has a distinct direction and a vibration perpendicular to its direction. Normal or unpolarized light vibrates in equal intensity in all directions. Polarized light vibrates in the same plane or direction. As the light passes through a birefringent substance, it splits into two beams, one beam rotated 90 degrees to the other. Isotropic substances such as blood cells do not have this refractive property, and the light passes through unchanged. A substance that rotates the plane of polarized light 90 degrees in a clockwise direction is said to have positive birefringence. In contrast, a substance that rotates the plane in a counterclockwise direction has negative birefringence.

Polarized light is obtained by using two polarizing filters. The light emerging from one filter vibrates in one plane, and a second filter placed at a 90-degree angle blocks all incoming light, except that rotated by the birefringent substance. The filters are in opposite directions called a "crossed configuration." Between cross-polarizing filters, birefringent crystals are visible in characteristic patterns (Figure 6–4).

Bright-field microscopes can be adapted for ***polarizing microscopy***. Two polarizing filters must be installed in a crossed configuration. The first filter, the polarizing filter, is placed in the condenser filter holder; the second filter, the analyzer, is placed in the head between the objectives and the ocular. The polarizing filter is rotated to allow light vibrating in one direction only to reach the object. If the object does not have birefringent properties, no light will reach the analyzer filter and the object will appear black. Refracted rays from a birefringent object will reach the analyzer, causing the object to appear white or colored against the black background.

Polarizing microscopy is used in urinalysis to confirm the identification of fat droplets, oval fat bodies, and fatty casts that produce a characteristic Maltese cross pattern. Birefringent uric acid crystals can be distinguished from cystine crystals, monohydrate calcium oxalate crystals from nonpolarizing RBCs, and calcium phosphate crystals differentiated from nonpolarizing bacteria by their polarizing characteristics. As discussed in Chapter 12, polarized microscopy is a valuable tool for the identification of synovial fluid crystals.

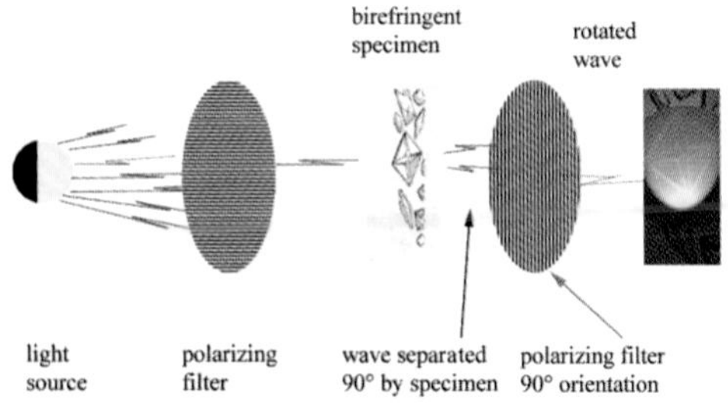

FIGURE 6–4 Diagram of polarized light.

Interference-Contrast Microscopy

Interference-contrast microscopy provides a three-dimensional image showing very fine structural detail by splitting the light ray so that the beams pass through different areas of the specimen. The light interference produced by the varied depths of the specimen is compared, and a three-dimensional image is visualized. The advantage of interference-contrast microscopy is that an object will appear bright against a dark background but without the diffraction halo associated with phase-contrast microscopy. More extensive modifications to the bright-field microscope are required to perform this technique. Therefore, it is not routinely used in the urinalysis laboratory.

Two types of interference-contrast microscopy are available: modulation contrast (Hoffman) and differential interference contrast (Nomarski). Bright-field microscopes can be adapted for both methods. In the modulation-contrast microscope, a split aperature is placed below the condenser, a polarizer is placed below the split aperature, and an amplitude filter is placed in back of each objective. The differential interference-contrast microscope uses prisms. A polarizing filter to output plane polarized light and a two-layered Nomarski-modified Wollaston prism that separates individual rays of light into ray pairs are placed between the light source and the condenser. The lower Wollaston prism is built into the condenser of the microscope. The upper prism is placed above the objective and recombines the rays. Above the top Wollaston prism, another polarizing filter is placed that causes wave interference to occur and produce the three-dimensional image (Figure 6–5).[25] These two types of microscopy provide layer-by-layer imaging of a specimen and enhanced detail for specimens with either a low or high refractive index.

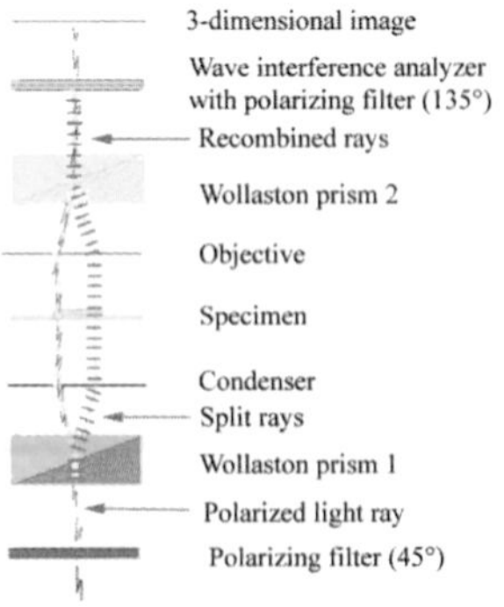

FIGURE 6–5 Differential interference-contrast (Nomarski) microscopy. (Adapted from b-online@botamk.um-hamburg.de © Peter V. Sengbusch.)

Sediment Constituents

The normal urine sediment may contain a variety of formed elements. Even the appearance of small numbers of the usually pathologically significant RBCs, WBCs, and ***casts*** can be normal. Likewise, many routine urines will contain nothing more than a rare epithelial cell or mucous strand. Students often have difficulty adjusting to this, because in the classroom setting, sediments containing abnormalities and multiple elements are usually stressed. They must learn to trust their observations after looking at the recommended number of fields. Cellular elements are also easily distorted by the widely varying concentrations, pH, and presence of metabolites in urine, making identification more difficult.

Actual normal numerical values are not clearly defined. As discussed previously, sediment preparation methods determine the actual concentration of the sediment and, therefore, the number of elements that may be present in a microscopic field. Commonly listed values include zero to two or three RBCs per hpf, zero to five to eight WBCs per hpf, and zero to two hyaline casts per lpf. Even these figures must be taken in context with other factors, such as recent stress and exercise, menstrual contamination, and the presence of other sediment constituents. To put this in better perspective, the sediment constituents are now discussed individually with reference to the accompanying figures.

RED BLOOD CELLS

In the urine, RBCs appear as smooth, non-nucleated, biconcave disks measuring approximately 7 μm in diameter (Figure 6–6). They must be identified using high-power (40×) magnification. RBCs are routinely reported as the average number seen in 10 hpfs (400×).

In concentrated (hypersthenuric) urine, the cells shrink due to loss of water and may appear **crenated** or irregularly shaped (Figure 6–7). In dilute (hyposthenuria) urine, the cells absorb water, swell, and lyse rapidly, releasing their hemoglobin, leaving only the cell membrane. These large empty cells are called **ghost cells** and can be easily missed if specimens are not examined under reduced light.

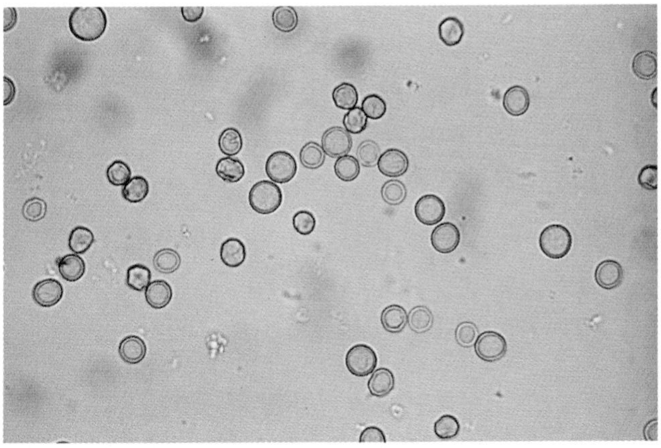

FIGURE 6–6 Normal RBCs (×400).

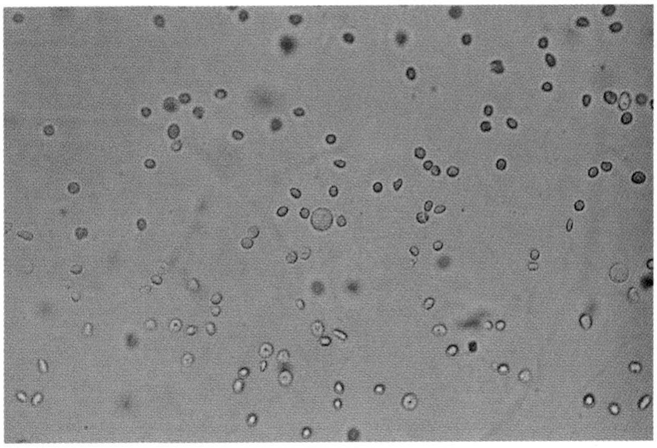

FIGURE 6–7 Microcytic and crenated RBCs (×400).

Of all the sediment elements, RBCs cause students the most difficulty in recognition. Reasons for this difficulty include their lack of characteristic structures, variations in size, and close resemblance to other sediment constituents. RBCs are frequently confused with yeast cells, oil droplets, and air bubbles. Yeast cells will usually exhibit budding (Figure 6–8). Oil droplets and air bubbles are highly refractile when the fine adjustment is focused up and down (Figure 6–9). They may also appear in a different plane than other sediment constituents (Figure 6–10). The rough appearance of crenated RBCs may resemble the granules seen in WBCs; however, they will be much smaller than WBCs. Should the identification continue to be doubtful, adding acetic acid to a portion of the sediment will lyse the RBCs, leaving the yeast, oil droplets, and WBCs intact. Supravital staining may also be helpful.

Studies have focused on the morphology of urinary RBCs as an aid in determining the site of renal bleeding. RBCs that vary in size, have cellular protrusions, or are fragmented are termed **dysmorphic** (Figure 6–11) and have been associated primarily with glomerular bleeding. The number and appearance of the dysmorphic cells must also be considered because abnormal urine concentration will

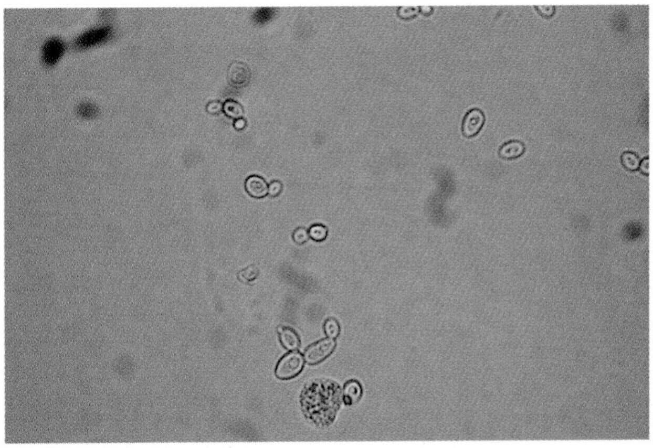

FIGURE 6–8 Yeast. The presence of budding forms aid in distinguishing from RBCs (×400).

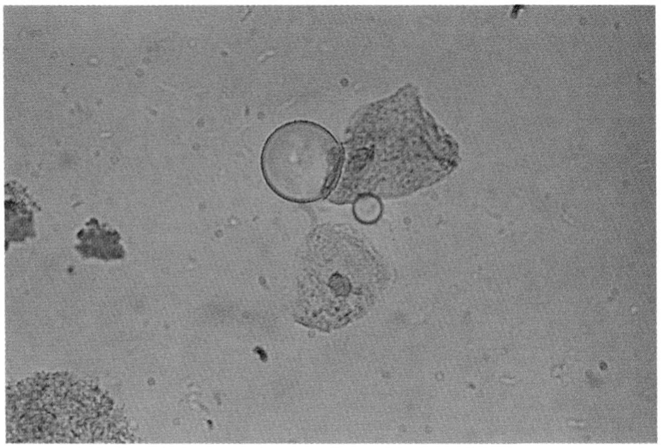

FIGURE 6–9 KOVA-stained squamous epithelial cells and oil droplets (×400).

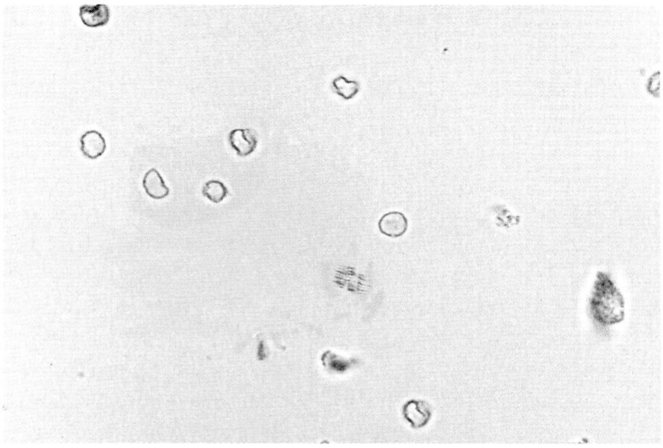

FIGURE 6–11 Dysmorphic RBCs (×400).

affect RBC appearance, and small numbers of dysmorphic cells are found with nonglomerular hematuria.[29,31] Dysmorphic RBCs also have been demonstrated after strenuous exercise, indicating a glomerular origin of this phenomenon.[6] The dysmorphic cell most closely associated with glomerular bleeding appears to be the acanthocyte with multiple protrusions, which may be difficult to observe under brightfield microscopy.[16,34] Further analysis of sediments containing dysmorphic RBCs using Wright's stained preparations shows the cells to be hypochromic and better delineates the presence of cellular blebs and protrusions. The cells also have been characterized using planar morphology.[13]

The presence of RBCs in the urine is associated with damage to the glomerular membrane or vascular injury within the genitourinary tract. The number of cells present is indicative of the extent of the damage or injury. Patient histories often mention the presence of macroscopic versus microscopic hematuria.

When macroscopic hematuria is present, the urine will appear cloudy with a red to brown color. The microscopic analysis may be reported in terms of greater than 100 per hpf or as specified by laboratory protocol. Macroscopic hematuria is frequently associated with advanced glomerular damage but is also seen with damage to the vascular integrity of the urinary tract caused by trauma, acute infection or inflammation, and coagulation disorders.

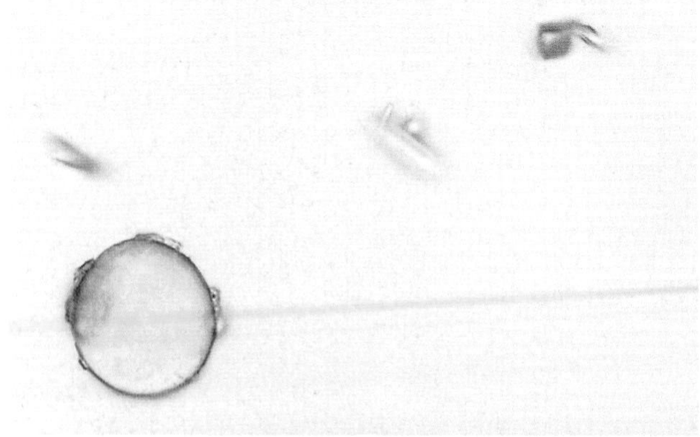

FIGURE 6–10 Air bubble. Notice no formed elements are in focus (×100).

The observation of microscopic hematuria can be critical to the early diagnosis of glomerular disorders and malignancy of the urinary tract and to confirm the presence of renal calculi. The presence of not only RBCs but also hyaline, granular and RBC casts may be seen following strenuous exercise. These abnormalities are nonpathologic and disappear after rest.[11] The possibility of menstrual contamination must also be considered in specimens from female patients.

As discussed previously, the presence or absence of RBCs in the sediment cannot always be correlated with specimen color or a positive chemical test result for blood. The presence of hemoglobin that has been filtered by the glomerulus will produce a red urine with a positive chemical test result for blood in the absence of microscopic hematuria. Likewise, a specimen appearing macroscopically normal may contain a small but pathologically significant number of RBCs when examined microscopically.

WHITE BLOOD CELLS

WBCs are larger than RBCs, measuring an average of about 12 μm in diameter.

Summary of Microscopic RBCs

Appearance:	Non-nucleated biconcave disks Crenated in hypertonic urine Ghost cells in hypotonic urine Dysmorphic with glomerular membrane damage
Sources of identification error:	Yeast cells Oil droplets Air bubbles
Reporting:	Average number per 10 high-power fields
Complete urinalysis correlations:	Color Reagent strip blood reaction

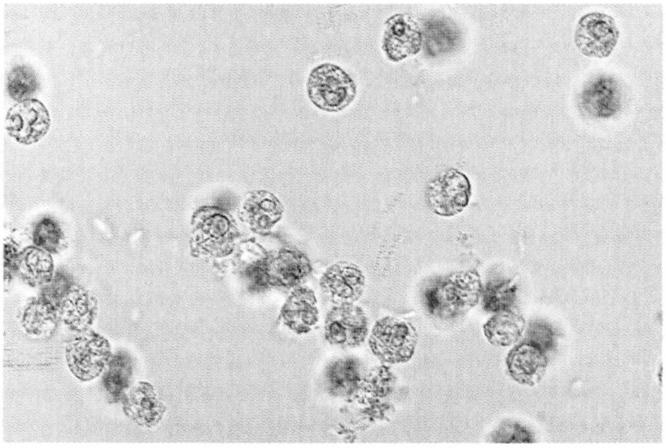

FIGURE 6–12 WBCs. Notice the multilobed nucleoli (×400).

The predominant WBC found in the urine sediment is the neutrophil. Neutrophils are much easier to identify than RBCs because they contain granules and multilobed nuclei (Figures 6–12 and 6–13). However, they are still identified using high power microscopy and are also reported as the average number seen in 10 hpfs. Neutrophils lyse rapidly in dilute alkaline urine and begin to lose nuclear detail.

Neutrophils exposed to hypotonic urine absorb water and swell. Brownian movement of the granules within these larger cells produces a sparkling appearance, and they are referred to as "glitter cells." When stained with Sternheimer-Malbin stain, these large cells stain light blue as opposed to the violet color usually seen with neutrophils. They are of no pathologic significance.

Eosinophils

The presence of urinary eosinophils is primarily associated with drug-induced interstitial nephritis; however, small numbers of eosinophils may be seen with urinary tract infection (UTI) and renal transplant rejection. Evaluation of a concentrated, stained urine sediment is required for performing a urinary eosinophil test. Sediment may be concentrated by routine centrifugation alone or with cytocentrifugation. The preferred eosinophil stain is Hansel's; however, Wright's stain can also be used. The percentage of eosinophils in 100 to 500 cells is determined. Eosinophils are not normally seen in the urine; therefore, the finding of more than 1 percent eosinophils is considered significant.[4]

Mononuclear Cells

Lymphocytes, monocytes, macrophages, and histiocytes may be present in small numbers and are usually not identified in the wet preparation urine microscopic. Because lymphocytes are the smallest WBCs, they may resemble RBCs. They may be seen in increased numbers in the early stages of renal transplant rejection. Monocytes, macrophages, and histiocytes are large cells and may appear vacuolated or contain inclusions. Specimens containing an increased amount of mononuclear cells that cannot be identified as epithelial cells should be referred for cytodiagnostic urine testing.

The primary concern in the identification of WBCs is the differentiation of mononuclear cells and disintegrating neutrophils from renal tubular epithelial (**RTE**) cells. RTE cells are usually larger than WBCs and more polyhedral in shape with an eccentrically located nucleus. WBCs in the process of ameboid motion may be difficult to distinguish from epithelial cells because of their irregular shape. Supravital staining or the addition of acetic acid can be used to enhance nuclear detail (Figure 6–14), if necessary.

Usually, fewer than five leukocytes per hpf are found in normal urine; however, higher numbers may be present in female urine.[21] Although leukocytes, like RBCs, may enter the urine through glomerular or capillary trauma, they are also capable of ameboid migration through the tissues to sites of infection or inflammation. An increase in urinary WBCs is called pyuria and indicates the presence of an infection or inflammation in the genitourinary system. Bacterial infections, including pyelonephritis, cystitis, prostatitis, and urethritis, are frequent causes of pyuria. However, pyuria is also present in nonbacterial disorders, such as glomerulonephritis, lupus erythematosus, interstitial nephritis, and tumors. Reporting the presence of bacteria in specimens containing leukocytes is important.

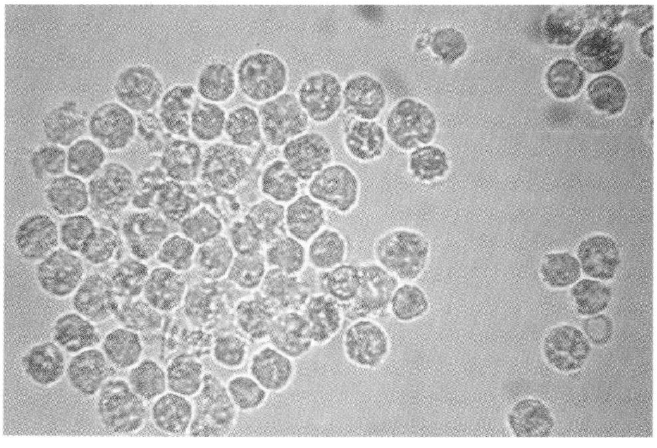

FIGURE 6–13 WBC clump (×400).

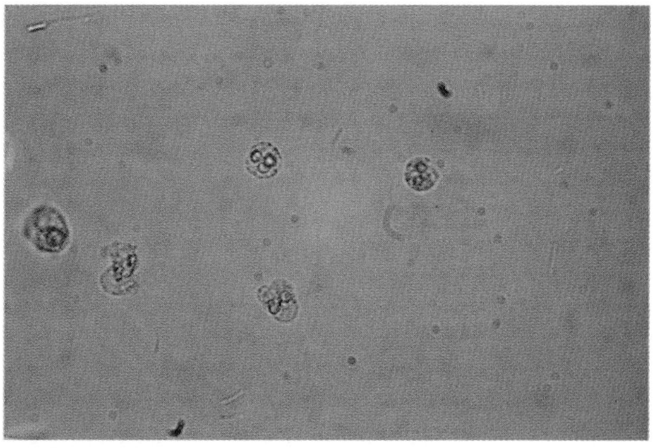

FIGURE 6–14 WBCs with acetic acid nuclear enhancement (×400).

Summary of Microscopic WBCs

Appearance:	Larger than red blood cells Granulated, multilobed neutrophils Glitter cells in hypotonic urine Mononuclear cells with abundant cytoplasm
Sources of identification error:	Renal tubular epithelial cells
Reporting:	Average number per 10 high-power fields
Complete urinalysis correlations:	Leukocyte esterase Nitrite Specific gravity pH

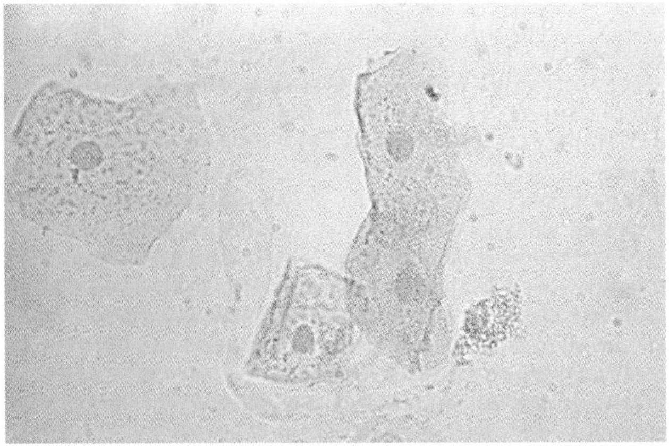

FIGURE 6–16 KOVA-stained squamous epithelial cells (×400).

EPITHELIAL CELLS

It is not unusual to find epithelial cells in the urine, because they are derived from the linings of the genitourinary system. Unless they are present in large numbers or in abnormal forms, they represent normal sloughing of old cells. Three types of epithelial cells are seen in urine: squamous, transitional (urothelial), and renal tubular (Figure 6–15). They are classified according to their site of origin within the genitourinary system.

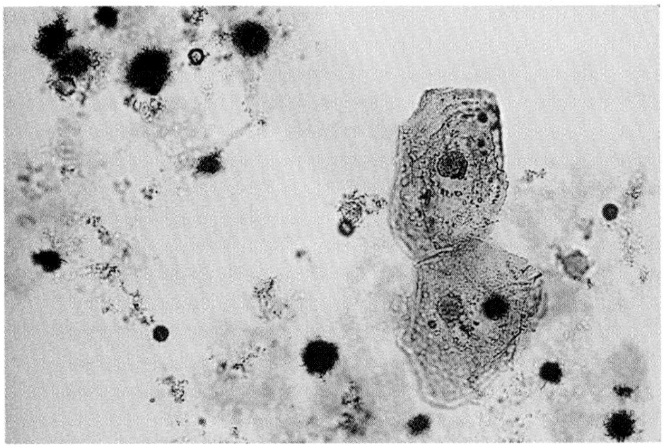

FIGURE 6–17 Phenazopyridine-stained sediment showing squamous epithelial cells and phenazopyridine crystals formed following refrigeration (×400).

Squamous Epithelial Cells

Squamous cells are the largest cells found in the urine sediment. They contain abundant, irregular cytoplasm and a prominent nucleus about the size of a RBC (Figures 6–16 and 6–17). They are often the first structures observed when the sediment is examined under low-power magnification. Usually at least a few squamous epithelial cells are present in the sediment and can serve as a good reference for focusing of the microscope (Figure 6–18). After examination of the appropriate number of fields, squamous ep-

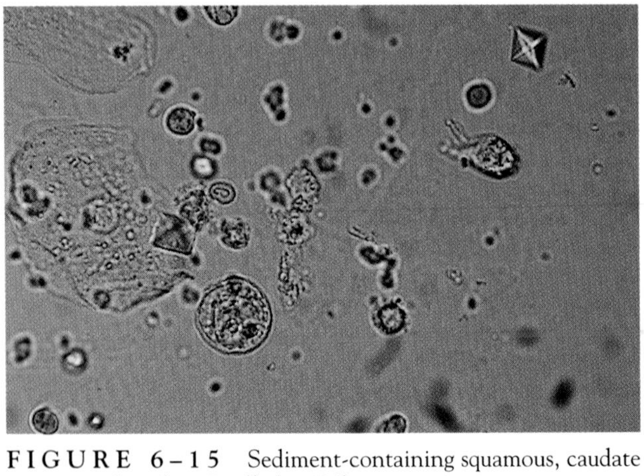

FIGURE 6–15 Sediment-containing squamous, caudate transitional, and RTE cells (×400).

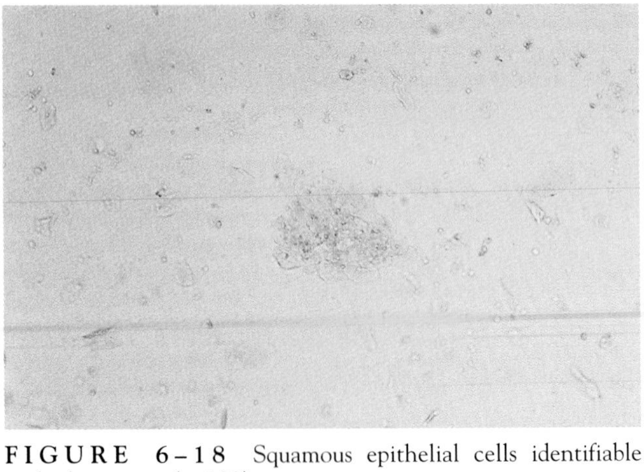

FIGURE 6–18 Squamous epithelial cells identifiable under low power (×100).

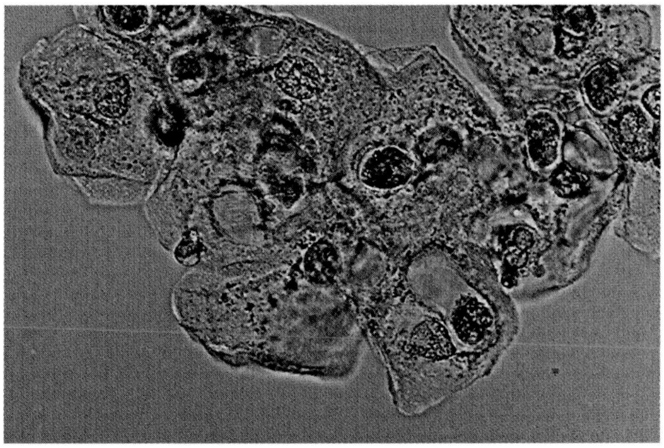

FIGURE 6–19 Clump of squamous epithelial cells (×400).

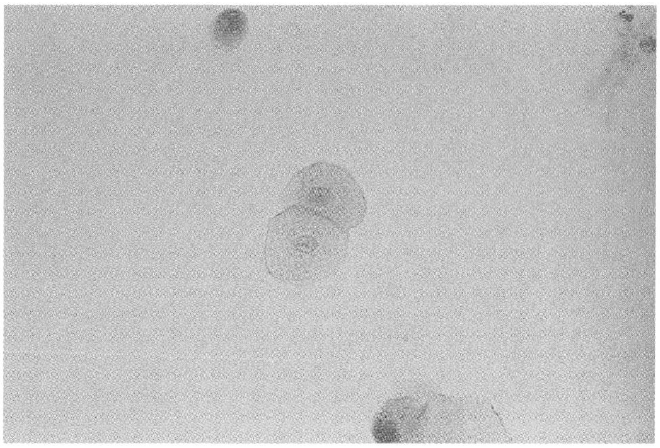

FIGURE 6–20 KOVA-stained spherical transitional epithelial cells (×400).

ithelial cells are commonly reported in terms of rare, few, moderate, or many. They are reported in terms of low-power or high-power magnification based on laboratory protocol.

Difficulty identifying squamous cells is rare. However, they may occasionally appear folded, possibly resembling a cast, and will begin to disintegrate in urine that is not fresh. In sediments containing large amounts of squamous cells, it may be more difficult to enumerate smaller pathologic elements, such as RBCs and WBCs, and they should be carefully examined (Figure 6–19).

Squamous epithelial cells originate from the linings of the vagina and female urethra and the lower portion of the male urethra. They represent normal cellular sloughing and have no pathologic significance. Increased amounts are more frequently seen in urine from female patients. Specimens collected using the midstream clean-catch technique will contain less squamous cell contamination.

A variation of the squamous epithelial cell is the clue cell, which does have pathologic significance. Clue cells are indicative of vaginal infection by the bacterium *Gardnerella vaginalis*. They appear as squamous epithelial cells covered with the *Gardnerella* coccobacillus. To be considered a clue cell, the bacteria should cover most of the cell surface and extend beyond the edges of the cell. This gives the cell a granular, irregular appearance. Routine testing for clue cells is performed by examining a vaginal wet preparation for the presence of the characteristic cells. However, small numbers of clue cells may be present in the urinary sediment. Microscopists should remain alert for their presence as urinalysis may be the first test performed on the patient.

Transitional Epithelial (Urothelial) Cells

Transitional epithelial cells are smaller than squamous cells and appear in several forms, including spherical, polyhedral, and caudate (Figures 6–20 and 6–21). These differences are caused by the ability of transitional epithelial cells to absorb large amounts of water. Cells in direct contact with the urine absorb water, becoming spherical in form and much larger than the polyhedral and caudate cells. All forms have distinct, centrally located nuclei. Transitional cells are identified and enumerated using high-power magnification. Like squamous cells they are usually reported as rare, few, moderate, or many following laboratory protocol.

Spherical forms of transitional epithelial cells are sometimes difficult to distinguish from RTE cells. The presence of a centrally located rather than eccentrically placed nucleus and supravital staining can aid in the differentiation.

Transitional epithelial cells originate from the lining of the renal pelvis, calyces, ureters, and bladder and upper portion of the male urethra. They are usually present in small numbers in normal urine, representing normal cellular sloughing. Increased numbers of transitional cells seen singly, in pairs, or in clumps (**syncytia**) are present following invasive urologic procedures such as catheterization and are of no clinical significance (Figure 6–22). An increase in transitional cells exhibiting abnormal morphology such as vacuoles and irregular nuclei may be indicative of malignancy or viral infection. The specimen should be referred for cytologic examination.

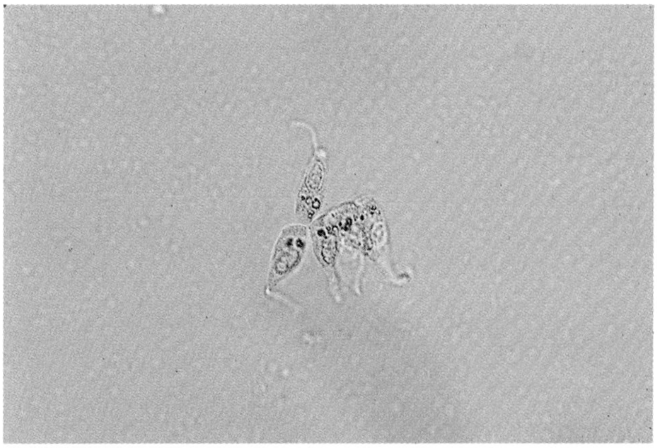

FIGURE 6–21 Caudate-shaped transitional epithelial cells (×400).

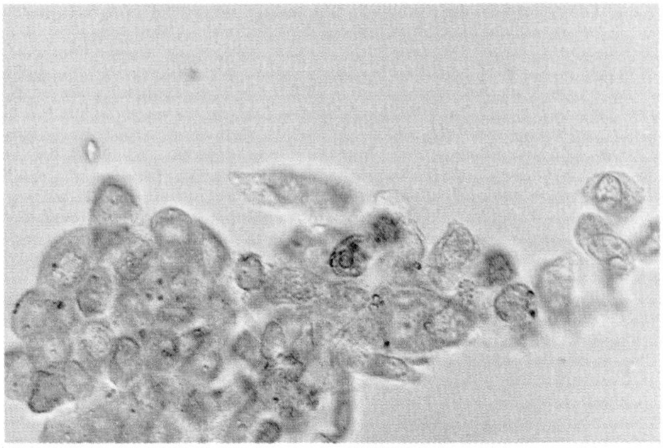

FIGURE 6-22 Syncytia of transitional epithelial cells (×400).

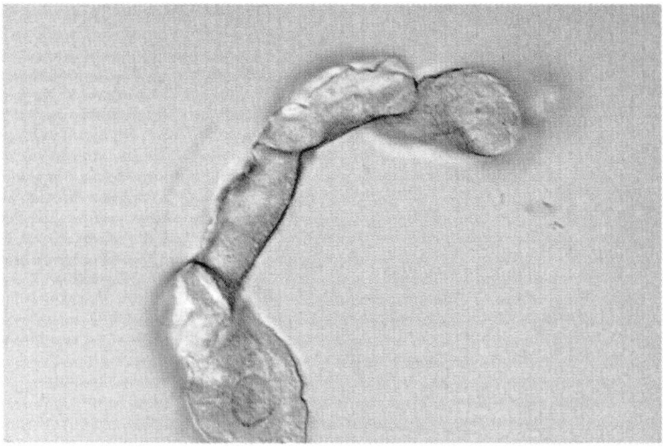

FIGURE 6-24 RTE cells, columnar-shaped (×400).

Renal Tubular Epithelial Cells

RTE cells vary in size and shape depending on the area of the renal tubules from which they originate. The size of the cells tends to diminish as they progress from large, rectangular cells in the proximal convoluted tubule to cuboidal or columnar cells not much larger than WBCs in the collecting duct (Figures 6–23 and 6–24).

Cells from the proximal convoluted tubule have coarsely granulated cytoplasm, whereas those from the collecting ducts are very finely granulated. Cells from the collecting ducts that occur in groups of three or more are called renal fragments and may indicate more severe renal damage (Figure 6–25). RTE cells must be identified and enumerated using high-power magnification. Depending on laboratory protocol, they may be reported as rare, few, moderate, or many or as the actual number per high-power field. Classification of RTE cells as to site of origin is not considered a part of the routine sediment analysis and often requires special staining techniques. The presence of more than two RTE cells per high-power field indicates tubular injury, and specimens should be referred for cytologic urine testing.[27] The presence of a small, dense, eccentrically placed nucleus is characteristic of RTE cells (Figure 6–26).

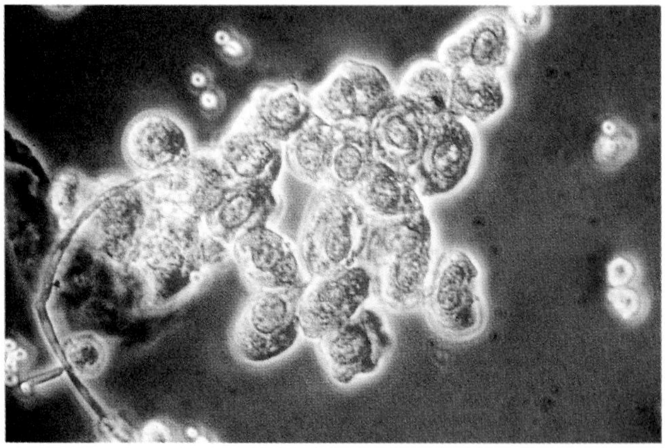

FIGURE 6-25 Clump of RTE cells under phase microscopy (×400).

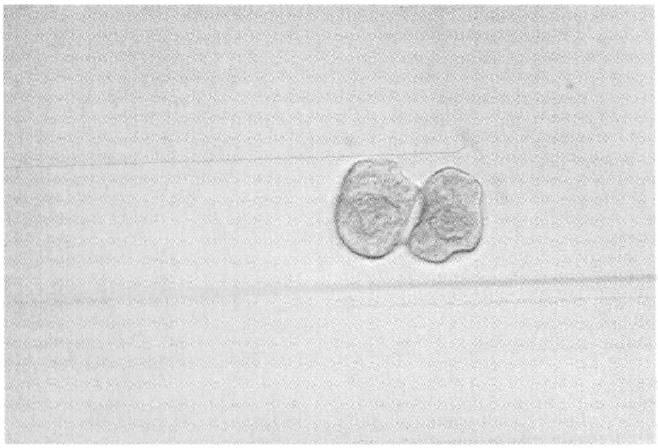

FIGURE 6-23 RTE cells, cuboidal-shaped (×400).

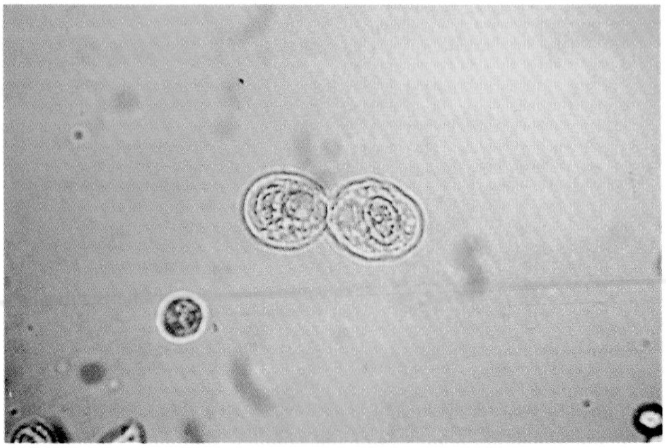

FIGURE 6-26 RTE cells. Notice the eccentrically placed nucleii (×400).

Identification of RTE cells can be difficult because of the variations in their appearance. The rectangular, coarsely granular cells from the proximal convoluted tubule often resemble granular casts. Structures should be carefully examined for the presence of a nucleus, which would not be present in a cast. The eccentric nuclear placement in RTE cells can aid in distinguishing them from similarly appearing polyhedral and spherical forms of transitional epithelial cells. Unfortunately, because RTE cells are often present as a result of tissue destruction (necrosis), the nucleus is not easily visible in the unstained sediment. Another aid in identification is that RTE cells are not totally round; therefore, the presence of a flattened edge helps in their differentiation from spherical transitional cells and mononuclear leukocytes.

RTE cells are the most clinically significant of the epithelial cells. The presence of increased amounts is indicative of necrosis of the renal tubules with the possibility of affecting overall renal function.

Conditions producing tubular necrosis include exposure to heavy metals, drug-induced toxicity, hemoglobin and myoglobin toxicity, viral infections (hepatitis B), pyelonephritis, allergic reactions, malignant infiltrations, and acute allogenic transplant rejection. RTE cells may also be seen as secondary effects of glomerular disorders.

Because one of the functions of RTE cells is reabsorption of the glomerular filtrate, it is not unusual for them to contain substances from the filtrate. RTE cells absorb bilirubin present in the filtrate as the result of liver damage, such as occurs with viral hepatitis, and will appear a deep yellow color. As discussed in Chapter 5, hemoglobin present in the filtrate is absorbed by the RTE cells and converted to hemosiderin. Therefore, following episodes of hemoglobinuria (transfusion reactions, paroxysmal nocturnal hemoglobinuria, etc.), the RTE cells may contain the characteristic yellow-brown hemosiderin granules. The granules may also be seen free-floating in the sediment. Confirmation of the presence of hemosiderin is performed by staining the sediment with Prussian blue. The iron-containing hemosiderin granules will stain blue.

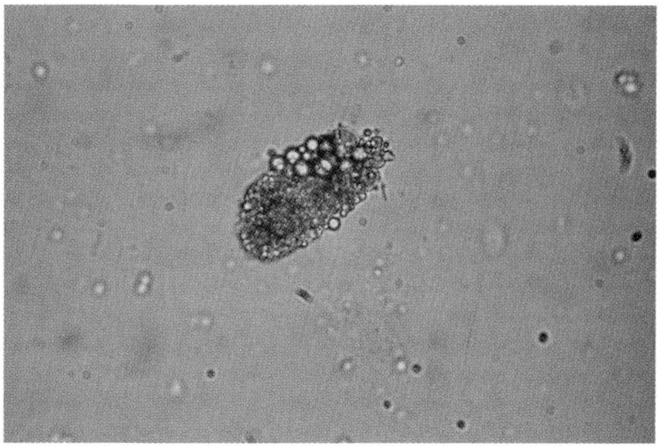

FIGURE 6–28 Columnar-shaped oval fat body (×400).

Oval Fat Bodies

RTE cells will absorb lipids that are present in the glomerular filtrate. They will then appear highly refractile, and the nucleus may be more difficult to observe. These lipid-containing RTE cells are called oval fat bodies (Figures 6–27 and 6–28). They are usually seen in conjunction with free-floating fat droplets.

Identification of oval fat bodies is confirmed by staining the sediment with Sudan III or Oil Red O fat stains and examining the sediment using polarized microscopy. The droplets are composed of triglycerides, neutral fats, and cholesterol. Fat stains will stain triglycerides and neutral fats, producing orange-red droplets (Figure 6–29). Examination of the sediment using polarized light results in the appearance of characteristic Maltese cross formations in droplets containing cholesterol (Figure 6–30). Sediments negative for fat after staining should still be checked using polarized light in case only cholesterol is present. Likewise, staining should be performed on sediments negative under polarized light. Oval fat bodies are reported as the average number per hpf.

Free-floating fat droplets will also stain or polarize depending on their composition. They may be observed floating on the top of the specimen. Care should be taken not to

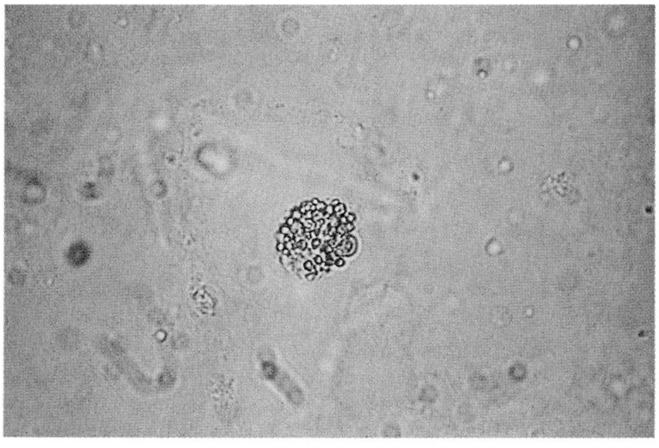

FIGURE 6–27 Oval fat body (×400).

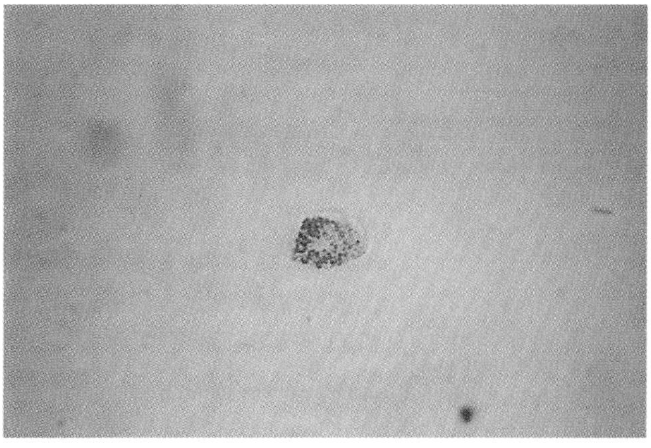

FIGURE 6–29 Sudan III-stained oval fat body (×400).

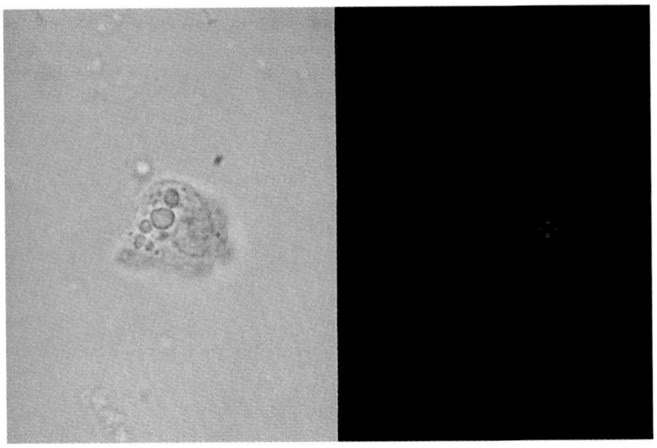

FIGURE 6–30 Oval fat body under bright-field and polarized microscopy. Notice the Maltese cross formation (×400).

confuse the droplets with starch and crystal particles that also polarize. Specimen contamination by vaginal preparations and lubricants used in specimen collection must be considered when only free-floating fat droplets are present.

Lipiduria is most frequently associated with damage to the glomerulus caused by the nephrotic syndrome (see Chap. 8). It is also seen with severe tubular necrosis, diabetes mellitus, and in trauma cases that cause release of bone marrow fat from the long bones. In lipid-storage diseases, large fat-laden histiocytes may also be present. They can be differentiated from oval fat bodies by their large size.

In cases of acute tubular necrosis, RTE cells containing large, nonlipid-filled vacuoles may be seen along with normal renal tubular cells and oval fat bodies. Referred to as "bubble cells," they appear to represent injured cells in which the endoplasmic reticulum has dilated prior to cell death.[8]

Summary of Epithelial Cells

Squamous Cells	
Appearance:	Largest cells in the sediment with abundant, irregular cytoplasm and prominent nucleii
Sources of error:	Rarely encountered, folded cells may resemble casts
Reporting:	Rare, few, moderate, or many per low-power field
Complete urinalysis correlations:	Clarity
Transitional Cells	
Appearance:	Spherical, polyhedral, or caudate with centrally located nucleus
Sources of error:	Spherical forms resemble RTE cells
Reporting:	Rare, few, moderate, or many per high-power field
Complete urinalysis correlations:	Clarity Blood, if malignancy associated
RTE Cells	
Appearance:	Rectangular, polyhedral, cuboidal, or columnar with an eccentric nucleus, possibly bilirubin stained or hemosiderin laden
Sources of error:	Spherical transitional cells Granular casts
Reporting:	Average number per 10 high-power fields
Complete urinalysis correlations:	Leukocyte esterase and nitrite (pyelonephritis) Color Clarity Protein Bilirubin (hepatitis) Blood
Oval Fat Bodies	
Appearance:	Highly refractile RTE cells
Sources of error:	Confirm with fat stains and polarized microscopy
Reporting:	Average number per high-power field
Complete urinalysis correlations:	Clarity Blood Protein Free fat droplets/fatty casts

BACTERIA

Bacteria are not normally present in urine. However, unless specimens are collected under sterile conditions (catheterization), a few bacteria are usually present as a result of vaginal, urethral, external genitalia, or collection-container contamination. These contaminant bacteria will multiply rapidly in specimens that remain at room temperature for extended periods, but are of no clinical significance. They may produce a positive nitrite test result and also frequently result in a pH above 8, indicating an unacceptable specimen.

Bacteria may be present in the form of cocci (spherical) or bacilli (rods). Owing to their small size, they must be observed and reported using high-power magnification. They are reported as few, moderate, or many per high-power field. To be considered significant for UTI, bacteria should be accompanied by WBCs. Many laboratories report bacteria only when observed in fresh specimens in conjunction with WBCs (Figure 6–31). The presence of motile organisms in a drop of fresh urine collected under sterile conditions correlates well with a positive urine culture. Observing bacteria for motility also is useful in differentiating them from similarly appearing amorphous phosphates and urates. Use of phase microscopy aids in the visualization of bacteria.

The presence of bacteria can be indicative of either lower or upper UTI. Specimens containing increased bacteria and leukocytes are routinely followed up with a specimen for quantitative urine culture. The bacteria most frequently associated with UTI are the Enterobacteriaceae (referred to as gram-negative rods); however, the cocci-shaped *Staphylococcus* and *Enterococcus* are also capable of causing UTI. The actual bacteria producing an UTI cannot be identified with the microscopic examination.

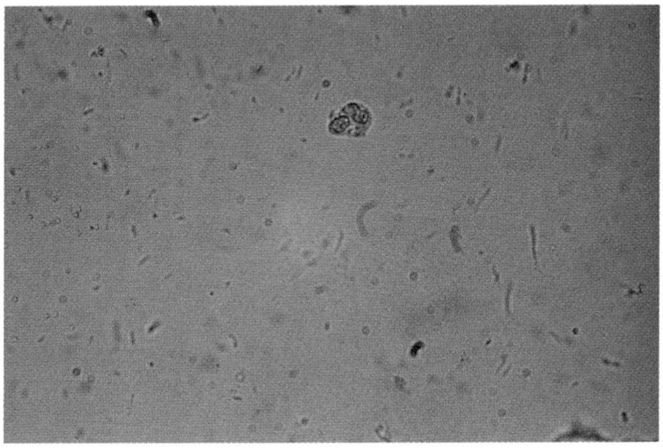

FIGURE 6–31 KOVA-stained bacteria and WBC (×400).

YEAST

Yeast cells appear in the urine as small, refractile oval structures that may or may not contain a bud. In severe infections, they may appear as branched, mycelial forms (Figure 6–32). Yeast cells are reported as rare, few, moderate, or many per hpf.

Differentiation between yeast cells and RBCs can sometimes be difficult. Careful observation for budding yeast cells should be helpful, as shown in Figure 6–8.

Yeast cells, primarily *Candida albicans*, are seen in the urine of diabetic, immunocompromised patients and in women with vaginal moniliasis. The acidic, glucose-containing urine of patients with diabetes provides an ideal medium for the growth of yeast. Like bacteria, a small amount of yeast entering a specimen as a contaminant will multiply rapidly if the specimen is not examined while fresh. A true yeast infection should be accompanied by the presence of WBCs.

PARASITES

The most frequent parasite encountered in the urine is *Trichomonas vaginalis*. The *Trichomonas* trophozoite is a pear-shaped flagellate with an undulating membrane. It is easily identified in wet preparations and the urine sediment by its rapid darting movement in the microscopic field. *Trichomonas* is usually reported as rare, few, moderate, or many per hpf.

When not moving, *Trichomonas* is more difficult to identify and may resemble a WBC, transitional, or RTE cell. Use of phase microscopy may enhance visualization of the flagella or undulating membrane.

T. vaginalis is a sexually transmitted pathogen associated primarily with vaginal inflammation. Infection of the male urethra and prostate is asymptomatic.

The ova of the bladder parasite *Schistosoma haematobium* will appear in the urine. However, this parasite is seldom seen in the United States.

Fecal contamination of a urine specimen also can result in the presence of ova from intestinal parasites in the urine sediment. The most common contaminant is ova from the pinworm *Enterobius vermicularis*.

SPERMATOZOA

Spermatozoa are easily identified in the urine sediment by their oval, slightly tapered heads and long, flagella-like tails (Figure 6–33). Urine is toxic to spermatozoa; therefore, they rarely exhibit the motility observed when examining a semen specimen.

Spermatozoa are occasionally found in the urine of both men and women following sexual intercourse, masturbation, or nocturnal emission. They are rarely of clinical significance except in cases of infertility or retrograde ejaculation in which sperm is expelled into the bladder instead of the urethra. A positive reagent strip test for protein may be seen when increased amounts of semen are present.

Laboratory protocols vary with regard to reporting or not reporting the presence of spermatozoa in a urine specimen. Laboratories not reporting its presence cite the lack of clinical significance and possible legal consequences. Laboratories supporting the reporting of spermatozoa cite the possible clinical significance and the minimal possibility of legal consequences.[2]

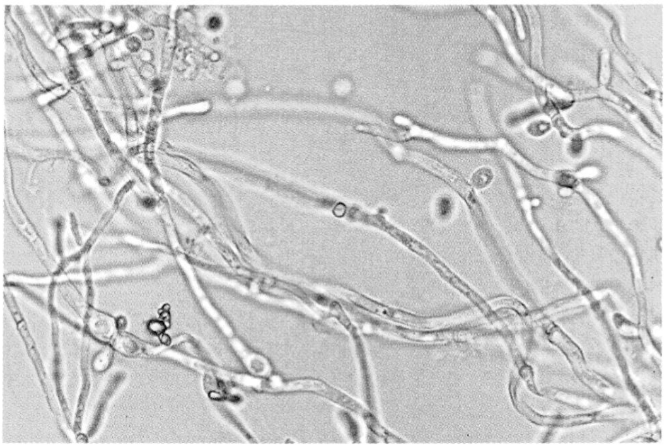

FIGURE 6–32 Yeast showing mycelial forms (×400).

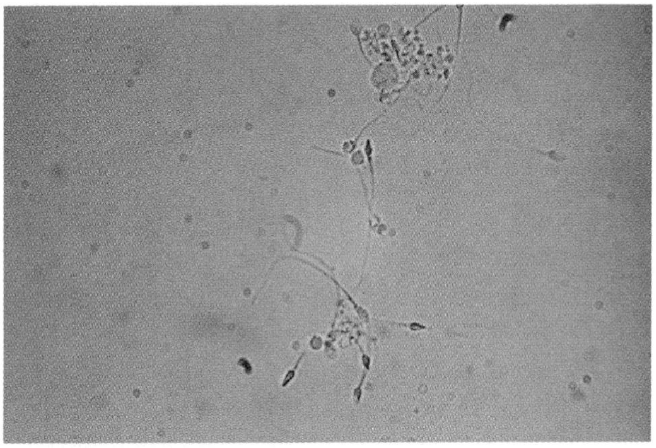

FIGURE 6–33 Spermatozoa (×400).

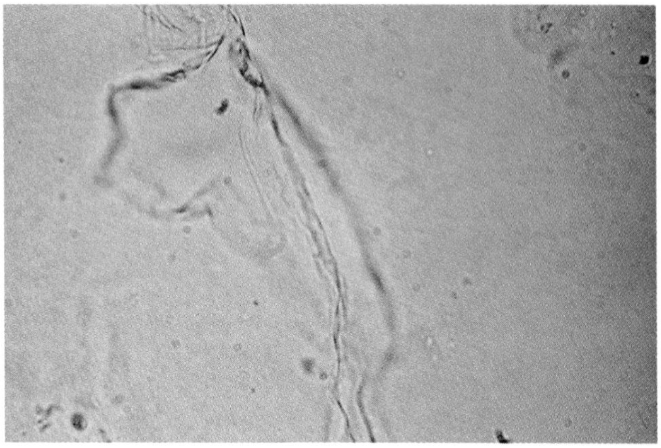

FIGURE 6–34 Mucous threads (×400).

MUCUS

Mucus is a protein material produced by the glands and epithelial cells of the lower genitourinary tract and the RTE cells. Immunologic analysis has shown that ***Tamm-Horsfall protein*** is a major constituent of mucus.

Mucus appears microscopically as thread-like structures with a low refractive index (Figure 6–34). Subdued light is required when using bright-field microscopy. Care must be taken not to confuse clumps of mucus with hyaline casts. The differentiation can usually be made by observing the irregular appearance of the mucous threads. Mucous threads are reported as rare, few, moderate, or many per lpf.

Mucus is more frequently present in female urine specimens. It has no clinical significance when present in either female or male urine.

Summary of Miscellaneous Structures

Bacteria	
Appearance:	Small spherical and rod-shaped structures
Sources of error:	Amorphous phosphates and urates
Reporting:	Few, moderate, or many per high-power field, the presence of WBCs may be required
Complete urinalysis correlations:	pH Nitrite LE WBCs
Yeast	
Appearance:	Small, oval, refractile structures with buds and/or mycelia
Sources of error:	RBCs
Reporting:	Rare, few, moderate, or many per high-power field, the presence of WBCs may be required
Complete urinalysis correlations:	Glucose LE WBCs
Trichomonas	
Appearance:	Pear-shaped, motile, flagellated
Sources of error:	WBCs, renal tubular epithelial cells
Reporting:	Rare, few, moderate, or many per high-power field
Complete urinalysis correlations:	LE WBCs
Spermatozoa	
Appearance:	Tapered oval head with long, thin tail
Sources of error:	None
Reporting:	Present, based on laboratory protocol
Complete urinalysis correlations:	Protein
Mucus	
Appearance:	Single or clumped threads with a low refractive index
Sources of error:	Hyaline casts
Reporting:	Rare, few, moderate, or many per low-power field
Complete urinalysis correlations:	None

CASTS

Casts are the only elements found in the urinary sediment that are unique to the kidney. They are formed within the lumens of the distal convoluted tubules and collecting ducts, providing a microscopic view of conditions within the nephron. Their shape is representative of the tubular lumen, with parallel sides and somewhat rounded ends, and they may contain additional elements present in the filtrate.

Examination of the sediment for the detection of casts is performed using lower power magnification. When the glass cover-slip method is used, low-power scanning should be performed along the edges of the cover slip. Observation under subdued light is essential, because the cast matrix has a low refractive index. Similar to many other sediment constituents, the cast matrix dissolves quickly in dilute, alkaline urine. Once detected, casts must be further identified as to composition using high-power magnification. They are reported as the average number per 10 lpfs.

Cast Composition and Formation

The major constituent of casts is Tamm-Horsfall protein, a glycoprotein excreted by the RTE cells of the distal convoluted tubules and upper collecting ducts. Other proteins present in the urinary filtrate such as albumin and immunoglobulins are also incorporated into the cast matrix. Under normal conditions, Tamm-Horsfall protein is excreted at a relatively constant rate. The rate of excretion appears to increase under conditions of stress and exercise, which may account for the transient appearance of hyaline casts when these conditions are present. The protein gels more readily under conditions of urine-flow stasis, acidity, and the presence of sodium and calcium. The extent of protein glycosylation is also important.[17] Tamm-Horsfall protein is found in both normal and abnormal urine and, as discussed previously, is a major constituent of mucus. It is not detected by reagent strip protein methods. Therefore, the increased urinary protein frequently associated with the presence of casts is caused by underlying renal conditions.

Scanning electron microscope studies have provided a step-by-step analysis of the formation of the Tamm-Horsfall protein matrix:[9]

1. Aggregation of Tamm-Horsfall protein into individual protein fibrils attached to the RTE cells
2. Interweaving of protein fibrils to form a loose fibrillar network (urinary constituents may become enmeshed in the network at this time)
3. Further protein fibril interweaving to form a solid structure
4. Possible attachment of urinary constituents to the solid matrix
5. Detachment of protein fibrils from the epithelial cells
6. Excretion of the cast

As the cast forms, urinary flow within the tubule decreases as the lumen becomes blocked. The accompanying dehydration of the protein fibrils and internal tension may account for the wrinkled and convoluted appearance of older hyaline casts.[18] The width of the cast depends on the size of the tubule in which it is formed. Broad casts may result from tubular distention or, in the case of extreme urine stasis, from formation in the collecting ducts. Formation of casts at the junction of the ascending loop of Henle and the distal convoluted tubule may produce structures with a tapered end. These have been referred to as cylindroids, but they have the same significance as casts. In fact, the presence of urinary casts is termed ***cylindruria***. The appearance of a cast is also influenced by the materials present in the filtrate at the time of its formation and the length of time it remains in the tubule. Any elements present in the tubular filtrate, including cells, bacteria, granules, pigments, and crystals, may become embedded in or attached to the cast matrix. The types of casts found in the sediment represent different clinical conditions and will be discussed separately in this section.

Hyaline Casts

The most frequently seen cast is the hyaline type, which consists almost entirely of Tamm-Horsfall protein. The presence of zero to two hyaline casts per lpf is considered normal, as is the finding of increased numbers following strenuous exercise, dehydration, heat exposure, and emotional stress.[11] Pathologically, hyaline casts are increased in acute glomerulonephritis, pyelonephritis, chronic renal disease, and congestive heart failure.[3]

Hyaline casts appear colorless in unstained sediments and have a refractive index similar to that of urine; thus, they can easily be overlooked if specimens are not examined under subdued light (Figure 6–35). Sternheimer-Malbin stain produces a pink color in hyaline casts. Increased visualization can be obtained by phase microscopy (Figures 6–36 and 6–37).

FIGURE 6–35 Hyaline cast and amorphous urate pseudocast (×400).

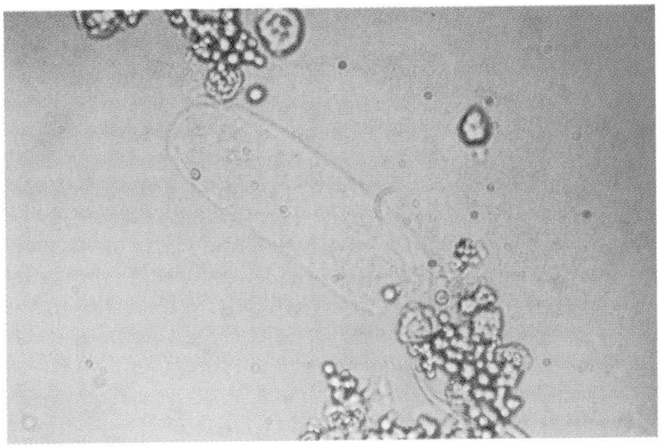

FIGURE 6–36 Hyaline cast (×400).

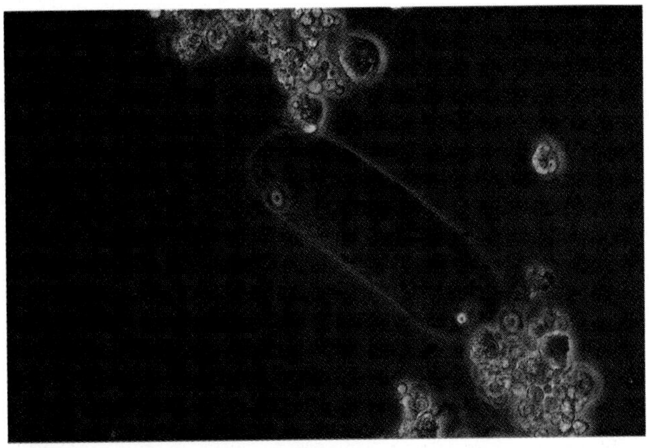

FIGURE 6–37 Hyaline cast under phase microscopy (×400).

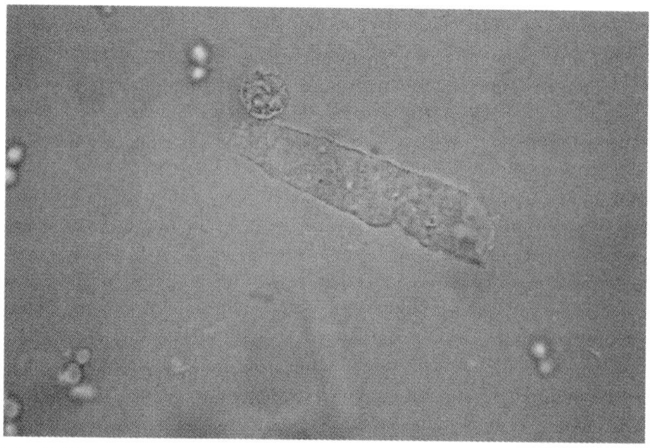

FIGURE 6–38 Convoluted hyaline cast (×400).

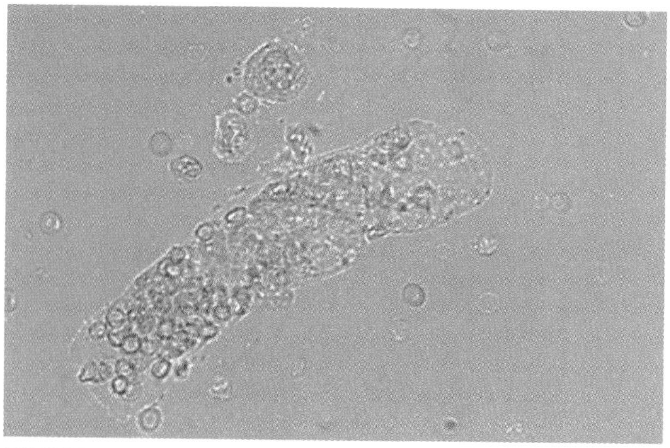

FIGURE 6–40 RBC cast. Notice the presence of hypochromic and dysmorphic free RBCs (×400).

The morphology of hyaline casts is varied, consisting of normal parallel sides and rounded ends, cylindroid forms, and wrinkled or convoluted shapes that indicate aging of the cast matrix (Figure 6–38). The presence of an occasional adhering cell or granule may also be observed (Figure 6–39) but does not change the cast classification.

Red Blood Cell Casts

Whereas the finding of RBCs in the urine indicates bleeding from an area within the genitourinary tract, the presence of RBC casts is much more specific, showing bleeding within the nephron. RBC casts are primarily associated with damage to the glomerulus (glomerulonephritis) that allows passage of the cells through the glomerular membrane; however, any damage to the nephron capillary structure can cause their formation. RBC casts associated with glomerular damage are usually associated with proteinuria and dysmorphic erythrocytes. RBC casts have also been observed in healthy individuals following participation in strenuous contact sports.[11]

RBC casts are easily detected under low power by their orange-red color. They are more fragile than other casts and may exist as fragments or have a more irregular shape as the result of tightly packed cells adhering to the protein matrix (Figures 6–40 and 6–41). Examination under high-power magnification should concentrate on determining that a cast matrix is present, thereby differentiating the structure from a clump of RBCs. Because of the serious diagnostic implications of RBC casts, the actual presence of RBCs must also be verified to prevent the inaccurate reporting of nonexistent RBC casts. It is highly improbable that RBC casts will be present in the absence of free-standing RBCs and a positive reagent strip test for blood.

As a RBC cast ages, cell lysis begins and the cast will develop a more homogenous appearance, but will retain the characteristic orange-red color from the released hemoglobin (Figure 6–42). These casts may be distinguished as blood casts, indicating greater stasis of urine flow. However, because all casts containing blood have the same clinical significance, this is not considered necessary.[3] Both types of casts are reported as the number of RBC casts per lpf.

In the presence of massive hemoglobinuria or myoglobinuria, homogenous orange-red or red-brown casts may be observed. Granular, dirty, brown casts representing hemo-

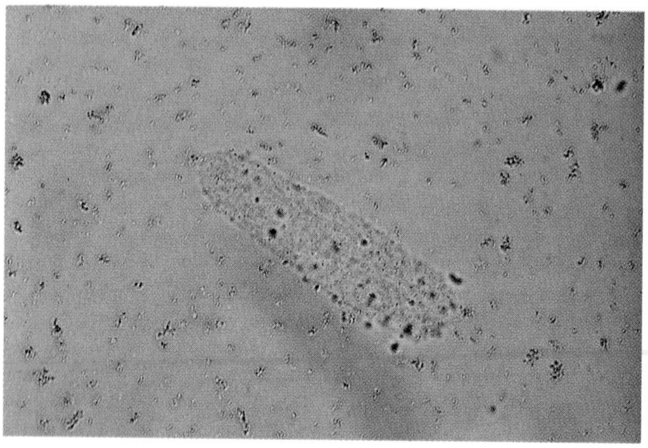

FIGURE 6–39 Hyaline cast containing occasional granules (×400).

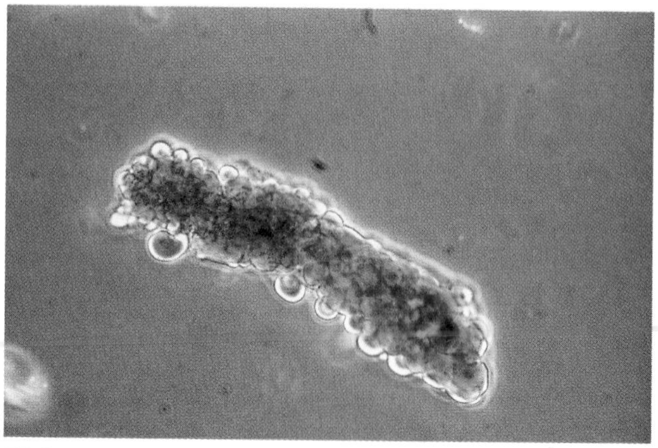

FIGURE 6–41 KOVA-stained RBC cast under phase microscopy (×400).

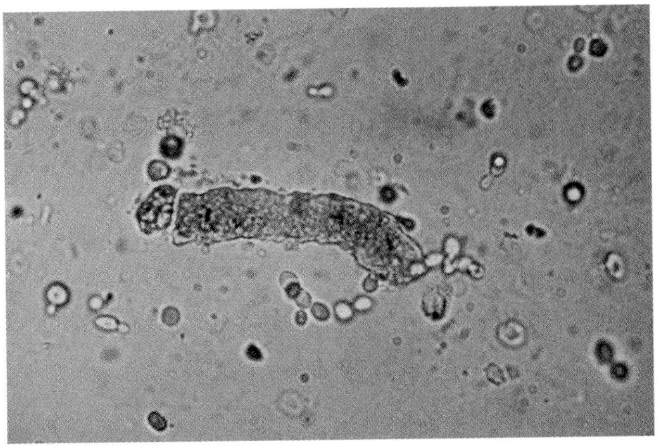

FIGURE 6–42 Cast containing hemoglobin pigment. A comparison of RBCs and yeast also can be made (×400).

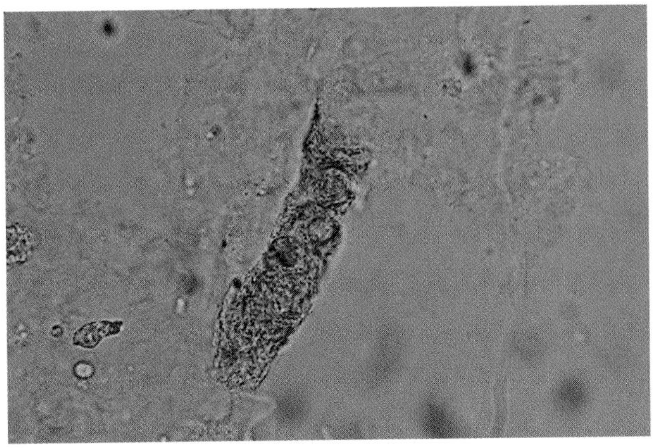

FIGURE 6–44 Disintegrating WBC cast (×400).

globin degradation products such as methemoglobin also may be present (Figure 6–43). They are associated with the acute tubular necrosis often caused by the toxic effects of massive hemoglobinuria that can lead to renal failure. These dirty, brown casts must be present in conjunction with other pathologic findings such as RTE cells and a positive reagent strip test for blood.

White Blood Cell Casts

The appearance of WBC casts in the urine signifies infection or inflammation within the nephron. They are most frequently associated with pyelonephritis and are a primary marker for distinguishing pyelonephritis (upper UTI) from lower UTIs. However, they will also be present in nonbacterial inflammations such as acute interstitial nephritis and may accompany RBC casts in glomerulonephritis.

WBC casts are visible under low-power magnification but must be positively identified using high power. Most frequently WBC casts are composed of neutrophils; therefore, they may appear granular, and, unless disintegration has occurred, multilobed nuclei will be present (Figure 6–44). Supravital staining may be necessary to demonstrate the characteristic nuclei (Figure 6–45). It is particularly helpful for differentiating WBC casts from RTE casts. Observation of free WBCs in the sediment is also essential. Bacteria will be present in cases of pyelonephritis, but will not be present with acute interstitial nephritis; however, eosinophil casts may be present in appropriately stained specimens.

Casts tightly packed with WBCs may have irregular borders. These structures should be carefully examined to determine that a cast matrix is present. WBCs frequently form clumps, and these do not have the same significance as casts.

Bacterial Casts

Bacterial casts containing bacilli both within and bound to the protein matrix are seen in pyelonephritis.[19] They may be pure bacterial casts or mixed with WBCs.

Identification of bacterial casts can be difficult, because packed casts will resemble granular casts. Their presence should be considered when WBC casts and many free WBCs and bacteria are seen in the sediment. Confirmation of bacterial casts is best made by performing a Gram stain on the dried or cytocentrifuged sediment.

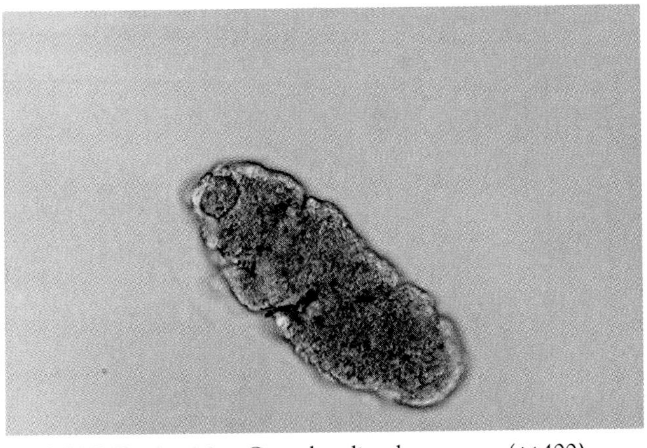

FIGURE 6–43 Granular, dirty brown cast (×400).

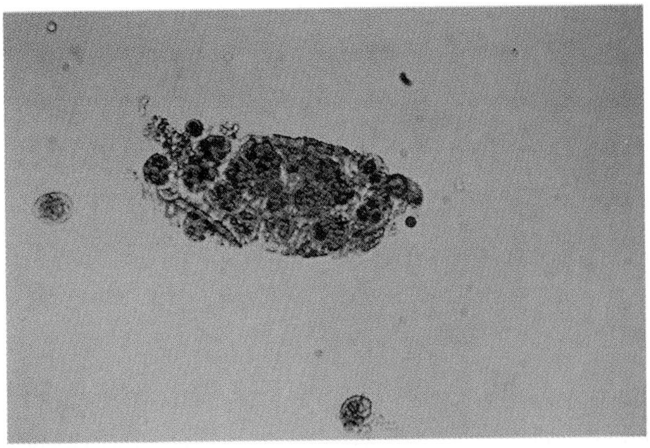

FIGURE 6–45 KOVA-stained WBC cast (×400).

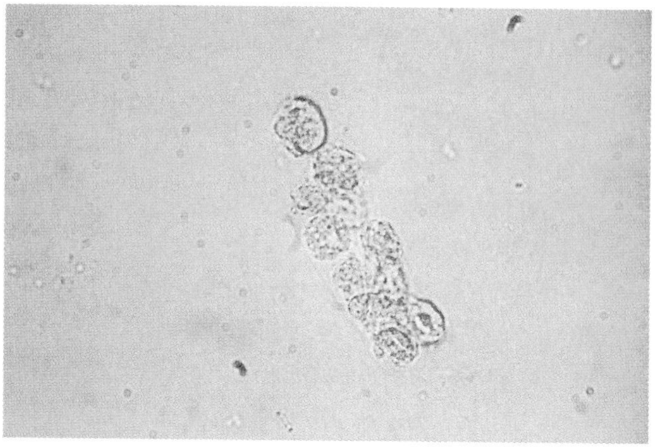

FIGURE 6–46 RTE cell cast (×400).

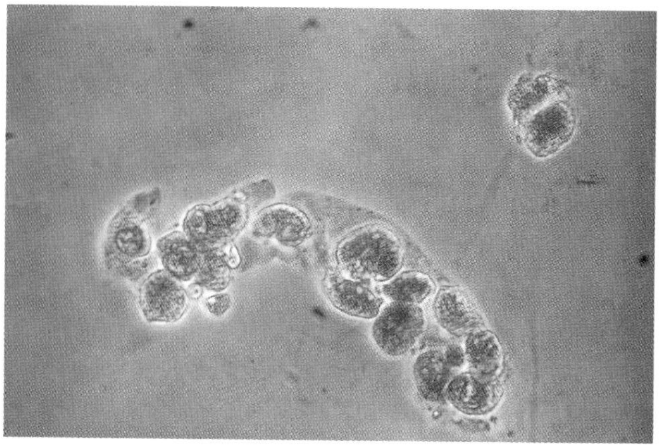

FIGURE 6–48 KOVA-stained RTE cell cast under phase microscopy (×400).

Epithelial Cell Casts

Casts containing RTE cells represent the presence of advanced tubular destruction, producing urinary stasis along with disruption of the tubular linings. Similarly to RTE cells, they are associated with heavy metal and chemical or drug-induced toxicity, viral infections, and allograft rejection. They will also accompany WBC casts in cases of pyelonephritis.

As discussed previously, the fibrils of Tamm-Horsfall protein that make up the cast matrix remain attached to the RTE cells that produce them; therefore, the observation of an occasional tubular cell attached to a hyaline cast can be expected. When tubular damage is present, some cells may be incorporated into the cast matrix, but the majority will be very noticeably attached to the cast surface.

Owing to the formation of casts in the distal convoluted tubule, the cells visible on the cast matrix are the smaller, cuboidal, and columnar-shaped cells (Figure 6–46). They may be difficult to differentiate from WBCs, particularly if degeneration has occurred. Staining and the use of phase microscopy can be helpful to enhance the nuclear detail needed for identification (Figures 6–47 and 6–48). Fragments of epithelial tissue also may be attached to the cast matix. Bilirubin-stained RTE cells will be seen in cases of hepatitis.

Fatty Casts

Fatty casts are seen in conjunction with oval fat bodies and free fat droplets in disorders causing lipiduria. They are most frequently associated with the nephrotic syndrome, but are also seen in toxic tubular necrosis, diabetes mellitus, and crush injuries.

Fatty casts are highly refractile under bright-field microscopy. The cast matrix may contain few or many fat droplets, and intact oval fat bodies may be attached to the matrix (Figures 6–49 through 6–51). Confirmation of fatty casts is performed using polarized microscopy and Sudan III or Oil Red O fat stains. As discussed previously, cholesterol will demonstrate characteristic Maltese cross formations under polarized light, and triglycerides and neutral fats will stain orange with fat stains. Fats do not stain with Sternheimer-Malbin stains.

Mixed Cellular Casts

Considering that a variety of cells may be present in the urinary filtrate, observing casts containing multiple cell types is not uncommon. Mixed cellular casts most frequently encountered include RBC and WBC casts in

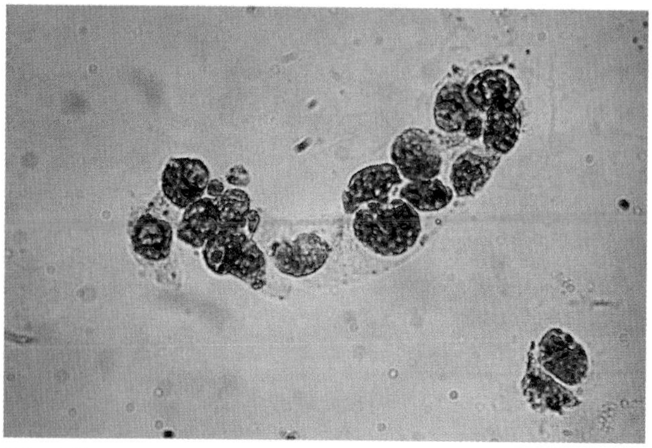

FIGURE 6–47 KOVA-stained RTE cell cast (×400).

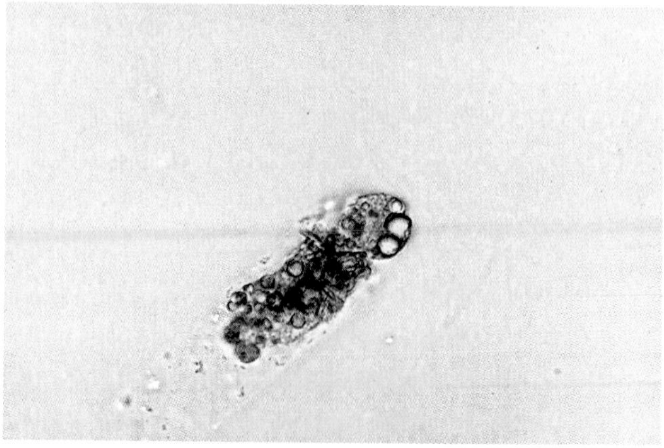

FIGURE 6–49 Fatty cast showing adherence of fat droplets to cast matrix (×400).

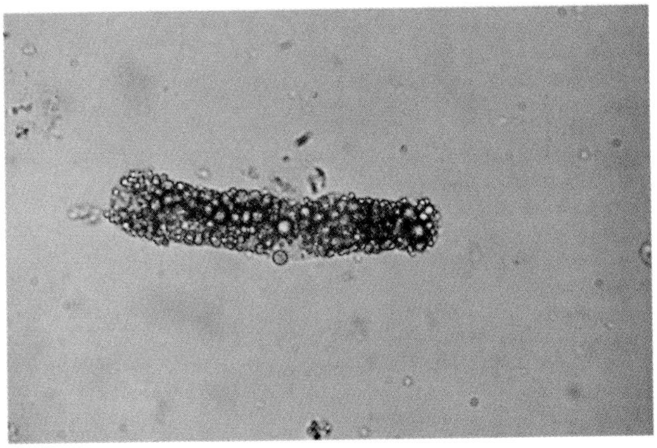

FIGURE 6–50 Fatty cast (×400).

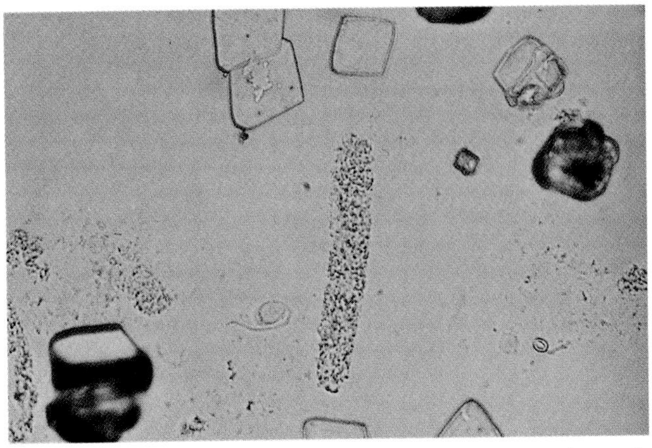

FIGURE 6–52 Finely granular cast and uric acid crystals (×400).

glomerulonephritis and WBC and RTE cell casts, or WBC and bacterial casts in pyelonephritis.

The presence of mixed elements in a cast may make identification more difficult. Staining or phase microscopy will aid in the identification. When mixed casts are present, there should also be homogenous casts of at least one of the cell types, and they will be the primary diagnostic marker. For example, in glomerulonephritis, the predominant casts will be RBC, and in pyelonephritis, the predominant casts will be WBC. Bacteria are often incorporated into WBC casts and provide little additional diagnostic significance. Laboratory protocol should be followed in the reporting of mixed cellular casts.

Granular Casts

Coarsely and finely granular casts are frequently seen in the urinary sediment and may be of pathologic or nonpathologic significance. It is not considered necessary to distinguish between coarsely and finely granular casts.

The origin of the granules in nonpathologic conditions appears to be from the lysosomes excreted by RTE cells during normal metabolism.[10] It is not unusual to see hyaline casts containing one or two of these granules. Increased cellular metabolism occurring during periods of strenuous exercise accounts for the transient increase of granular casts that accompany the increased hyaline casts (Figure 6–52).[11] In disease states, granules may represent disintegration of cellular casts and tubule cells or protein aggregates filtered by the glomerulus (Figures 6–53 and 6–54). Scanning electron microscope studies have confirmed that granular casts seen in conjunction with WBC casts contain WBC granules of varying sizes.[20] Urinary stasis allowing the casts to remain in the tubules must be present for granules to result from disintegration of cellular casts.

Granular casts occurring as a result of cellular disintegration may contain an occasional recognizable cell. Granular casts are easily visualized under low-power microscopy. However, final identification should be performed using high power to determine the presence of a cast matrix.

Artifacts, such as clumps of small crystals and fecal debris, may occur in shapes resembling casts and must be differentiated. As mentioned previously, columnar RTE cells may also resemble granular casts, and staining for nuclear detail may be required.

When granular casts remain in the tubules for extended periods, the granules further disintegrate, and the cast matrix develops a waxy appearance. The structure becomes

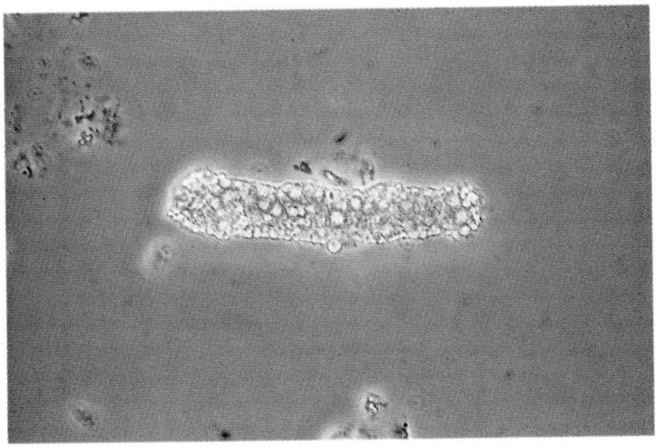

FIGURE 6–51 Fatty cast under phase microscopy (×400).

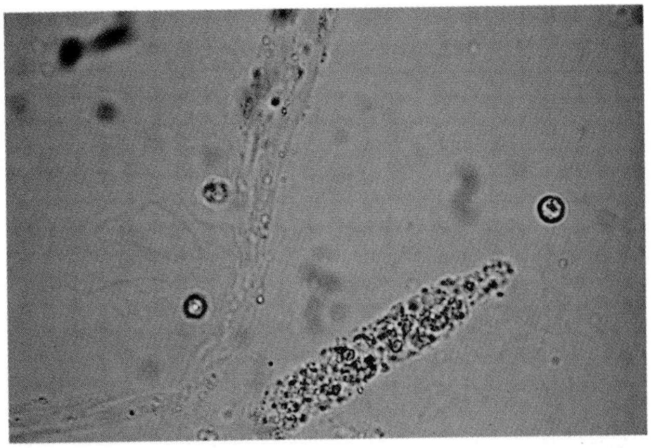

FIGURE 6–53 Granular disintegrating cellular cast (×400).

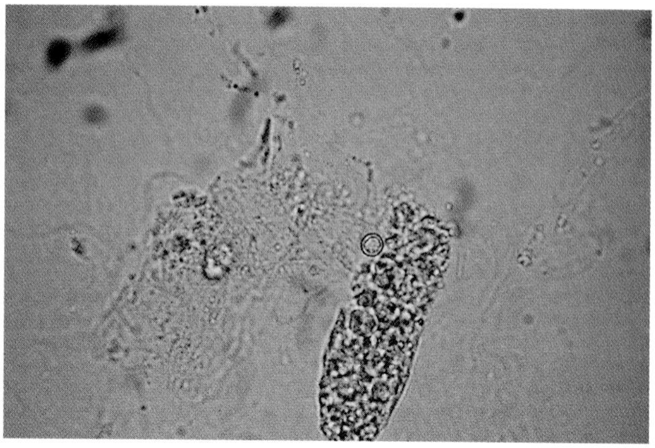

FIGURE 6–54 Coarsely granular cast, squamous epithelial cell, and mucus (×400).

more rigid, the ends of the casts may appear jagged or broken, and the diameter becomes broader (Figure 6–55).

Waxy Casts

Waxy casts are representative of extreme urine stasis, indicating chronic renal failure. They are usually seen in conjunction with other types of casts associated with the condition that has caused the renal failure.

The brittle, highly refractive cast matrix from which these casts derive their name is believed to be caused by degeneration of the hyaline cast matrix and any cellular elements or granules contained in the matrix.[10,18]

Waxy casts are more easily visualized than hyaline casts because of their higher refractive index. As a result of the brittle consistency of the cast matrix, they often appear fragmented with jagged ends and have notches in their sides (Figures 6–56 through 6–58). With supravital stains, waxy casts stain a homogenous, dark pink.

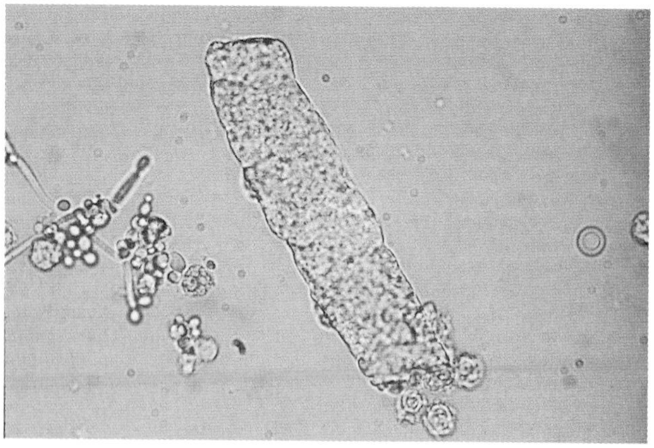

FIGURE 6–55 Granular cast degenerating into waxy cast (×400).

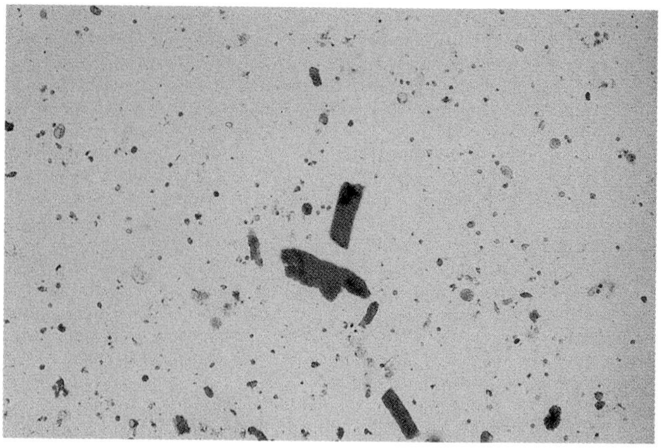

FIGURE 6–56 KOVA-stained waxy casts (×100).

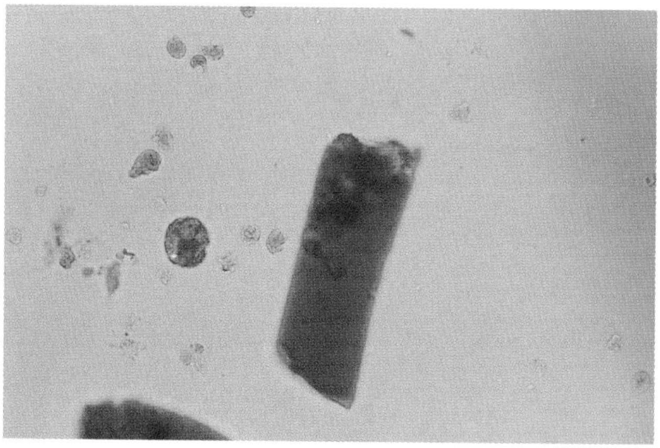

FIGURE 6–57 KOVA-stained waxy cast (×400).

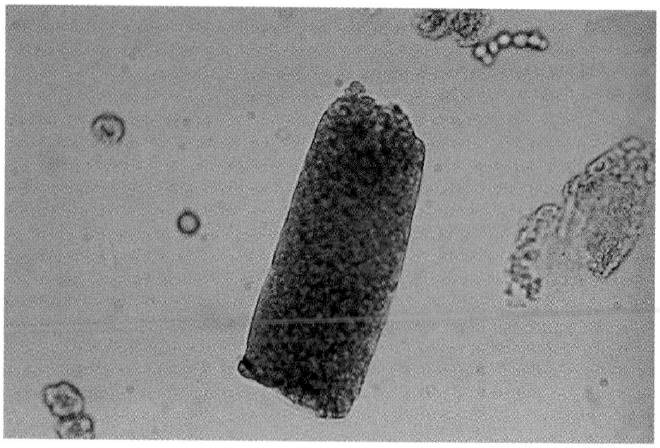

FIGURE 6–58 KOVA-stained broad waxy cast (×400).

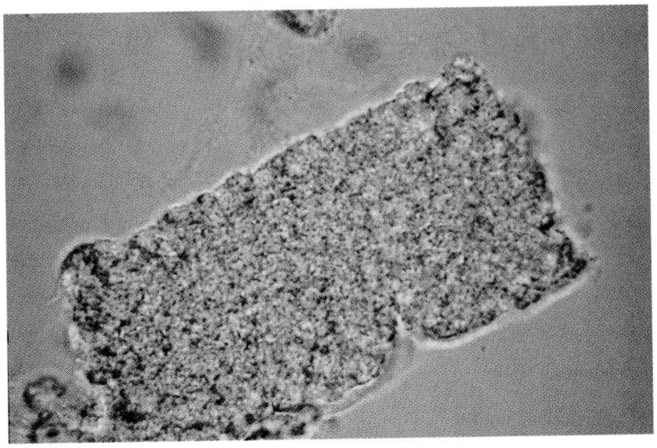

FIGURE 6–59 Broad granular cast becoming waxy (×400).

Broad Casts

Often referred to as *renal failure casts*, broad casts like waxy casts represent extreme urine stasis. As a mold of the distal convoluted tubules, the presence of broad casts indicates destruction (widening) of the tubular walls. Also, when the flow of urine to the larger collecting ducts becomes severely compromised, casts will form in this area and appear broad.

All types of casts may occur in the broad form. However, considering the accompanying urinary stasis, the most commonly seen broad casts are granular and waxy (Figure 6–59). Bile-stained broad, waxy casts are seen as the result of the tubular necrosis caused by viral hepatitis (Figure 6–60).

URINARY CRYSTALS

Crystals frequently found in the urine are rarely of clinical significance. They may appear as true geometrically formed structures or as amorphous material. The primary reason for the identification of urinary crystals is to detect the presence of the relatively few abnormal types that may represent such disorders as liver disease, inborn errors of

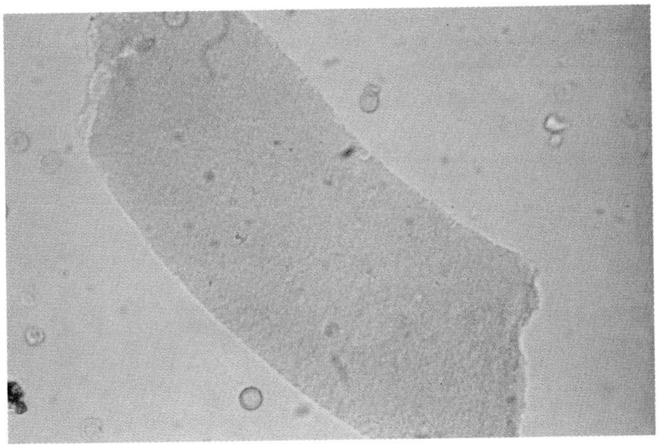

FIGURE 6–60 Broad bile-stained waxy cast (×400).

Summary of Urine Casts

Hyaline	
Appearance:	Colorless homogenous matrix
Sources of error:	Mucus, fibers, hair
Reporting:	Average number per low-power field
Complete urinalysis correlations:	Protein
Clinical significance:	Glomerulonephritis Pyelonephritis Chronic renal disease Congestive heart failure Stress and exercise
RBCs	
Appearance:	Orange-red color, cast matrix containing RBCs
Sources of error:	RBC clumps
Reporting:	Average number per low-power field
Complete urinalysis correlations:	RBCs Blood Protein
Clinical significance:	Glomerulonephritis Strenuous exercise
WBCs	
Appearance:	Cast matrix containing WBCs
Sources of error:	WBC clumps
Reporting:	Average number per low-power field
Complete urinalysis correlations:	WBCs Protein LE
Clinical significance:	Pyelonephritis Acute interstitial nephritis
Bacterial	
Appearance:	Bacilli bound to protein matrix
Sources of error:	Granular casts
Reporting:	Average number per low-power field
Complete urinalysis correlations:	WBC cast WBCs LE Nitrite Protein Bacteria
Clinical significance:	Pyelonephritis
Epithelial Cell	
Appearance:	RTE cells attached to protein matrix
Sources of error:	WBC cast
Reporting:	Average number per low-power field
Complete urinalysis correlations:	Protein RTE cells
Clinical significance:	Renal tubular damage

(Continued)

Summary of Urine Casts *(continued)*

Granular	
Appearance:	Coarse and fine granules, and protein aggregates in a protein matrix
Sources of error:	Clumps of small crystals Columnar RTE cells
Reporting:	Average number per low-power field
Complete urinalysis correlations:	Protein Cellular casts RBCs WBCs
Clinical significance:	Glomerulonephritis Pyelonephritis Stress and exercise
Waxy	
Appearance:	Highly refractile cast with jagged ends and notches
Sources of error:	Fibers and fecal material
Reporting:	Average number per low-power field
Complete urinalysis correlations:	Protein Cellular casts Granular casts WBCs RBCs
Clinical significance:	Stasis of urine flow Chronic renal failure
Fatty	
Appearance:	Fat droplets and oval fat bodies attached to protein matrix
Sources of error:	Fecal debris
Reporting:	Average number per low-power field
Complete urinalysis correlations:	Protein Free fat droplets Oval fat bodies
Clinical significance:	Nephrotic syndrome Toxic tubular necrosis Diabetes mellitus Crush injuries
Broad	
Appearance:	Wider than normal cast matrix
Sources of error:	Fecal material
Reporting:	Average number per low-power field
Complete urinalysis correlations:	Protein WBCs RBCs Granular casts Waxy casts
Clinical significance:	Extreme urine stasis Renal failure

metabolism, or renal damage caused by crystallization of **iatrogenic** compounds within the tubules. Crystals are usually reported as rare, few, moderate, or many per hpf. Abnormal crystals may be averaged and reported per lpf.

Crystal Formation

Crystals are formed by the precipitation of urine solutes, including inorganic salts, organic compounds, and medications (iatrogenic compounds). Precipitation is subject to changes in temperature, solute concentration, and pH, which affect solubility.

Solutes precipitate more readily at low temperatures. Therefore, the majority of crystal formation takes place in specimens that have remained at room temperature or been refrigerated prior to testing. Crystals are extremely abundant in refrigerated specimens and often present problems because they obscure clinically significant sediment constituents.

As the concentration of urinary solutes increases, their ability to remain in solution decreases resulting in crystal formation. The presence of crystals in freshly voided urine is most frequently associated with concentrated (high specific gravity) specimens.

A valuable aid in the identification of crystals is the pH of the specimen because this will determine the type of chemicals precipitated. In general, organic and iatrogenic compounds crystallize more easily in an acid pH, whereas inorganic salts are less soluble in neutral and alkaline solutions. An exception is calcium oxalate, which precipitates in both acid and neutral urine.

General Identification Techniques

The most commonly seen crystals have very characteristic shapes and colors; however, variations do occur and can present identification problems, particularly when they resemble abnormal crystals. As discussed previously, the first consideration when identifying crystals is the urine pH. In fact, crystals are routinely classified not only as normal and abnormal, but also as to their appearance in acidic or alkaline urine. All abnormal crystals are found in acid urine.

Additional aids in crystal identification include the use of polarized microscopy and solubility characteristics of the crystals. The geometric shape of a crystal determines its birefringence and, therefore, its ability to polarize light. Although the size of a particular crystal may vary (slower crystallization produces larger crystals), the basic structure remains the same. Therefore, polarization characteristics for a particular crystal are constant for identification purposes.

Just as changes in temperature and pH contribute to crystal formation, reversal of these changes can cause crystals to dissolve. These solubility characteristics can be used to aid in identification. Amorphous urates that frequently form in refrigerated specimens and obscure sediments may dissolve if the specimen is warmed. Amorphous phosphates require acetic acid to dissolve, and this is not practical, as formed elements, such as RBCs, will also be destroyed. When solubility characteristics are needed for identification, the sediment should be aliquoted to pre-

TABLE 6–6 **Major Characteristics of Normal Urinary Crystals[14]**

Crystal	pH	Color	Solubility	Appearance
Uric acid	Acid	Yellow-brown	Alkali soluble	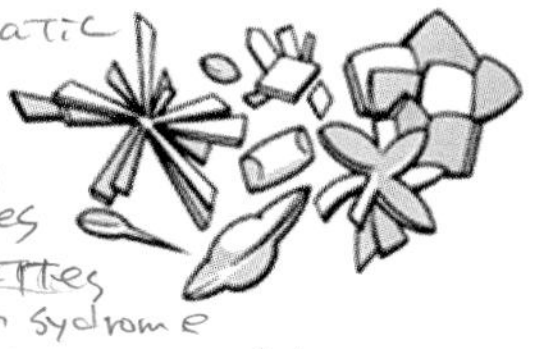
Amorphous urates	Acid	Brick dust or yellow brown	Alkali and heat	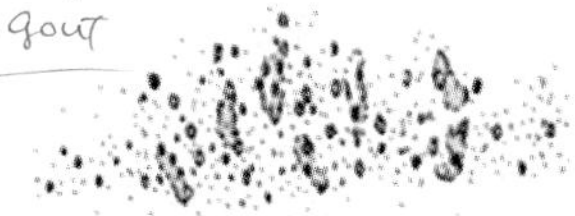
Calcium oxalate	Acid/neutral (alkaline)	Colorless (envelopes)	Dilute HCl	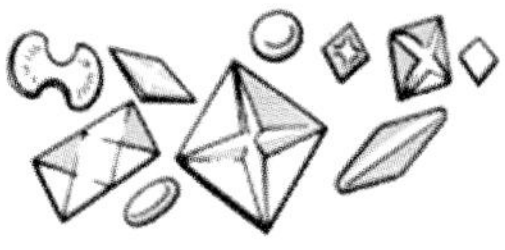
Amorphous phosphates	Alkaline Neutral	White–colorless	Dilute acetic acid	
Calcium phosphate	Alkaline Neutral	Colorless	Dilute acetic acid	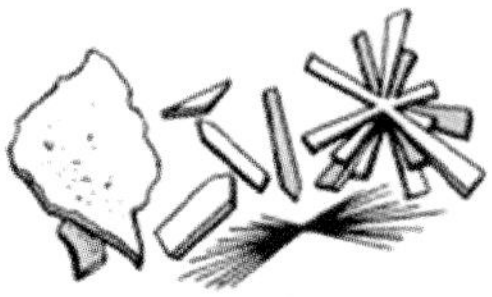
Triple phosphate	Alkaline	Colorless ("coffin lids")	Dilute acetic acid	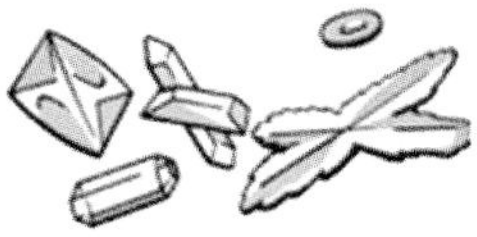
Ammonium biurate	Alkaline	Yellow-brown ("thorny apples")	Acetic acid with heat	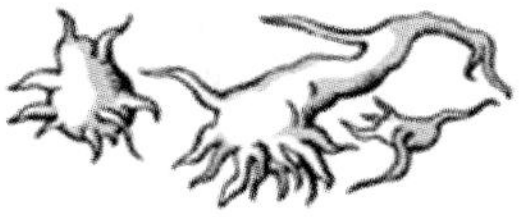
Calcium carbonate	Alkaline	Colorless (dumbbells)	Gas from acetic acid	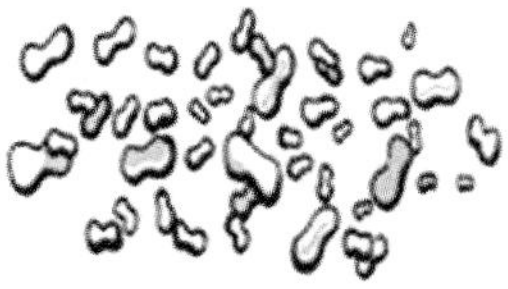

vent destruction of other elements. In Table 6–6, solubility characteristics for the most commonly encountered crystals are provided.

Normal Crystals Seen in Acidic Urine

The most common crystals seen in acidic urine are urates, consisting of amorphous urates, uric acid, acid urates, and sodium urates. Microscopically most urate crystals appear yellow to reddish-brown and are the only normal crystals found in acidic urine that appear colored.

Amorphous urates appear microscopically as yellow-brown granules (Figure 6–61). They may occur in clumps resembling granular casts. Amorphous urates are frequently encountered in specimens that have been refrigerated and produce a very characteristic pink sediment. Accumulation of the pigment, uroerythrin, on the surface of the granules is the cause of the pink color. Amorphous urates are found

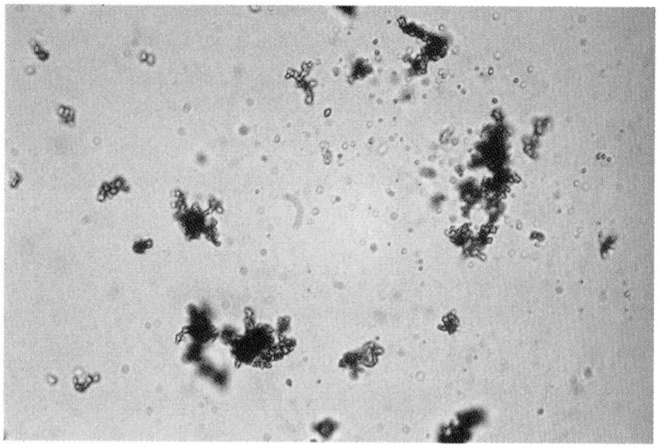

FIGURE 6–61 Amorphous urates (×400).

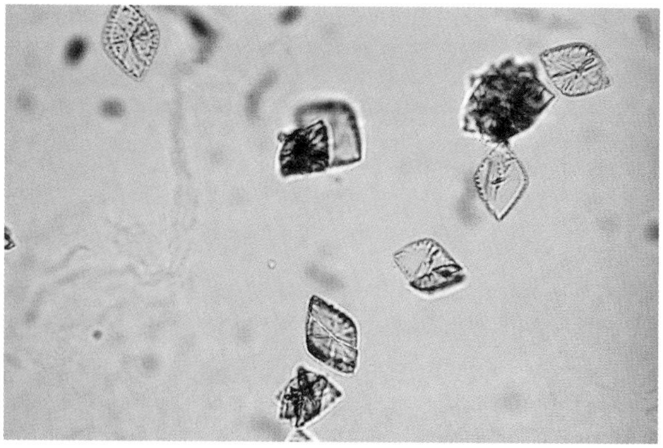

FIGURE 6–63 Uric acid crystals (×400).

in acidic urine with a pH greater than 5.5, whereas uric acid crystals can appear when the pH is lower.

Uric acid crystals are seen in a variety of shapes, including rhombic, four-sided flat plates (whetstones), wedges, and rosettes. They usually appear yellow-brown in color, but may be colorless and have a six-sided shape, similar to cystine crystals (Figures 6–62 and 6–63). Uric acid crystals are highly birefringent under polarized light, which aids in distinguishing them from cystine crystals (Figures 6–64 and 6–65). Increased amounts of uric acid crystals, particularly in fresh urine, are associated with increased levels of purines and nucleic acids and are seen in patients with leukemia who are receiving chemotherapy, Lesch-Nyhan syndrome (see Chap. 9), and, sometimes, with gout.

Acid urates and sodium urates are rarely encountered and, like amorphous urates, are seen in less acidic urine. They are frequently seen in conjunction with amorphous urates and have little clinical significance. Acid urates appear as larger granules and may have spicules similar to the ammonium biurate crystals seen in alkaline urine. Sodium urate crystals are needle-shaped and are seen in synovial fluid during episodes of gout but do appear in the urine.

Calcium oxalate crystals are frequently seen in acid urine, but they can be found in neutral urine and even

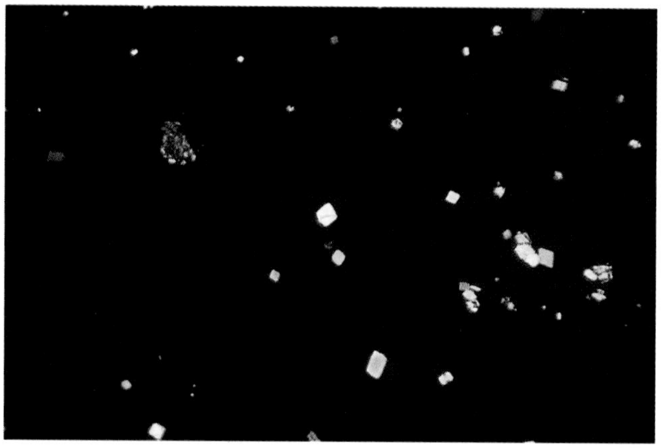

FIGURE 6–64 Uric acid crystals under polarized light (×100).

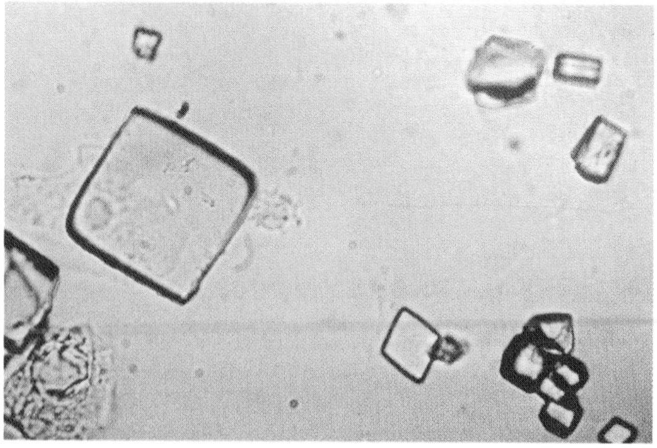

FIGURE 6–62 Uric acid crystals (×400).

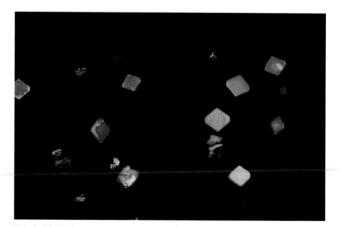

FIGURE 6–65 Uric acid crystals under polarized light (×400).

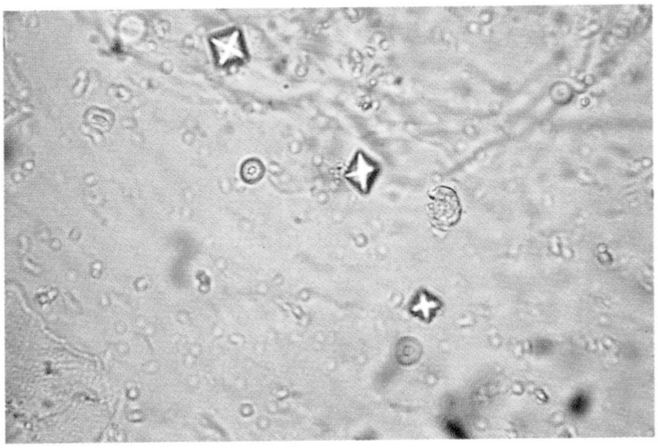

FIGURE 6–66 Classic dihydrate calcium oxalate crystals (×400).

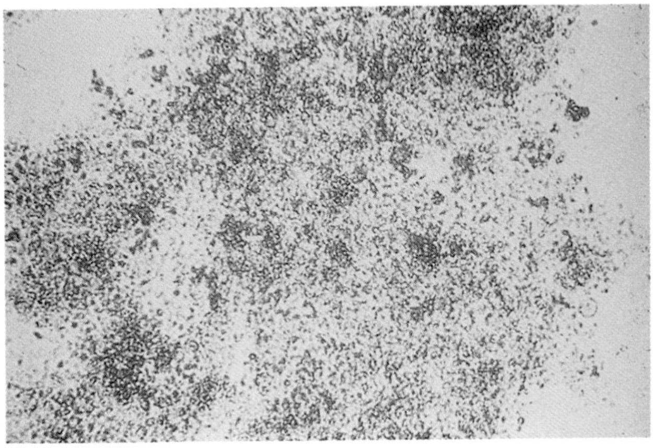

FIGURE 6–68 Amorphous phosphates (×400).

rarely in alkaline urine. The most common form of calcium oxalate crystals is the dihydrate that is easily recognized as a colorless, octahedral envelope or as two pyramids joined at their bases (Figure 6–66). Less characteristic and less frequently seen is the monohydrate form (Figure 6–67). Monohydrate calcium oxalate crystals are oval or dumbbell shaped. Both the dihydrate and monohydrate forms are birefringent under polarized light. This may be helpful to distinguish the monohydrate form from nonpolarizing RBCs. Calcium oxalate crystals are sometimes seen in clumps attached to mucous strands and may resemble casts.

The finding of clumps of calcium oxalate crystals in fresh urine may be related to the formation of renal calculi, because the majority of renal calculi are composed of calcium oxalate. They are also associated with foods high in oxalic acid, such as tomatoes and asparagus, and ascorbic acid, because oxalic acid is an end product of ascorbic acid metabolism. The primary pathologic significance of calcium oxalate crystals is the very noticeable presence of the monohydrate form in cases of ethylene glycol (antifreeze) poisoning. Massive amounts of crystals are frequently produced.

Normal Crystals Seen in Alkaline Urine

Phosphates represent the majority of the crystals seen in alkaline urine and include amorphous phosphate, triple phosphate, and calcium phosphate. Other normal crystals associated with alkaline urine are calcium carbonate and ammonium biurate. Amorphous phosphates are granular in appearance, similar to amorphous urates (Figure 6–68). When present in large quantities following specimen refrigeration, they cause a white precipitate that does not dissolve on warming. They can be differentiated from amorphous urates by the color of the sediment and the urine pH.

Triple phosphate (ammonium magnesium phosphate) crystals are commonly seen in alkaline urine. In their routine form, they are easily identified by their colorless, prism shape that resembles a "coffin lid" (Figures 6–69 and 6–70). As they disintegrate, the crystals may develop a feathery appearance. Triple phosphate crystals are birefringent under polarized light. They have no clinical significance; however, they are often seen in highly alkaline urine associated with the presence of urea-splitting bacteria (Figure 6–71).

Calcium phosphate crystals are not frequently encountered. They may appear as colorless, flat rectangular plates

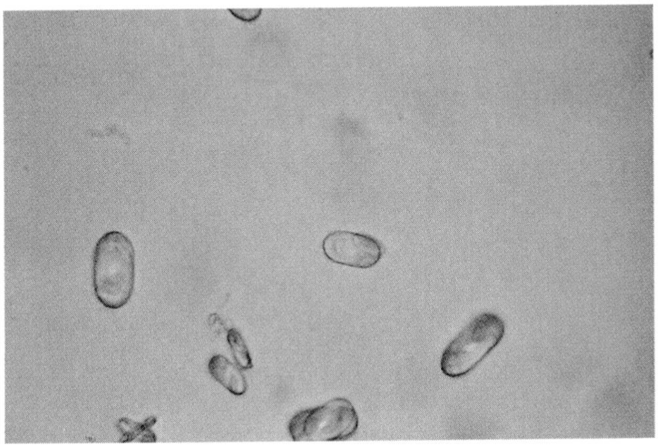

FIGURE 6–67 Monohydrate calcium oxalate crystals (×400).

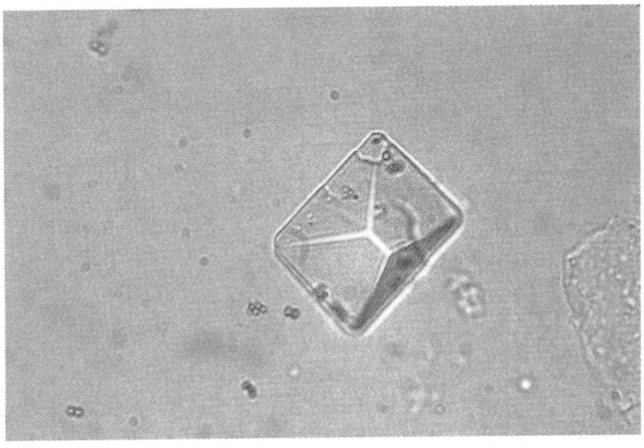

FIGURE 6–69 Triple phosphate crystal (×400).

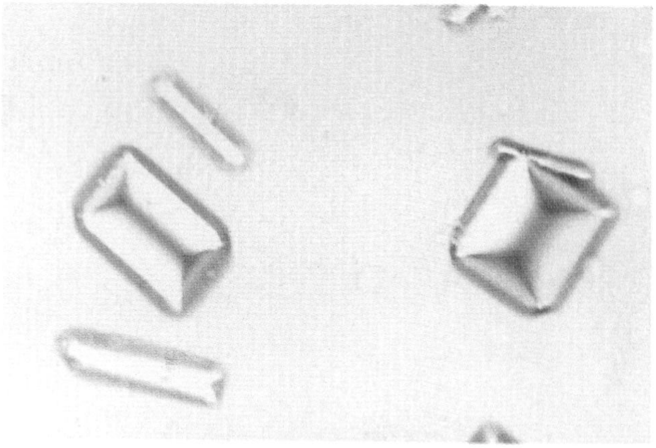

FIGURE 6-70 "Coffin lid" and other forms of triple phosphate crystals (×400).

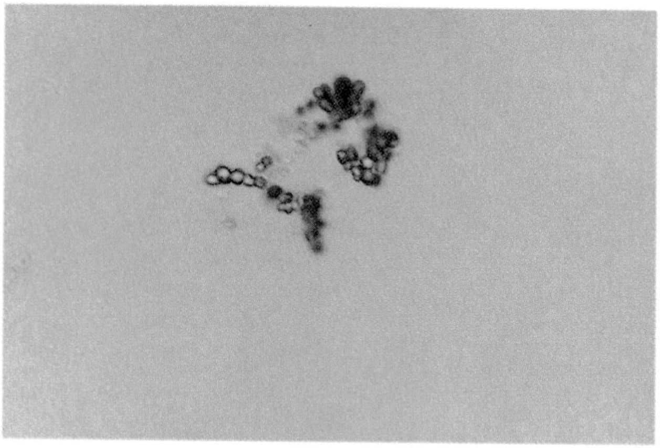

FIGURE 6-72 Calcium carbonate crystals (×400). (Courtesy of Kenneth L. McCoy, MD.)

or thin prisms often in rosette formations. The rosette forms may be confused with sulfonamide crystals when the urine pH is in the neutral range. Calcium phosphate crystals will dissolve in dilute acetic acid and sulfonamides will not. They have no clinical significance although calcium phosphate is a common constituent of renal calculi.

Calcium carbonate crystals are small and colorless, with dumbbell or spherical shapes (Figure 6–72). They may occur in clumps that resemble amorphous material, but they can be distinguished by the formation of gas after the addition of acetic acid. They are also birefringent, which differentiates them from bacteria. Calcium carbonate crystals have no clinical significance.

Ammonium biurate crystals exhibit the characteristic yellow-brown color of the urate crystals seen in acid urine. They are frequently described as "thorny apples" because of their appearance as spicule-covered spheres (Figure 6–73). Except for their occurrence in alkaline urine, ammonium biurate crystals resemble other urates in that they dissolve at 60°C and will convert to uric acid crystals when glacial acetic acid is added. Ammonium biurate crystals are almost always encountered in old specimens and may be associated with the presence of the ammonia produced by urea-splitting bacteria.

Abnormal Urine Crystals

Abnormal urine crystals are found in acid urine or rarely in neutral urine. Most abnormal crystals have very characteristic shapes. However, their identity should be confirmed by chemical tests (Table 6–7) or by patient information (medications). Iatrogenic crystals can be caused by a variety of compounds, particularly when they are administered in high concentrations. They may be of clinical significance when they precipitate in the renal tubules. The most commonly encountered iatrogenic crystals are discussed in this section.

CYSTINE CRYSTALS

Cystine crystals are found in the urine of persons who inherit a metabolic disorder that prevents reabsorption of cystine by the renal tubules (cystinuria). Persons with cystinuria have a tendency to form renal calculi, particularly at an early age.

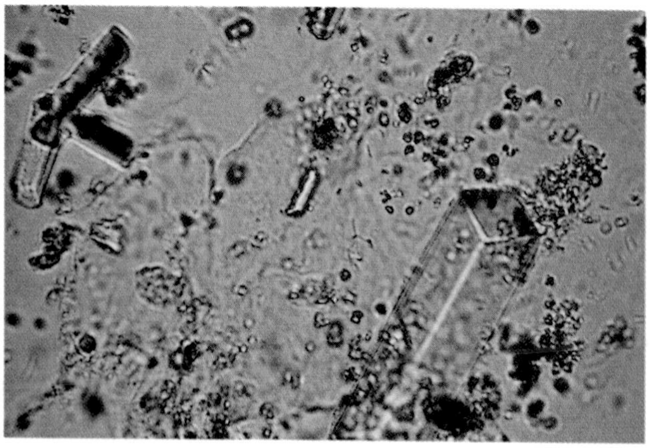

FIGURE 6-71 Triple phosphate crystals and amorphous phosphates (×400).

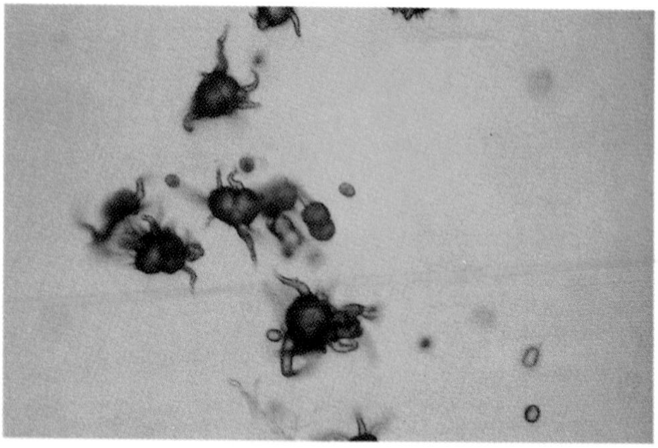

FIGURE 6-73 Ammonium biurate crystals (×400).

TABLE 6–7 **Major Characteristics of Abnormal Urinary Crystals**[14]

Crystal	pH	Color	Solubility	Appearance
Cystine	Acid	Colorless	Ammonia, dilute HCl	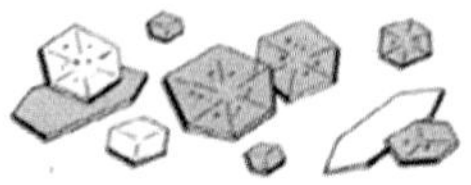
Cholesterol	Acid	Colorless (notched plates)	Chloroform	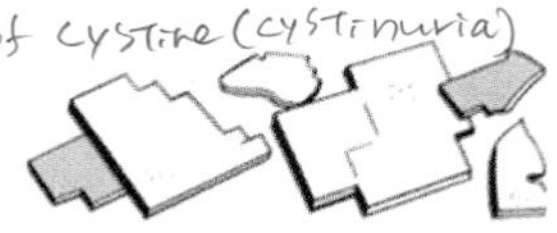
Leucine	Acid/ neutral	Yellow	Hot alkali or alcohol	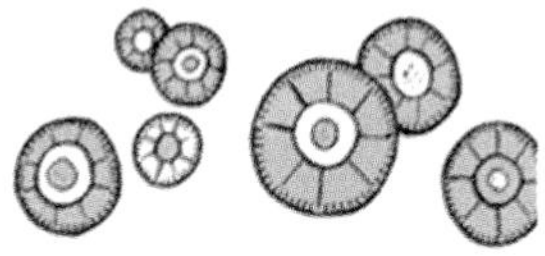
Tyrosine	Acid/ neutral	Colorless–yellow	Alkali or heat	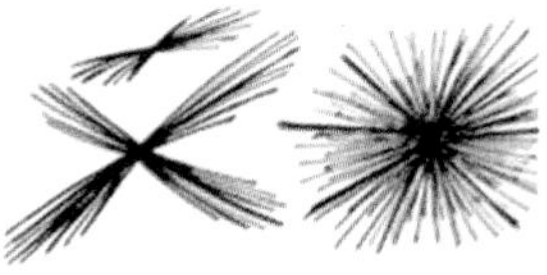
Bilirubin	Acid	Yellow	Acetic acid, HCl, NaOH, ether, chloroform	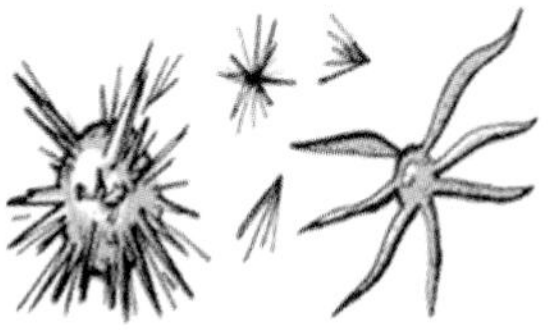
Sulfonamides	Acid/ neutral	Varied	Acetone	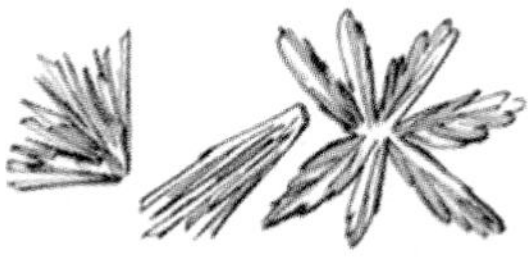
Radiographic dye	Acid	Colorless	10% NaOH	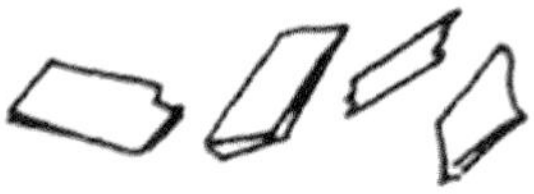
Ampicillin	Acid/ neutral	Colorless	Refrigeration forms bundles	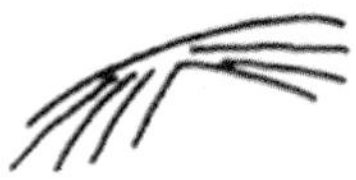

Cystine crystals appear as colorless, hexagonal plates and may be thick or thin (Figures 6–74 and 6–75). Disintegrating forms may be seen in the presence of ammonia. They may be difficult to differentiate from colorless uric acid crystals. Uric acid crystals are very birefringent under polarized microscopy, whereas only thick cystine crystals have polarizing capability. Positive confirmation of cystine crystals is made using the cyanide-nitroprusside test (see Chap. 9).

CHOLESTEROL CRYSTALS

Cholesterol crystals are rarely seen unless specimens have been refrigerated, because the lipids remain in droplet form. However, when observed, they have a most characteristic appearance, resembling a rectangular plate with a notch in one or more corners (Figure 6–76). They are associated with disorders producing lipiduria, such as the nephrotic syndrome, and are seen in conjunction with fatty casts and oval fat bodies. Cholesterol crystals are highly birefringent with polarized light (Figure 6–77).

RADIOGRAPHIC DYE CRYSTALS

Crystals of radiographic contrast media have a very similar appearance to cholesterol crystals and also are highly birefringent.

Differentiation is best made by comparison of the other urinalysis results and the patient history. As mentioned previously, cholesterol crystals should be accompanied by

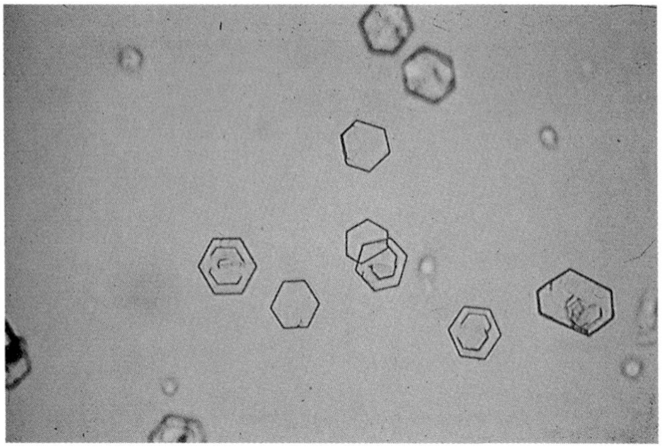

FIGURE 6–74 Cystine crystals (×400).

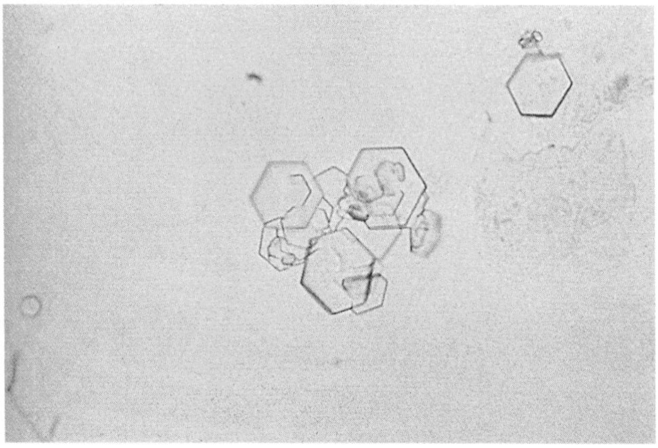

FIGURE 6–75 Cystine crystals (×400).

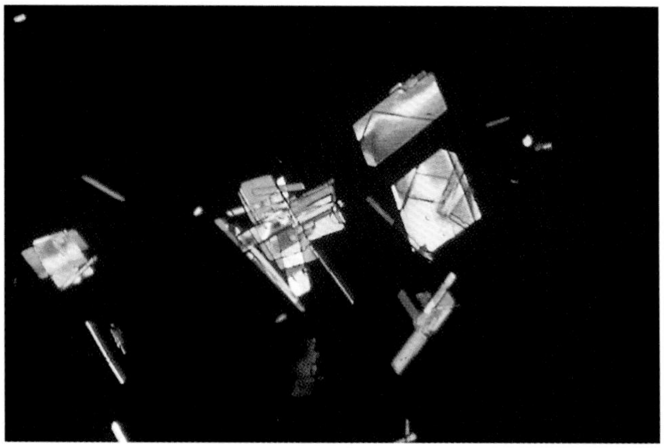

FIGURE 6–77 Cholesterol crystals under polarized light (×400).

birefringent

other lipid elements and heavy proteinuria. Likewise, the specific gravity of a specimen containing radiographic contrast media is markedly elevated when measured by refractometer.

CRYSTALS ASSOCIATED WITH LIVER DISORDERS

In the presence of severe liver disorders, three rarely seen crystals may be found in the urine sediment. They are crystals of tyrosine, leucine, and bilirubin.

Tyrosine crystals appear as fine colorless to yellow needles that frequently form clumps or rosettes (Figures 6–78 and 6–79). They are usually seen in conjunction with leucine crystals in specimens with positive chemical test results for bilirubin. Tyrosine crystals may also be encountered in inherited disorders of amino-acid metabolism (see Chap. 9).

Leucine crystals are yellow-brown spheres that demonstrate concentric circles and radial striations (Figure 6–80). They are seen less frequently than tyrosine crystals and, when present, should be accompanied by tyrosine crystals.

Bilirubin crystals are present in hepatic disorders producing large amounts of bilirubin in the urine. They appear as clumped needles or granules with the characteristic yel-

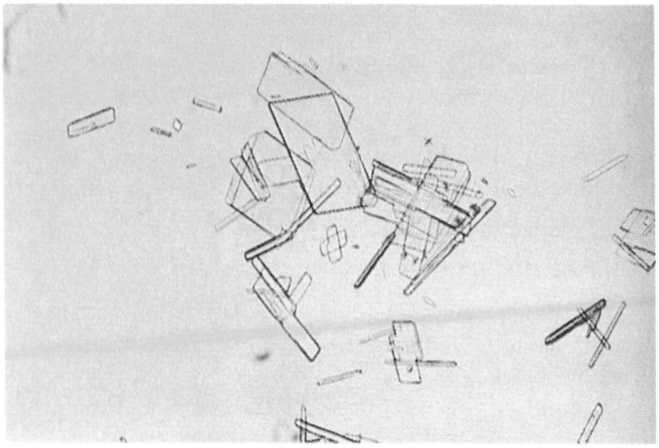

FIGURE 6–76 Cholesterol crystals. Notice the notched corners (×400).

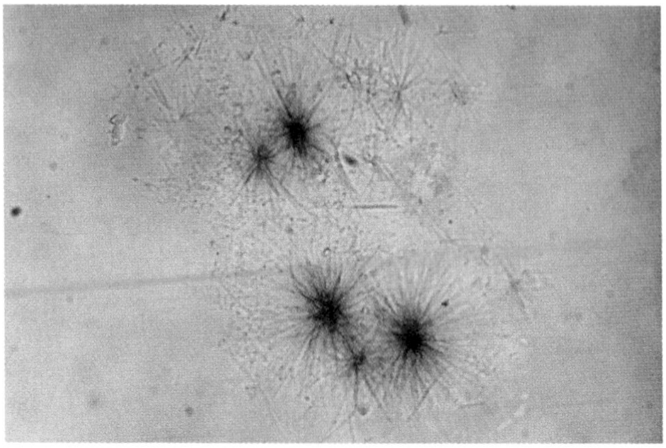

FIGURE 6–78 Tyrosine crystals in fine needle clumps (×400).

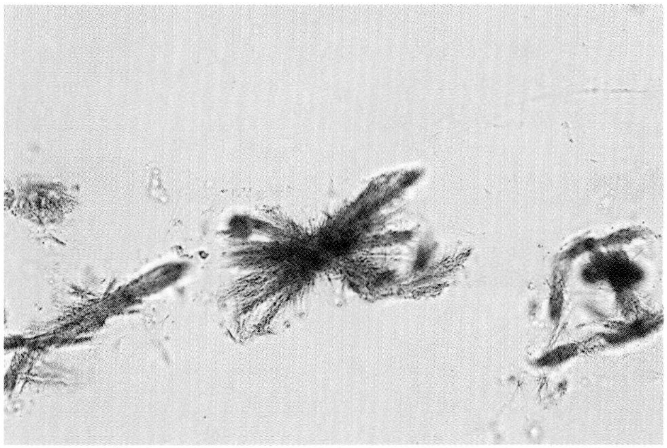

FIGURE 6–79 Tyrosine crystals in rosette forms (×400).

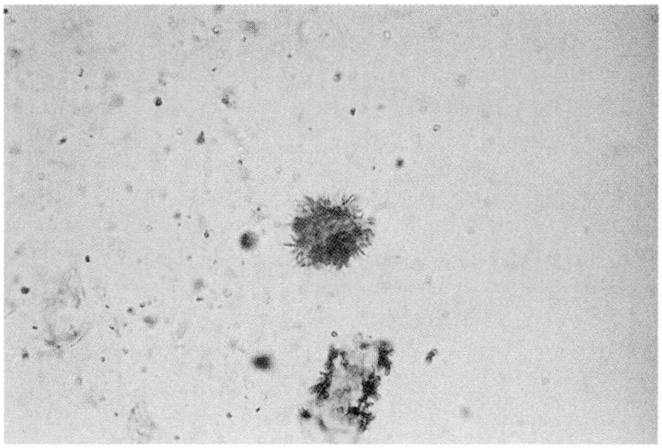

FIGURE 6–81 Bilirubin crystals. Notice the classic bright yellow color (×400).

low color of bilirubin (Figure 6–81). A positive chemical test result for bilirubin would be expected. In disorders, such as viral hepatitis, that produce renal tubular damage, bilirubin crystals may be found incorporated into the matrix of casts.

SULFONAMIDE CRYSTALS

Until the development of more soluble sulfonamides, the finding of these crystals in the urine of patients being treated for UTIs was common. Inadequate patient hydration was and still is the primary cause of sulfonamide crystallization. The appearance of sulfonamide crystals in fresh urine can suggest the possibility of tubular damage if crystals are forming in the nephron.

A variety of sulfonamide medications are currently on the market; therefore, one can expect to encounter a variety of crystal shapes and colors. Shapes most frequently encountered include needles, rhombics, whetstones, sheaves of wheat, and rosettes with colors ranging from colorless to yellow-brown (Figures 6–82 and 6–83). A check of the patient's medication history aids in the identification confirmation. If necessary, a diazo reaction can be performed for further confirmation.

AMPICILLIN CRYSTALS

Precipitation of antibiotics is not frequently encountered except for the rare observation of ampicillin crystals following massive doses of this penicillin compound without adequate hydration. Ampicillin crystals appear as colorless needles that tend to form bundles following refrigeration (Figure 6–84). Knowledge of the patient's history can aid in the identification.

URINARY SEDIMENT ARTIFACTS

Contaminants of all types can be found in urine, particularly in those specimens collected under improper conditions or in dirty containers. The most frequently encountered artifacts include starch, oil droplets, air bubbles, pollen grains, fibers, and fecal contamination. Because artifacts frequently resemble pathologic elements such as RBCs and casts, artifacts can present a major problem to students. They are often very highly refractile or occur in a different microscopic plane than the true sediment constituents. The reporting of artifacts is not necessary.

Starch granules are a frequent contaminant because corn starch is the powder used in powdered gloves. The

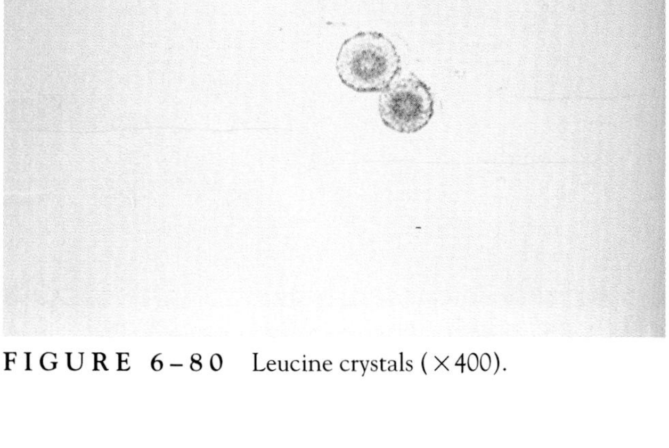

FIGURE 6–80 Leucine crystals (×400).

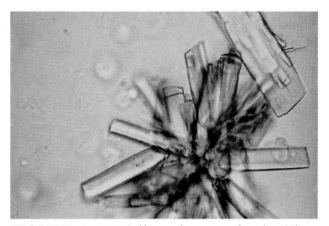

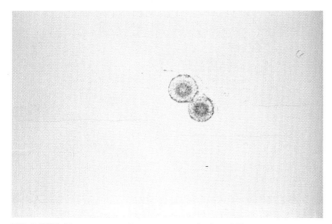

FIGURE 6–82 Sulfa crystals in rosette form (×400).

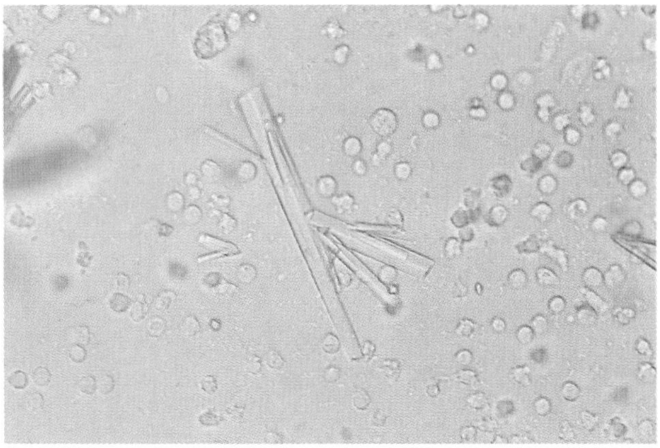

FIGURE 6–83 Sulfa crystals, WBCs, and bacteria seen in UTI (×400).

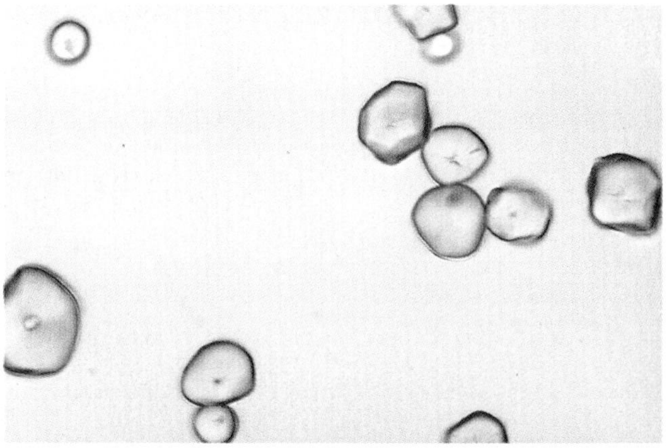

FIGURE 6–85 Starch granules. Notice the dimpled center (×400).

granules are highly refractile spheres, usually with a dimpled center (Figure 6–85). They resemble fat droplets when polarized, producing a Maltese cross formation. Starch granules may also occasionally be confused with RBCs. Differentiation between starch and pathologic elements can be made by considering other urinalysis results including chemical tests for blood or protein and the presence of oval fat bodies or fatty casts.

Oil droplets and air bubbles also are highly refractile and may resemble RBCs to the inexperienced laboratory personnel. Oil droplets may result from contamination by immersion oil or lotions and creams. Air bubbles occur when the specimen is placed under a cover slip. The presence of these artifacts should be considered in the context of the other urinalysis results.

Pollen grains are seasonal contaminants that appear as spheres with a cell wall and occasional concentric circles (Figure 6–86). Like many artifacts, their large size may cause them to be out of focus with true sediment constituents.

Hair and fibers from clothing and diapers may initially be mistaken for casts (Figures 6–87 and 6–88), although

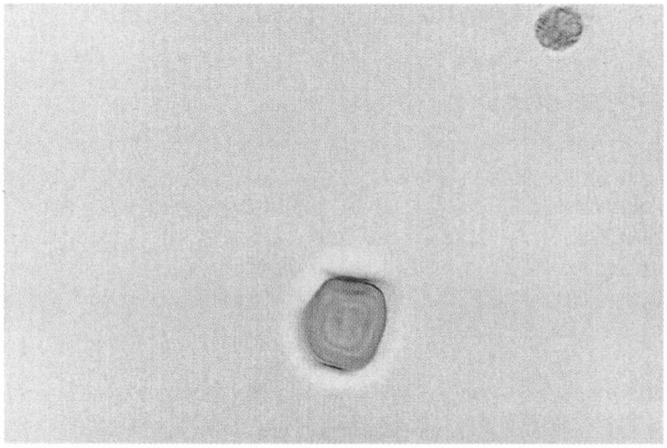

FIGURE 6–86 Pollen grain. Notice the concentric circles (×400).

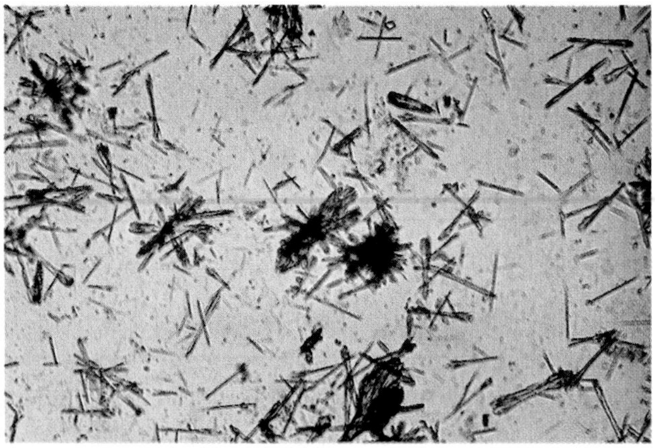

FIGURE 6–84 Ampicillin crystals following refrigeration (×400).

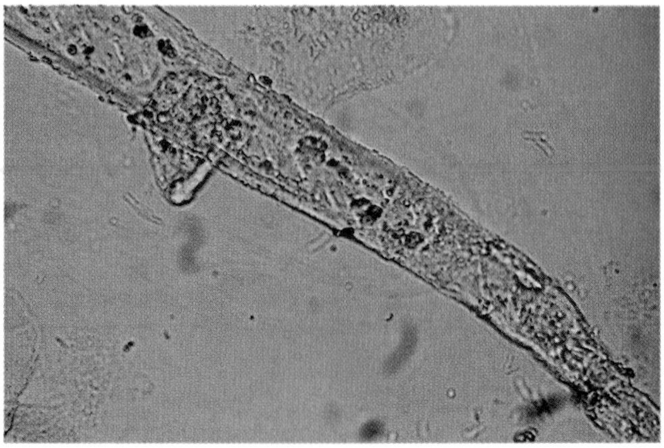

FIGURE 6–87 Fiber-resembling cast (×400).

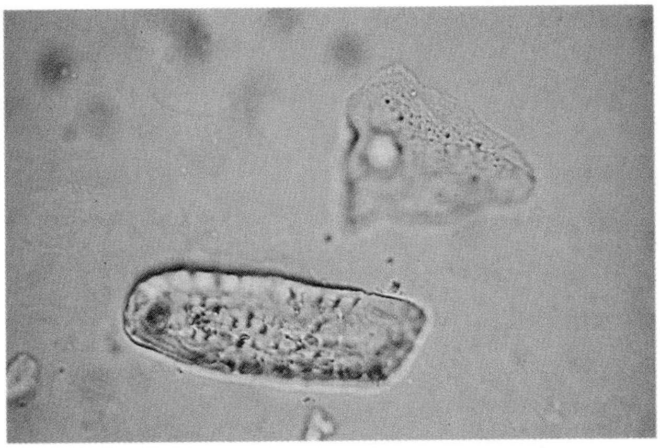

FIGURE 6–88 Diaper fiber resembling cast. Notice the refractility (×400).

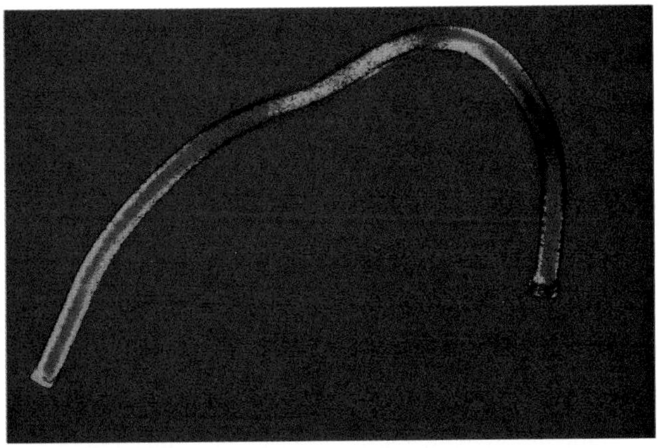

FIGURE 6–89 Fiber under polarized light (×100).

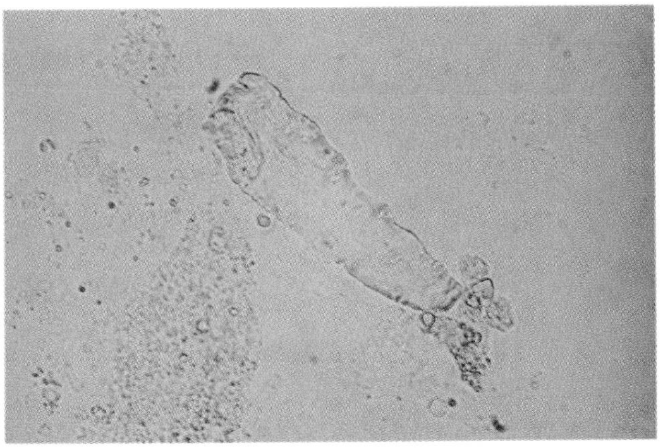

FIGURE 6–90 Vegetable fiber resembling waxy cast (×400).

they are usually much longer and more refractile. Examination under polarized light can frequently differentiate between fibers and casts (Figure 6–89). Fibers will often polarize, whereas, casts, other than fatty casts, do not.

Improperly collected specimens or rarely the presence of a fistula between the intestinal and urinary tracts may produce fecal specimen contamination. Fecal artifacts may appear as plant and meat fibers or as brown amorphous material in a variety of sizes and shapes (Figure 6–90).

REFERENCES

1. Addis, T: The number of formed elements in the urinary sediment of normal individuals. J Clin Invest 2(5):409–415, 1926.
2. Baer, DM: Tips from clinical experts: Reporting of spermatozoa in microscopic urine exams. MLO 12:12, 1997.
3. Cannon, DC: The identification and pathogenesis of urine casts. Lab Med 10(1):8–11. 1979.
4. Corwin, HL, Bray, RA, and Haber, MH: The detection and interpretation of urinary eosinophils. Arch Pathol Lab Med 113:1256–1258, 1989.
5. Cramer, AD, et al: Macroscopic screening urinalysis. Lab Med Sept:623–627, 1989.
6. Fassett, EG, et al: Urinary red cell morphology during exercise. Am J Clin Pathol 285(6353):1455–1457, 1982.
7. Ferris, JA: Comparison and standardization of the urine microscopic examination. Lab Med 14(10):659–662, 1983.
8. Graber, M, et al: Bubble cells: Renal tubular cells in the urinary sediment with characteristics of viability. J Am Soc Nephrol 1(7): 999–1004, 1991.
9. Haber, MH: Urinary Sediment: A Textbook Atlas. American Society of Clinical Pathologists, Chicago, 1981.
10. Haber, MH, and Lindner, LE: The surface ultrastructure of urinary casts. Am J Clin Pathol 68(5):547–552, 1977.
11. Haber, MH, Lindner, LE, and Ciofalo, LN: Urinary casts after stress. Lab Med 10(6):351–355, 1979.
12. Hamoudi, AC, Bubis, SC, and Thompson, C: Can the cost savings of eliminating urine microscopy in biochemically negative urines be extended to the pediatric population? Am J Clin Pathol 86(5): 658–660,1986.
13. Harr, R: Characterization of hematuria by plantar morphometry. Clin Lab Sci 8(6):353–359, 1995.
14. Henry, JB, Lauzon, RB, and Schumann, GB: basic examination of urine. In Henry, JB (ed): Clinical Diagnosis and Management by Laboratory Methods. WB Saunders, Philadelphia, 1996.
15. High, SR, Rowe, JA, and Maksem, JA: Macroscopic urinalysis. Lab Med 19:174–176, 1988.
16. Kohler, H, Wandel, E, and Brunch, B: Acanthocyturia—A characteristic marker for glomerular bleeding. Int Soc Nephrol 40:115–120, 1991.
17. Kumar, S, and Muchmore, A: Tamm-Horsfall protein—Uromodulin, 1950–1990. Kidney Int 37:1395–1399, 1990.
18. Lindner, LE, and Haber, MH: Hyaline casts in the urine: Mechanism of formation and morphological transformations. Am J Clin Pathol 80(3):347–352, 1983.
19. Lindner, LE, Jones, RN, and Haber, MH: A specific cast in acute pyelonephritis. Am J Clin Pathol 73(6):809–811, 1980.
20. Lindner, LE, Vacca, D, and Haber, MH: Identification and composition of types of granular urinary casts. Am J Clin Pathol 80(3): 353–358, 1983.
21. McGuchen, M, Cohen, L, and MacGregor, RR: Significance of pyuria in urinary sediment. J Urol 120:452–456, 1978.
22. Microscope Techniques—Phase Contrast: http://www.micro.magnet.fsuj.edu/ primer/ techniques/phase.html.
23. Mynahan, C: Evaluation of macroscopic urinalysis as a screening procedure. Lab Med 15(3):176–179, 1984.
24. National Committee for Clinical Laboratory Standards Approved Guideline GP16-A: Urinalysis and Collection, Transportation, and Preservation of Urine Specimens. NCCLS, Villanova, PA, 1995.

25. Polarizing and Interference Contrast Microscopy: http://www.rrz.uni-hamburg.de/biologic/b.
26. Product Profile: Sedi-Stain. Clay Adams, Division of Becton Dickinson & Company, Parsippany, NJ. 1974.
27. Schumann, GB: Utility of urinary cytology in renal diseases. Semin Nephrol 5(34) Sept, 1985.
28. Schumann, GB, and Tebbs, RD: Comparison of slides used for standardized routine microscopic urinalysis. J Med Technol 3(1):54–58, 1986.
29. Simpson, LO: Effects of normal and abnormal urine on red cell shape. Nephron 60(3):383–384, 1992.
30. Smalley, DL, and Bryan, JA: Comparative evaluation of biochemical and microscopic urinalysis. Am J Med Technol 49(4): 237–239, 1983.
31. Stapleton, FB: Morphology of urinary red blood cells: A simple guide in localizing the site of hematuria. Pediatr Clin North Am 34(3): 561–569, 1987.
32. Sternheimer, R, and Malbin, R: Clinical recognition of pyelonephritis with a new stain for urinary sediments. Am J Med 11:312–313, 1951.
33. Tetrault, GA: Automated reagent strip urinalysis. Utility in reducing work load of urine microscopy and culture. Lab Med 25:162–167, 1994.
34. Tomita, M, et al: A new morphological classification of urinary erythrocytes for differential diagnosis of hematuria. Clin Nephrol 37(2):84–89, 1992.

STUDY QUESTIONS

1. State an advantage and a disadvantage of performing urine microscopics based on macroscopic screening.
2. List the seven parameters commonly used as markers in macroscopic screening. Which is most likely to result in a nonclinically significant microscopic? Why?
3. What is the unique advantage to laboratory personnel provided by the Cen-Slide and R/S 2000 microscopic systems?
4. State three conditions that can occur prior to a specimen being poured into a centrifuge tube that can produce false-negative microscopic results.
5. Why should a laboratory be consistent in the volume of urine used to prepare the sediment? State two methods of reporting the microscopic if less than the usual volume of urine is available.
6. Why should specimen centrifugation be standardized in terms of relative centrifugal force rather than revolutions per minute?
7. State an error in centrifugation technique that could produce falsely decreased sediment constituents and an error that could compromise laboratory safety.
8. Calculate the sediment concentration factor if 15 mL of urine is centrifuged and 14.5 mL of specimen is decanted. If only 14 mL of specimen is decanted, how would this affect the sediment?
9. State two technical errors in sediment preparation that could produce decreased sediment constituents.
10. Discuss the advantages of using commercial-system slides for sediment examination.
11. What magnifications should be used for sediment examination? What is the purpose of each magnification?
12. Name three errors that may result in significant sediment constituents not being observed.
13. How are casts routinely reported? RBCs andWBCs?
14. Using a microscope with a hpf area of 0.090 mm^2, cover-slip area of 400 mm^2, a sediment concentration factor of 12, and a sediment volume of 0.02 mL, how many RBCs per milliliter are present if an average of 10 RBCs are counted per 10 hpfs?
15. What are the components of Sternheimer-Malbin stain?
16. State two methods for enhancing nuclear detail and two methods for detecting lipids.
17. What is the purpose of Hansel's stain?
18. How does cytodiagnostic urinalysis differ from routine microscopic examination?
19. A microscope has a 10× magnification eyepiece and a 40× magnification objective lens. What is the total magnification of the specimen? List two elements found in a urine specimen that would be identified at this magnification.
20. Name the type of microscopy that identifies birefringent substances.
21. List the requirements that are necessary to adapt a bright-field microscope for phase microscopy. What adjustment must be made for maximum contrast?
22. What type of microscopy uses optical path differences within the specimen to provide three-dimensional images and layer-by-layer imaging of a specimen?
23. True or False. When using bright-field microscopy, the condenser should be lowered when reduced lighting is required.
24. Contrast the appearance of RBCs in hypersthenuric and hyposthenuric urine.
25. Name three artifacts that may be mistaken for RBCs. What are their distinguishing characteristics?
26. Indicate whether macroscopic or microscopic hematuria would be expected if the following are present: renal calculi, coagulation disorders, advanced glomerular disease, malignancy, and acute infection.
27. Describe the appearance of dysmorphic RBCs. What is their significance?
28. What is the primary WBC seen in urine? When is it necessary to identify the presence of eosinophils?
29. Describe a glitter cell. What is the significance of these cells?
30. How can WBCs be differentiated from RTE cells?

31. List and briefly describe the three types of epithelial cells seen in urine, and state their sites of origin.

32. Name and describe a clinically significant form of squamous epithelial cells.

33. State a pathologic and a nonpathologic cause of increased urothelial cells.

34. Why is the finding of increased RTE cells clinically significant? Why do they sometimes contain bilirubin or hemosiderin granules?

35. Describe the origin of oval fat bodies.

36. If a structure believed to be an oval fat body stains orange with Sudan III but does not produce a Maltese cross formation with polarized light, can it be an oval fat body? Explain your answer.

37. What is the most common significance of bacteriuria in the absence of WBCs?

38. Why is glucose included as a macroscopic urine screening parameter?

39. Why do casts vary in size and composition? What is the primary constituent that all casts have in common?

40. State the primary condition required for the formation of casts.

41. Explain the difference in the clinical significance of free RBCs or WBCs versus RBC casts and WBC casts in the urine sediment.

42. What is the primary significance of a bacterial cast? What other constituents should be present in the sediment?

43. Describe two methods by which granular casts are formed.

44. Describe and discuss the significance of the urine sediment following strenuous exercise.

45. What do waxy and broad casts have in common?

46. List three factors that contribute to the formation of urinary crystals, and explain the significance of each.

47. State two techniques that can be used to aid in the identification of crystals.

48. Match the following crystals seen in acid urine with their description/identifying characteristic:

Crystal	Description/ Characteristic
a. _____ Amorphous urates	1. Yellow-brown whetstone
b. _____ Uric acid	2. Ovoid
c. _____ Monohydrate calcium oxalate	3. Thin needles
d. _____ Dehydrate calcium oxalate	4. Envelopes
	5. Yellow-brown granules

49. Match the following crystals seen in alkaline urine with their description/identifying characteristic:

Crystal	Description/ Characteristic
a. _____ Amorphous phosphate	1. Thorny apple
b. _____ Triple phosphate	2. White precipitate
c. _____ Ammonium biurate	3. Pink precipitate
d. _____ Calcium phosphate	4. Dumbbell shape
e. _____ Calcium carbonate	5. "Coffin lids"
	6. Thin prisms

50. Match the following abnormal crystals with their description/identifying characteristics:

Crystal	Description/ Characteristic
a. _____ Cystine	1. Concentric circles and radial striations
b. _____ Cholesterol	2. Bright yellow clumps
c. _____ Tyrosine	3. Bundles following refrigeration
d. _____ Leucine	4. Notched corners
e. _____ Bilirubin	5. Hexagonal plates
f. _____ Ampicillin	6. Fine needles seen in liver disease
g. _____ Radiographic dye	7. Flat plates, high specific gravity
	8. Highly alkaline pH

CASE STUDIES AND CLINICAL SITUATIONS

1. An 85-year-old women with diabetes and a broken hip has been confined to bed for the past 3 months. Results of an ancillary blood glucose test are 250 mg/dL, and her physician orders additional blood tests and a routine urinalysis. The urinalysis report is as follows:

COLOR: Pale yellow	KETONES: Negative
CLARITY: Hazy	BLOOD: Moderate
SP. GRAVITY: 1.020	BILIRUBIN: Negative
pH: 5.5	UROBILINOGEN: Normal
PROTEIN: Trace	NITRITE: Negative
GLUCOSE: 100 mg/dL	LEUKOCYTES: 2+

Microscopic

20–25 WBCs/hpf	Many yeast cells and hyphae

a. Why are yeast infections common in patients with diabetes mellitus?
b. With a blood glucose level of 250 mg/dL, should glucose be present in the urine? Why or why not?
c. Is there a discrepancy between the negative nitrite and the positive leukocyte esterase results? Explain your answer.
d. What is the major discrepancy between the chemical and microscopic results?
e. Considering the patient's history, what is the most probable cause for the discrepancy?

2. A medical technology student training in a newly renovated STAT laboratory is having difficulty performing a microscopic urinalysis. Reagent strip testing indicates the presence of moderate blood and leukocytes, but the student is also observing some large unusual objects re-

sembling crystals and possible casts. The student is also having difficulty keeping all of the constituents in focus at the same time.
   a. Why is the student having difficulty focusing?
   b. What is a possible cause of the unusual microscopic constituents?
   c. Should the student be concerned about the unusual microscopic constituents? Explain your answer.
   d. What microscopy technique could be used to aid in differentiating a cast and an artifact?

3. A prisoner sentenced to 10 years for selling illegal drugs develops jaundice, lethargy, and hepatomegaly. A test for hepatitis B surface antigen is positive, and the patient is placed in the prison infirmary. When his condition appears to worsen and a low urinary output is observed, the patient is transferred to a local hospital. Additional testing detects a superinfection with delta hepatitis virus and decreased renal concentrating ability. Urinalysis results are as follows:

COLOR: Amber	KETONES: Negative
CLARITY: Hazy	BLOOD: Negative
SP. GRAVITY: 1.011	BILIRUBIN: Large
pH: 7.0	UROBILINOGEN: 8.0 EU
PROTEIN: 2+	NITRITE: Negative
GLUCOSE: Negative	LEUKOCYTES: Negative

Microscopic

2–4 WBCs/hpf	1–2 hyaline casts/lpf
1–3 RBCs/hpf	1–2 granular casts/lpf
Few squamous epithelial cells	2–4 bile-stained RTE cells/hpf
	0–1 RTE casts/lpf

0–1 bile-stained waxy casts/lpf

   a. Based on the urinalysis results, in what area of the nephron is damage occurring?
   b. Is this consistent with the patient's primary diagnosis? Explain your answer.
   c. What is causing the RTE cells and not the squamous epithelial cells to be bile stained?
   d. Why is the urobilinogen level elevated?
   e. State a disorder in which the urobilinogen level would be elevated, but the bilirubin result would be negative.

4. A 30-year-old woman being treated for a UTI brings a urine specimen to the Employee Health Clinic at 4:00 pm. The nurse on duty tells her that the specimen will be refrigerated and tested by the technologist the next morning. The technologist has difficulty interpreting the color of the reagent strip tests and reports only the following results:

COLOR: Amber	CLARITY: Slightly cloudy

Microscopic

3–5 RBCs/hpf	Few squamous epithelial cells
8–10 WBCs/hpf	Moderate unidentified orange crystals
Moderate bacteria	Moderate colorless crystals appearing in bundles

   a. What could have caused the technologist to have difficulty interpreting the reagent strip results?
   b. Could this specimen produce a yellow foam when shaken?
   c. How could it be checked for the presence of bilirubin? Would this really be necessary?
   d. What could the technologist do to aid in the identification of the crystals?
   e. What is the probable identification of the orange crystals?
   f. What is the probable identification of the colorless crystals?

5. A 2-year-old left unattended in the garage for 5 minutes is suspected of ingesting antifreeze (ethylene glycol). The urinalysis has a pH of 6.0 and is negative on the chemical examination. Two distinct forms of crystals are observed in the microscopic examination.
   a. What type of crystals would you expect to be present?
   b. What are the two crystal forms present?
   c. Describe the two forms.
   d. Which form would you expect to be predominant?

6. A female patient comes to the outpatient clinic with symptoms of UTI. She brings a urine specimen with her. Results of the routine analysis performed on this specimen are as follows:

COLOR: Yellow	KETONES: Negative
CLARITY: Hazy	BLOOD: Small
SP. GRAVITY: 1.015	BILIRUBIN: Negative
pH: 9.0	UROBILINOGEN: Normal
PROTEIN: Negative	NITRITE: Negative
GLUCOSE: Negative	LEUKOCYTE: 2+

Microscopic

1–3 RBCs/hpf	Heavy bacteria
8–10 WBCs/hpf	Moderate squamous epithelial cells

   a. What discrepancies are present between the chemical and microscopic test results?
   b. State a reason for the discrepancies.
   c. Identify a chemical result in the urinalysis that confirms your reason for the discrepancies.
   d. What course of action should the laboratory take to obtain accurate results for this patient?

7. A high-school student is taken to the emergency room with a broken leg that occurred during a football game. The urinalysis results are as follows:

COLOR: Dark yellow	KETONES: Negative
CLARITY: Hazy	BLOOD: Small
SP. GRAVITY: 1.030	BILIRUBIN: Negative
pH: 5.5	UROBILINOGEN: Normal
PROTEIN: 2+	NITRITE: Negative
GLUCOSE: Negative	LEUKOCYTE: Negative

Microscopic

0–2 RBCs/hpf	0–4 hyaline casts/lpf
0–3 WBCs/hpf	0–3 granular casts/lpf

Few squamous epithelial cells

   a. Are these results of clinical significance?

b. Explain the discrepancy between the chemical and microscopic blood results.
c. What is the probable cause of the granular casts?

8. As supervisor of the urinalysis section, you are reviewing results. State why or why not each of the following results would concern you.
a. The presence of waxy casts and a negative protein in urine from a 6-month-old girl
b. Increased transitional epithelial cells in a specimen obtained following cystoscopy
c. Tyrosine crystals in a specimen with a negative bilirubin test result
d. Cystine crystals in a specimen from a patient diagnosed with gout
e. Cholesterol crystals in urine with a specific gravity greater than 1.040
f. *Trichomonas vaginalis* in a male urine specimen
g. Amorphous urates and calcium carbonate crystals in a specimen with a pH of 6.0

CHAPTER 7

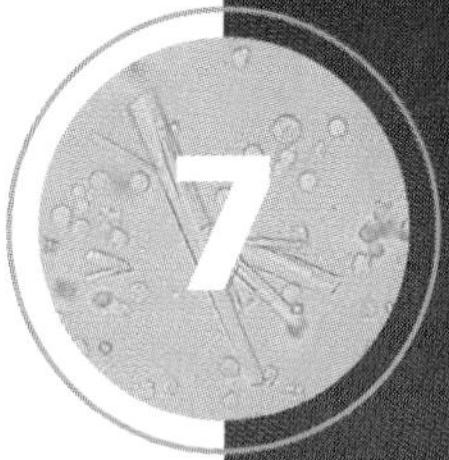

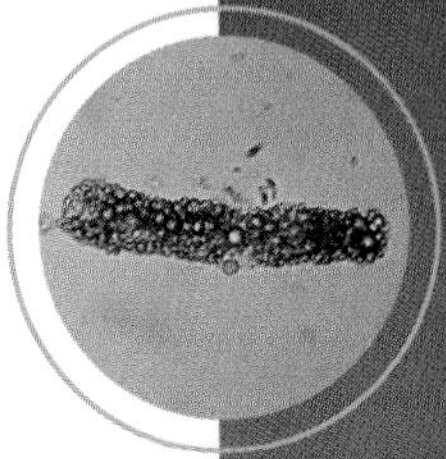

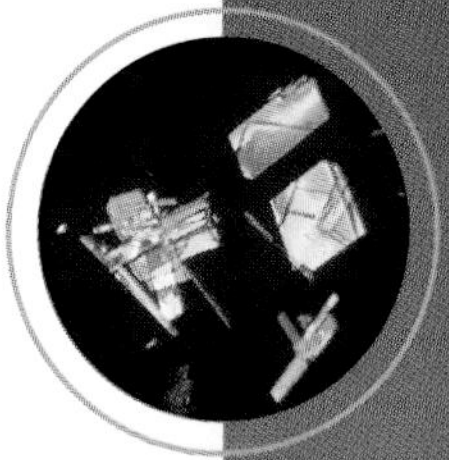

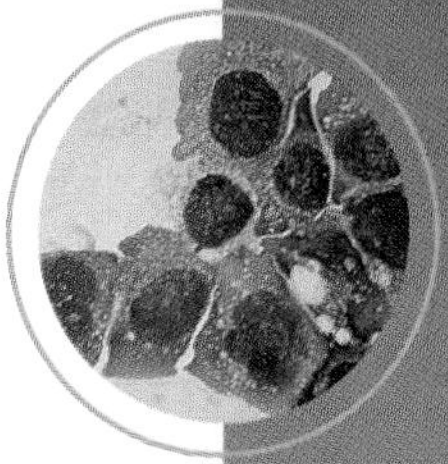

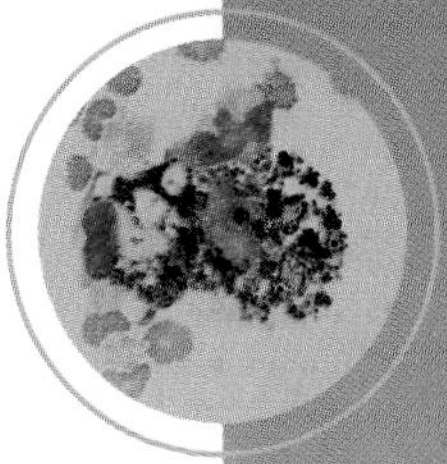

Quality Assurance and Management in the Urinalysis Laboratory

LEARNING OBJECTIVES

Upon completion of this chapter, the reader will be able to:

1. Discuss the quality assurance procedures and documentation for quality control of specimens, methodology, reagents, control materials, instrumentation, equipment, and reporting of results in the urinalysis laboratory.
2. Define the preanalytical, analytical, and postanalytical components of quality assurance.
3. Distinguish between the components of internal and external quality control.
4. List the elements required for quality assurance as regulated by the Clinical Laboratory Improvement Amendments (CLIA '88).
5. Describe the four levels of the CLIA '88 complexity model and how they relate to urinalysis testing.
6. Discuss the importance of continuous quality improvement and total quality management, including the recommendations of the Joint Commission on Accreditation of Healthcare Organizations.

KEY TERMS

accreditation
continuous quality improvement
external quality control
internal quality control
outcomes
process
proficiency testing
quality assurance
quality control
total quality management
turnaround time

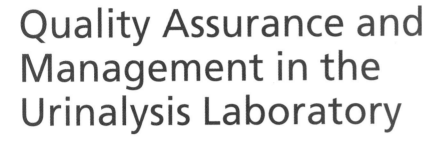

The term ***quality assurance*** (QA) refers to the overall process of guaranteeing quality patient care. In a clinical laboratory, a quality assurance program includes not only testing controls, referred to as ***quality control*** (QC), but also encompasses preanalytical factors (e.g., specimen collection, handling, and storage), analytical factors (e.g., reagent and test performance, instrument calibration and maintenance, personnel requirements, and technical competence), and postanalytical factors (e.g., reporting of results and interpretation), and documentation that the program is being meticulously followed.[8] Included in a QA program are procedure manuals, ***internal quality control*** and ***external quality control***, standardization, ***proficiency testing***, record keeping, equipment maintenance, safety programs, training and education of personnel, and a scheduled and documented review process. Essentially, QA is the continual monitoring of the entire test process from test ordering and specimen collection through reporting and interpreting results. Written policies and documented actions as they relate to the patient, the laboratory, ancillary personnel, and the health-care provider are required. Having written remedial actions mandating the steps to take when any part of the system fails is essential to a QA program.

During the discussion of the routine urinalysis in the preceding chapters, the methods of ensuring accurate results were covered on an individual basis for each of the tests. Because QA in the urinalysis laboratory—or any other laboratory department—is an integration of many factors, this section will provide a collection of the procedures essential for providing quality urinalysis.

Documentation of QA procedures is required for laboratory ***accreditation*** by either the Joint Commission on the Accreditation of Healthcare Organizations (**JCAHO**) or the College of American Pathologists (**CAP**) and for Medicare reimbursement. Guidelines published by CAP and the National Committee for Clinical Laboratory Standards provide very complete instructions for documentation and are used as a reference for the ensuing discussion of the specific areas of urinalysis QC and QA.[1,9] Documentation in the form of a procedure manual is required in all laboratories, and this format will be used as a basis for the following discussion.

Urinalysis Procedure Manual

A procedure manual containing all the procedures performed in the urinalysis section must be available for reference in the working area. The following information is included for each procedure: principle or purpose of the test, patient preparation, specimen type and method of collection, reagents, standards and controls, instrument calibration and maintenance protocols and schedules, step-by-step procedure, calculations, frequency and tolerance of controls and corrective actions, normal values and panic values, specific procedure notes, limitations of the method, method validation, references, effective date, author, and review schedule. Current package inserts should be available at the workplace.

St. JOSEPH HOSPITAL
PATHOLOGY DEPT
CLINICAL CHEMISTRY/ URINALYSIS SECTION

SPECIMEN ACCEPTABILITY/ LABELING

Prepared by: Carol Schmitt MT[ASCP]

Initial approval: Donna Wells MD

Procedure placed in use: June 1983

Revised: June 1999

Reason for Revision: Changes in format

Effective Date	Technical Approval	Medical Director Approval
Reviewed	[signature] 6/22/99	[signature] 6/22/99
Reviewed		
Reviewed		
Reviewed		
Reviewed		

FIGURE 7-1 Example of procedure review documentation. (From the Department of Pathology, St. Joseph Hospital, Omaha, NE, with permission.)

The evaluation of procedures and adoption of new methodologies is an ongoing process in the clinical laboratory. Whenever changes are made, the procedure should be reviewed and signed by a person with designated authority, such as the laboratory director or section supervisor (Figure 7-1). Documentation of an annual review of all procedures by the designated authority must also be substantiated.

PREANALYTICAL FACTORS

Preanalytical factors are the variables that occur before the actual testing of the specimen and include test requests, patient preparation, specimen collection, handling, and storage.[8] Health-care personnel outside the clinical laboratory control many of these factors such as ordering tests and specimen collection. Communication between departments and adequate training on the correct procedures for ordering a test and collecting the specimen will improve the ***turnaround time*** (TAT) of results, avoid duplication of test orders, and ensure a high-quality specimen.

Specimen Collection and Handling

Specific information on specimen collection and handling should be stated at the beginning of each procedure listed in the manual. Requisition forms and computerized entry forms should designate the type of urine specimen to be collected and the date and time of collection. The form should include space for recording 1) the actual date and time of specimen collection, 2) whether the specimen was refrigerated before transporting, 3) the time the specimen was received in the laboratory and the time the test was performed, 4) tests requested, 5) an area for specific instructions that might affect the results of the analysis, and 6) patient identification information.[9]

Patient preparation (e.g., fasting or elimination of interfering medications), the type and volume of specimen required, and the need for sterile or opaque containers must

TABLE 7–1 Policy for Handling Mislabeled Specimens

Do NOT assume any information about the specimen or patient.
Do NOT relabel an incorrectly labeled specimen.
Do NOT discard the specimen until investigation is complete.
Leave specimen EXACTLY as you receive it; put in the refrigerator for preservation until errors can be resolved.
Notify floor, nursing station, doctor's office, etc. of problem and why it must be corrected for analysis to continue.
Identify problem on specimen requisition with date, time, and your initials.
Make person responsible for specimen collection participate in solution of problem(s). Any action taken should be documented on the requisition slip.
Report all mislabeled specimens to the quality assurance board.

From Schweitzer, Schumann, and Schumann,[10] p. 568, with permission.

be included with the specific procedure. All specimens should be examined within 2 hours. If this is not possible, written instructions for the preservation of the specimen must be available.

Instructions of a general nature, such as procedures for the collection of clean-catch and timed specimens, processing of specimens, and any printed materials given to patients, are also included in the manual.

Criteria for specimen rejection for both physical characteristics and labeling errors must be present. In Table 7–1, an example of a policy for handling mislabeled specimens is provided. Written criteria for rejection of specimens must be documented and available to the physician and nursing staff.

Laboratory personnel must determine the suitability of a specimen and document any problems and corrective actions taken (Figure 7–2). An acceptable specimen requires verification of the patient's identification information on the requisition form and the container label, timely transport to the laboratory, the presence of refrigeration or recommended preservative if transport was delayed, and collection of an adequate amount of the correct urine specimen type in a noncontaminated, tightly closed container. After receipt in the laboratory, the specimen must be processed immediately or, if necessary, stored in a refrigerator and protected from light.[9]

ANALYTICAL FACTORS

The analytical factors are the processes that directly affect the testing of specimens. They include reagents, instrumentation and equipment, testing procedure, QC, **preventive maintenance (PM)**, access to procedure manuals, and competency of personnel performing the tests.[8]

Reagents

The manual should state the name and chemical formula of each reagent used, instructions for preparation, when necessary, or company source of prepared materials, storage requirements, and procedures for reagent QC. The type of water used for preparing reagents and controls must be specified. A bold-type statement of any safety or health precautions associated with reagents should be present. An example of this would be the heat produced in the Clinitest reaction.

All reagents and reagent strips must be properly labeled with the date of preparation or opening, purchase date, expiration date, and appropriate safety information. Reagent strips should be checked against known negative and positive control solutions on each shift or at a minimum once a day, and whenever a new bottle is opened. Reagents are checked daily or when tests requiring their use are requested. Results of all reagent checks are properly recorded.

Instrumentation and Equipment

Instructions regarding the operation, performance and frequency of calibration, limitations, and procedures to follow when limitations or linearity are exceeded, such as dilution procedures, must be clearly stated in the procedure manual. Instructions detailing the appropriate recording procedures must be included.

The most frequently encountered instruments in the urinalysis laboratory are refractometers, osmometers, automated reagent strip readers, and automated microscopy instruments. Refractometers are calibrated on each shift against distilled water (1.000) and a known control, such as 5 percent saline (1.022 ± 0.001) or 9 percent sucrose (1.034 ± 0.001), is run. Both the high and low commercial controls are available for the osmometer. All control values are recorded. Automated urinalysis systems and reagent strip readers are calibrated using manufacturer-supplied calibration materials following the protocol specified by the manufacturer. Both positive and negative control values must be run and recorded (Figure 7–3).

Equipment found in the urinalysis laboratory commonly includes refrigerators, centrifuges, microscopes, and water baths. Temperatures of refrigerators and water baths should be taken daily and recorded. Calibration of centrifuges is customarily performed every 3 months, and the appropriate relative centrifugal force for each setting is recorded. Centrifuges are routinely disinfected on a weekly basis. Microscopes should be kept clean at all times. A routine PM schedule for instruments and equipment should be prepared, and records are kept of all routine and nonroutine maintenance performed (Figure 7–4).

Deionized water used for reagent preparation is quality controlled by checking pH and purity meter resistance on a weekly basis and the bacterial count on a monthly schedule. All results must be recorded on the appropriate forms.

Testing Procedure

Detailed, concise testing instructions are written in a step-by-step manner. Instructions should begin with specimen preparation, such as time and speed of centrifugation, and include types of glassware needed, time limitations and stability of specimens and reagents, calculation formulas and a sample calculation, health and safety precautions, and procedures. Additional procedure information including reasons for special precautions, sources of error and interfering

Month/year ________/____

Core Laboratory
Errors/Corrections

				Origin of Error - place a check mark in one box																Check one									
				Collection				Processing			Mis-info			Tech sec.			Result rpt			Discov		When							
Error by: Initials	Recorded by: Initials	Date	Major Error/Incident rpt	Patient Identification	Specimen Identificatior	Specimen Integrity	Document Status	Aliquot ID	Requisition/Order	Specimen Processing	Nursing	Respiratory Therapy	Client	Performance	Interpretation	Math	Entry (tech)	Transcription (tech)	Clerical Personnel	By Lab	Non-lab	Immediately	Same Shift	After Shift	nrbc	Other non-error	Comments		Patient Name, Test
			/																										
			/																										
			/																										
			/																										
			/																										
			/																										
			/																										
			/																										
			/																										
			/																										
			/																										
			/																										
			/																										
			/																										
			/																										
			/																										
			/																										
			/																										
			/																										
			/																										

FIGURE 7–2 Sample of errors and corrections documentation form. (From the Department of Pathology, Methodist Hospital, Omaha, NE, with permission.)

QUALITY CONTROL - CLINITEK ATLAS **MONTH:____________20_____**

			KOVATROL LOT #:									SALINE								
			GLU	BIL	KET	SP GR	BLD	PH	PROT	NIT	LEU EST	GLU	BIL	KET	SP GR	BLD	PH	PROT	NIT	LEU EST
			mg/dl		mg/dl	1.0			mg/dl			mg/dl		mg/dl	1.0			mg/dl		
KOVATROL ASSAY VALUES																				
	TECH	DATE																		
REAGENT PACK																				
LOT #																				
EXP																				

FIGURE 7–3 Sample instrument QC recording sheet. (From the Department of Pathology, Methodist Hospital, Omaha, NE, with permission.)

IRIS 900 UDx BOEHRINGER MANNHEIM Super UA MAINTENANCE LOG

DAILY	OM SECTION	1	2	3	4	5	6	7	8	9	10	11	12	13	14	15	16	17	18	19	20	21	22	23	24	25	26	27	28	29	30	31
Check Waste Tray	4.2																															
Check Transport Tray	4.2																															
Execute Daily Wash	5.2																															
Empty Waste Tank	5.3																															
Check Water Level																																
Clean Instrument Surfaces																																
TECH INITIALS																																

WEEKLY	OM SECTION	1	2	3	4	5
Clean Rinse Bath	5.5					
Clean Sorter Stage	5.7					
Clean Mixing Rod/Displacement Rod	5.8					
Clean Di Water Reservoir	5.14					
BIWEEKLY						
Calibrate Reader	4.3					
TECH INITIALS						

AS NEEDED	OM SECTION	DATE
Clean Transport Plate	5.4	
Clean Sorter Drum	5.6	
Replace Waste Tray	5.9	
Floppy Disk Replacement and Disk Drive Cleaning	5.10	
Clean Sample Disk Compartment	5.11	
Replace Printer Paper	5.12	
Clean Sample Drip and Sample Disk Drip Trays	5.13	
Decontamination of Tubing Lines	5.15	
TECH INITIALS		

OM = Operator's Manual

FIGURE 7–4 Sample preventive maintenance documentation form. (Courtesy of International Remote Imaging Systems, Chatsworth, CA.)

substances, helpful hints, clinical situations that influence the test, alternative procedures, and acceptable TATs for STAT tests are listed under the title of Procedure Notes following the step-by-step procedure.[11]

Reference sources should be listed. Manufacturer's package inserts may be included but cannot replace the written procedure.

Quality Control

Quality control refers to the materials, procedures, and techniques that monitor the **accuracy**, **precision**, and **reliability** of a laboratory test.[5] QC procedures are performed to ensure that acceptable standards are being met during the process of patient testing. Specific QC information regarding the type of control specimen preparation and handling, frequency of use, tolerance levels, and methods of recording should be included in the step-by-step instructions for each test. QC is performed at scheduled times, such as at the beginning of each shift or prior to testing patient samples, and it must always be performed if reagents are changed, an instrument malfunction has occurred, or if test results are questioned by the physician. Both internal quality control and external quality control processes are practiced in the urinalysis laboratory.

Internal quality controls are used to verify the accuracy (ability to obtain the expected result) and precision (ability to obtain the same result on the same specimen) of a test and are exposed to the same conditions as the patient samples. Reliability is the ability to maintain both precision and accuracy. Commercial controls are available for the urine chemistry tests, specific gravity, and for certain microscopic constituents. Analysis of two levels of control material is recommended. Documentation of QC includes dating and initialing the material when it is first opened, recording the manufacturer's lot number and the expiration date each time a control is run and the test result obtained. Food and Drug Administration standards require that control material must test negative for the human immunodeficiency virus and hepatitis B virus. Internal controls are tested and interpreted in the laboratory by the same person performing the patient testing.

Control data are evaluated prior to release of patient results. Data obtained from repeated measurements will have a gaussian distribution or spread in the values that will indicate the ability to repeat the analysis and obtain the same value. The laboratory, after repeated testing, establishes the value for each analyte and the mean and standard deviation is calculated. The **control mean** is the average of all data points and the **standard deviation (SD)** is a measurement statistic that describes the average distance each data point in a normal distribution is from the mean. The **coefficient of variation (CV)** is the SD expressed as a percentage of the mean. The CV indicates whether the distribution of values about the mean is in a narrow versus broad range and should be less than 5 percent. Confidence intervals are the limits between which the specified proportion or percentage of results will lie. **Control ranges** are determined by setting confidence limits that are within ± 2 SD or ± 3 SD of the mean which indicates that 95.5 percent to 99.7 percent of the values are expected to be within that range.

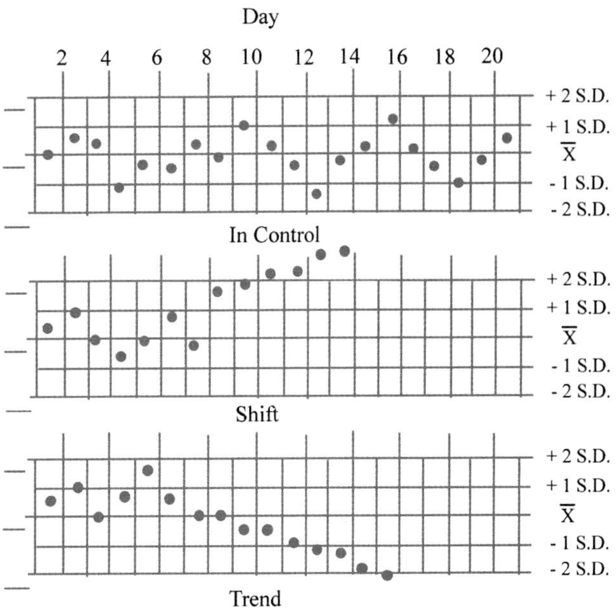

FIGURE 7–5 Levy-Jennings charts showing in-control results, trend, and shift.

Values are plotted on Levy-Jennings control charts to visually monitor control values. Immediate decisions about patient results are based on the ability of control values to remain within a preestablished limit. Changes in accuracy of results are indicated by either a **trend** that is a gradual changing in the mean in one direction or a **shift** that is an abrupt change in the mean (Figure 7–5). Changes in precision are shown by a large amount of scatter about the mean and an uneven distribution above and below the mean that are most often caused by errors in technique.

Corrective action, including the use of new reagents, reagent strips or controls and the verification of lot numbers and expiration dates, must be taken when control values are outside the tolerance limits. All corrective actions taken are documented. A protocol for corrective action is shown in Figure 7–6. A designated supervisor reviews all QC results.

External quality control is the testing of unknown samples received from an outside agency. It provides unbiased validation of the quality of patient test results. Proficiency testing such as that offered by the CAP provides this external quality control. Laboratories subscribing to this program receive lyophilized specimens for routine urinalysis and transparencies for sediment constituent identification. The results are returned to the CAP, where they are statistically analyzed with those from all participating laboratories, and a report is returned to the laboratory director. The laboratory accuracy is evaluated and compared with other laboratories using the same method of analysis. Corrective action must be taken for unacceptable results.

Laboratories may participate in a commercial QC program. Results from the same lot of QC material are sent to the manufacturer for statistical analysis and comparison with other laboratories using the same methodology.

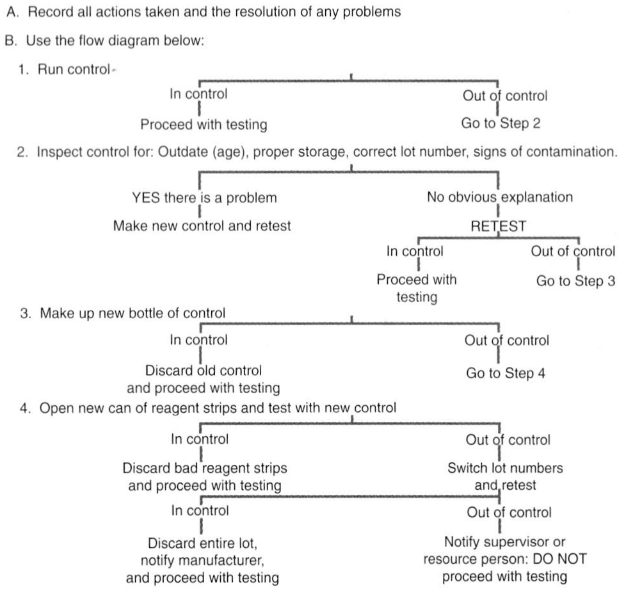

FIGURE 7–6 "Out-of-control" procedures. (From Schweitzer, Schumann, and Schumann,[10] with permission.)

MICROSCOPIC QUANTITATIONS

Quantitate an average of 10 representative fields. Do not quantitate budding yeast, mycelial elements, trichomonas, or sperm, but do note their presence with the appropriate LIS code.

Epithelial Cells/LPF	
None:	0
Rare:	0-5
Few:	5-20
Moderate:	20-100
Many:	>100
Casts/LPF	
None:	0
Numerical ranges:	0-2, 2-5, 5-10, >10
RBCs/HPF	
None:	0
Numerical ranges:	0-2, 2-5, 5-10, 10-25, 25-50, 50-100, >100
WBCs/HPF	
None:	0
Numerical ranges:	0-2, 2-5, 5-10, 10-25, 25-50, 50-100, >100
Crystals/HPF	
None:	0
Rare:	0-2
Few:	2-5
Moderate:	5-20
Many:	>20
Bacteria/HPF	
None:	0
Rare:	0-10
Few:	10-50
Moderate:	50-200
Many:	>200
Mucous Threads	
Rare:	0-1
Few:	1-3
Moderate:	3-10
Many:	>10

FIGURE 7–7 Sample standardized urine microscopic reporting format. (From University of Nebraska Medical Center, Omaha, NE, with permission.)

Personnel and Facilities

Quality control is only as good as the personnel performing and monitoring it. Personnel must understand the importance of QA, and the program should be administered in a manner such that personnel view it as a learning experience rather than as a threat.[10] Up-to-date reference materials and atlases should be readily available, and documentation of continuing education must be maintained.

An adequate, uncluttered, safe working area is also essential for both quality work and personnel morale. Universal precautions for handling body fluids must be followed at all times.

POSTANALYTICAL FACTORS

Postanalytical factors are processes that affect the reporting of results and correct interpretation of data.[8]

Reporting of Results

Standardized reporting formats and, when applicable, reference ranges should be included with each procedure covered in the procedure manual. A written procedure for reporting, reviewing, and correcting errors must be present.

Forms for reporting results should provide adequate space for writing and should present the information in a logical sequence. Standardized reporting methods will minimize health-care provider confusion when interpreting results (Figure 7–7).

Written procedures should be available for the reporting of critical values (Figure 7–8). In laboratories analyzing pediatric specimens, this should include the presence of ketones or sugars in newborns.

Summary of Quality Assurance Errors

Preanalytical

Patient misidentification
Wrong test ordered
Incorrect urine specimen type collected
Insufficient urine volume
Delayed transport of urine to the laboratory
Incorrect storage or preservation of urine

Analytical

Sample misidentification
Erroneous instrument calibration
Reagent deterioration
Poor testing technique
Instrument malfunction
Interfering substances present
Misinterpretation of quality control data

Postanalytical

Patient misidentification
Poor handwriting
Poor quality of instrument printer
Failure to send report
Failure to call critical values
Inability to identify interfering substances

ST.JOSEPH HOSPITAL
PATHOLOGY DEPT
CLINICAL CHEMISTRY/ URINALYSIS SECTION

CRITICAL RESULTS REPORTING IN URINALYSIS

Prepared by: Carol Schmitt MT[ASCP]

Initial approval: George McClellan MD

Procedure placed in use: January 1991

Revised: June 1999

Reason for Revision: format change

Effective Date	Technical Approval	Medical Director Approval
Reviewed	[signature] 6/22/99	[signature] 6/22/99
Reviewed		
Reviewed		
Reviewed		
Reviewed		

POSITIVE KETONES:

All positive ketones on pediatrics less than or equal to two years old shall be called to the appropriate nursing unit. The time of the call, initials of the "tech", and the name of the person receiving the call are to be documented in the computer as a chartable footnote appended to the result.

POSITIVE CLINITEST;

All positive Clinitest results on pediatrics less than or equal to two years old shall be called to the appropriate nursing unit. The time of the call, initials of the "tech", and the name of the person receiving the call are to be documented in the computer as a chartable footnote appended to the result.

This policy shall be reviewed by the Chemistry Section Supervisor and Chemistry Section Director annually or whenever changes are made.

FIGURE 7–8 Sample critical results–reporting procedure. (From the Department of Pathology, St. Joseph Hospital, Omaha, NE, with permission.)

Interpretation of Results

The specificity and the sensitivity for each test should be included in the procedure manual for correct interpretation of results. All known interfering substances should be listed for evaluation of patient test data. A well-documented QA program will ensure quality test results and patient care.

Regulatory Issues

Clinical Laboratory Improvement Amendments '88 stipulate that all laboratories that perform testing on human specimens for the purposes of diagnosis, treatment, monitoring, or screening must be licensed. This includes all independent and hospital laboratories, physician-office laboratories, rural health clinics, mobile health screening entities such as health fairs, and public health clinics. CLIA '88 defined categories of diagnostic laboratory tests and specified the training and educational levels required of personnel performing the tests. Tests are assigned to the following categories: waived, provider-performed microscopy, moderate complexity, and high complexity.

Waived tests are considered easy to perform and interpret, require no special training or educational background, require only a minimum of standardization and QC, and are not considered critical to immediate patient care. Urinalysis tests in this category are manual dipstick/chemical tablet testing and urine pregnancy tests. In Table 7–2, the current tests in this category are listed. Tests continue to be modified, enabling them to be approved for waived testing.

A modification of the CLIA categories created a new certificate category for provider-performed microscopy (**PPM**) procedures. This category includes certain microscopic procedures that can be performed in conjunction with any waived test to avoid disruption in the patient visit. Personnel standards authorize only physicians, physician's assistants, nurse practitioners, and dentists to perform the tests. Laboratories performing PPM must meet the moderate-complexity requirements for proficiency testing, patient test management, QC, and QA. Urine sediment examinations, wet mounts, and KOH preparations are examples of the tests in this category. A complete listing is provided in Table 7–3.

Moderate-complexity tests are more difficult to perform than are waived tests and require documentation of training in testing principles, instrument calibration, periodic proficiency testing and on-site inspections. In a hospital setting, even waived tests must adhere to the moderate-complexity test standards. Most chemistry and hematology tests are assigned to this category. Automated or semiautomated urinalysis tests and urine microscopic procedures are considered moderate-complexity tests.

High-complexity tests require sophisticated instrumentation and a high degree of interpretation by the testing per-

TABLE 7–2 **CLIA '88 Waived Tests**

Dipstick/chemical tablet urinalysis
Ovulation pregnancy tests (visual color comparison)
Urine pregnancy tests (visual color comparison)
Erythrocyte sedimentation rate (nonautomated)
Hemoglobin by copper sulfate and Hemocue
Fecal occult blood
Spun hematocrit
Blood glucose (using FDA-approved home-use instruments)
Group A streptococcus, mononucleosis, and *Helicobacter pylori* kits
Point-of-care cholesterol screening instruments
Prothrombin time

TABLE 7–3 **Provider-Performed Microscopy Category**

Urine sediment examination
Wet mounts (vaginal, cervical, skin, or prostatic secretions)
KOH preparations
Pinworm examinations
Fern test
Postcoital direct, qualitative examinations of vaginal mucus
Fecal leukocyte examination
Qualitative semen analysis
Nasal smear for granulocytes

sonnel. Many tests performed in microbiology, immunology, immunohematology, and cytology are in this category.

Clinical Laboratory Improvement Amendments '88 regulations specify required components for QA that include patient test management assessment, QC assessment, proficiency testing assessment, comparison of test results, relationship of patient information to patient test results, personnel assessment, communications, complaint investigation, QA review with staff, and QA records.[4]

Patient test management includes systems for patient preparation, correct specimen collection, sample identification, sample preservation, sample transportation, sample processing, and accurate result reporting. The testing facility must have available written procedures for each system to ensure that specimen integrity and identification are maintained throughout the entire testing process.

Quality control assessment requires that quality control records include date, results, testing personnel, and lot numbers for reagents and controls. Records must be retained for 2 years. Records should be reviewed daily and monthly to detect trends, shifts, inconsistent test systems, or operator difficulties.

Proficiency testing is required for all laboratories performing PPM moderate-complexity or high-complexity testing. An approved program will involve three events per year with five challenges per analyte that is regulated.[5] Samples must be tested in the same manner as patient samples. Communication or consultation with other laboratories is not permitted.

Personnel assessment includes education and training, continuing education, competency assessment, and performance appraisals. Each new employee must have documentation of training during orientation to the laboratory. A checklist of procedures must be documented with the date and initials of the person doing the training and of the employee being trained.

The qualifications of the personnel performing patient care are also regulated to ensure that only persons with appropriate education and training perform procedures. Health-care personnel become certified and/or licensed in their particular fields through the completion of specified educational requirements and/or satisfactory performance on standardized proficiency examinations. The level of education is documented in the employee personnel file. A record of all continuing education sessions should be kept in each personnel file. Currently no minimum hours of continuing education are mandated.

Technical competency assessment as mandated by CLIA '88 must be done for each employee for each procedure twice during the first year of employment and then annually. Methods for assessing competency include direct observation, review of QC records, review of proficiency testing records, and written assessments.[3]

Performance appraisals for each employee are done following the institution's protocol and evaluate the standards of performance as designated by the job description. The standards must be specific and measurable and may include evaluation of attitude as well as organizational and communication skills.

Clinical laboratory records must be maintained for 2 years. These records include patient test results, QC data, reagent logs, proficiency test data, competency assessment, education and training, equipment maintenance, service calls, documentation of problems, complaints, communication, inspection files, and certification records.

The Clinical Laboratory Improvement Amendments '88 are administered by the Health Care Financing Administration (**HCFA**). Accrediting agencies that have been approved by the federal government after demonstrating equivalency with CLIA '88 standards include the Commission on Laboratory Assessment (**COLA**), which is popular with physician office laboratories; the JCAHO; and CAP, which serves large laboratories. Compliance with accreditation regulations is ensured by periodic on-site visits to facilities by inspection teams and through performance on proficiency tests. If deficiencies are present, the facility must correct them within a specified time and be reinspected. Waived and PPM laboratories are not subject to routine inspection. Inspections must be scheduled and are done within the first 2 years of certification. The ultimate goal of these agencies is to promote ***continuous quality improvement*** (**CQI**).[3]

Continuous Quality Improvement

Quality control and QA programs are part of institutional CQI and ***total quality management*** (**TQM**). Whereas QA is designed to maintain an established level of quality, TQM and CQI are designed to develop methods to continually improve the quality of health care. Standards from the JCAHO address this concept by requiring documentation showing that effective, appropriate patient care is being provided, as shown by positive patient ***outcomes***. Areas addressed by the standards include availability of services, timeliness, continuity of care, effectiveness and efficiency of services, safety of service provided, and respect and care by the personnel providing services.

Total quality management is based on a team concept involving personnel at all levels working together to achieve a final outcome of customer satisfaction through implementation of policies and procedures identified by the CQI program. This concept applies scientific principles to management and uses graphical and statistical analysis of data as a basis for decision making.[13] TQM is a systematic problem-solving approach using visual tools to identify the steps in the process for meeting customer satisfaction of quality care in a timely manner at reduced costs. In the health-care setting, the patient is the ultimate customer; customers also include health-care providers, personnel in other departments, and the patient's family and friends. TQM is far-reaching and encompasses the quality and performance assessment of the infrastructure (physical, personnel, and management), ***processes***, outcomes, and customer satisfaction.

The focus of CQI is to improve patient outcomes by providing continual quality care in a constantly changing health-care environment. Performance is defined as what is done and how well it is done to provide health care. The level of performance in health care is the degree to which what is done is effective and appropriate for the individual patient and the degree to which it is available in a timely manner to patients who need it.[2] Characteristics of doing the right thing and doing the right thing well are termed the dimensions of performance.[12] Four phases of quality in doing the right things right can be demonstrated.[7] The first phase is "right things done wrong"—an example in urinalysis might be the acquisition of a very expensive and efficient instrument such as the 900 UDx Urine Pathology system but the personnel in the laboratory are not trained to use the instrument properly. The second phase is "wrong things done right"—an example would be the urinalysis instrument is insufficient for testing but the personnel in the laboratory make it work for them. The third phase is "wrong things done wrong"—an example would be an incorrectly calibrated 900UDx Urine Pathology system and no one in the laboratory knowing how to use the instrument. The fourth phase is "right things done right"—this is the ultimate goal and is represented by a properly calibrated 900UDx Urine Pathology system and all urinalysis laboratory personnel well trained to operate the instrument and interpret the results. The goal of CQI involves continuous performance improvement to ensure that "right things are done right" all of the time.

Helpful tools to assess CQI are flowcharts, cause and effect diagrams (fish-bone diagrams), pareto charts, histograms, run charts, and cause and effect diagrams. A flowchart is a picture of the process mapping out each individual step so that each group member can understand how it works. Cause and effect diagrams determine the cause of a problem and identify the different elements that contribute to the problem. They relate the interaction between equipment, methods, and customers. Pareto charts are based on the Pareto principle that states 80 percent of the trouble comes from 20 percent of the problems. Pareto charts are used to mainly identify the problems. The information in this type of graph displays the major contributors to a problem in descending order of importance. A run chart tracks individual data points recorded in a time sequence and compares the points to the average. It is useful to determine cyclic or seasonal differences. Control charts provide statistically determined limits drawn on both sides of the line indicating deviations from the average. Scatter diagrams are a visual plotting technique used to evaluate cause and effect correlations between two variables. Histograms display the shape of distribution of a variable indicating the amount of variation and are often used to summarize and communicate data.

Many models based on W. Edward Deming's 14 principles of CQI are available for implementing CQI. One example is the JCAHO 10-step process (Table 7–4). The most widely used plan for quality improvement in health care is the Plan-Do-Check-Act (**PDCA**) strategy.[7]

The "Plan" step is the process of making a change by identifying the customers and customer expectations, describing the current process, measuring and analyzing, focusing on improvement opportunities, identifying the root cause, and generating a solution. External customers are people such as the vendors or health-care providers who are not employed by one's organization. Internal customers are employees within the organization who are dependent on one's service. A nurse requesting a urinalysis result on a patient would be a customer of the laboratory. Customer needs and expectations are identified in the health-care field most often through complaint analysis, focus groups and interviews, satisfaction surveys, and JCAHO professional standards. An example would be "How to reduce the TAT for a patient's urinalysis test result?" Through the use of flowcharts, cause and effect diagrams, and Pareto charts (Figures 7–9 through 7–11), the data can visually be measured and analyzed, and the committee can arrive at a problem statement and focus on improvement opportunities. After generating theories of causes and collecting data, the root cause can be pinpointed, and, through focus groups with customers, discussions with staff, and brainstorming, a solution can be produced.

TABLE 7–4 **JCAHO 10-Step Process**

1. Appoint responsibility.
2. Outline the scope of care.
3. Identify key aspects of care.
4. Devise indicators.
5. Define thresholds of evaluation.
6. Collect and organize data.
7. Evaluate data.
8. Develop a corrective action plan.
9. Assess actions and document improvement.
10. Communicate relevant information.

The "Do" step is the process of testing the improvement by mapping out a trial run, implementing that run, collecting data, and analyzing the data. The person responsible for each step and the dates and time frames for the trial should be specified. Steps used to monitor implementation of the trial run and verification of results must be documented. As an example for the above urinalysis TAT, a trial run to shorten urinalysis testing TAT could be to transport the specimen from the patient location to the laboratory via a pneumatic tube system immediately upon collection.

The "Check" step involves evaluating the results and drawing conclusions as to the effect of the change. Tools to evaluate the solution are control charts, run or trend charts, simple observations, and surveys. From these results, it can be determined whether the process was a success, failure, or in need of minor modifications. An example would be to use a run chart to plot TATs from the time of collection of urine through the testing procedure to the time the report appeared in the patient chart for those specimens being transported by the pneumatic tube system.

The "Act" step is standardizing the change by modifying the standard procedure, policies, and performance expectations to reflect the changed process. These changes must be communicated effectively to the customers to ensure implementation and to avoid resistance to change. A plan must indicate ways the new procedure will be incorporated and how the customers will be supported throughout the change process and provide training to the people involved. In the previous urinalysis example, proper training

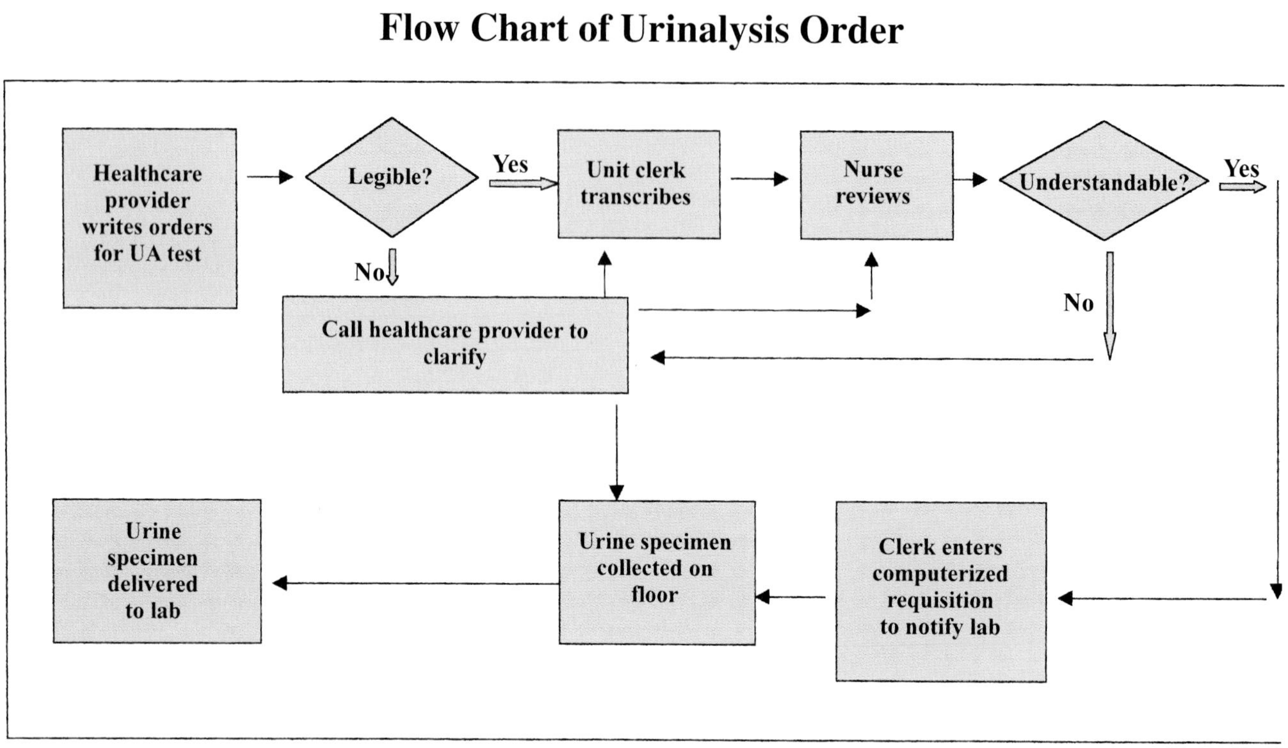

FIGURE 7–9 Flow chart demonstrating steps in the urinalysis collection procedure.

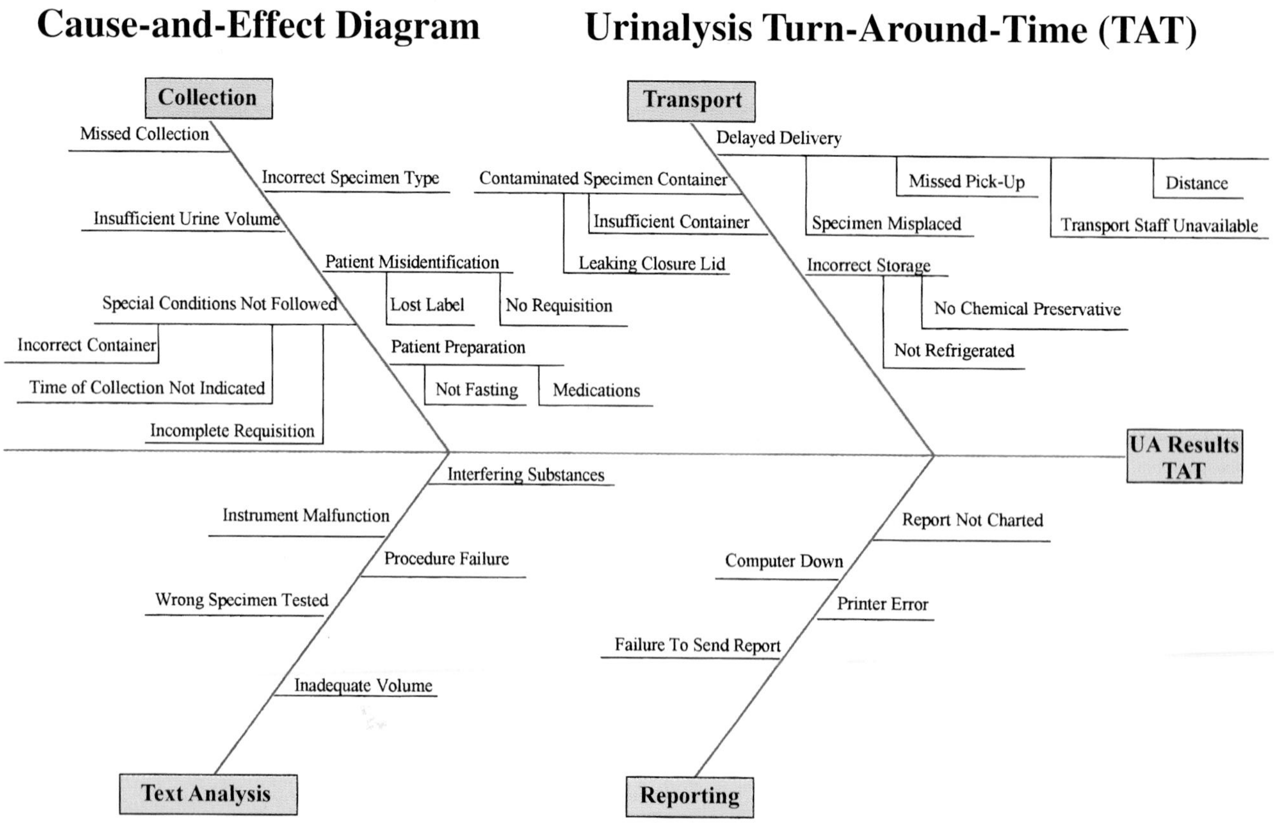

FIGURE 7–10 Cause-and-effect diagram for analyzing urinalysis TAT.

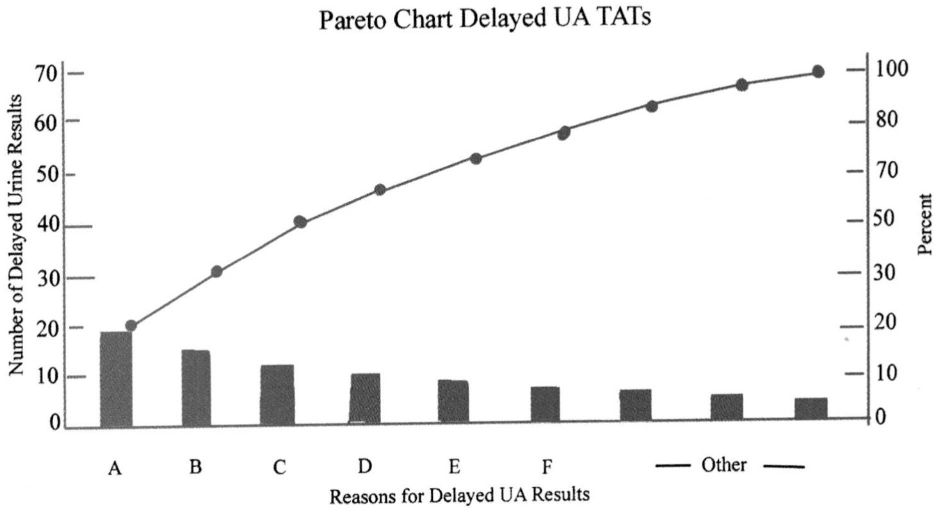

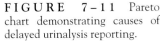

FIGURE 7-11 Pareto chart demonstrating causes of delayed urinalysis reporting.

on bagging the specimen to avoid leakage and on operating the pneumatic tube system would be necessary. Implementation of a regular schedule of measurement to monitor the change over an extended period confirms the success of the change or the gain.

The JCAHO 1996 *Comprehensive Accreditation Manual for Hospitals* recommends a method for improving organizational performance (**IOP**). Known as PDMAI, the plan provides standards PI.1 through PI.5 (plan, design, measure, assess, and improve) to outline a specific cycle for improving performance.[2,6,12] The five essential elements for performance improvement are as follows:

Plan (PI.1): The hospital has a planned, systematic, hospital-wide approach to process design and performance measurement, assessment, and improvement.

Design (PI.2): New processes are designed well.

Measure (PI.3): The organization has a systematic process in place to collect data.

Assess (PI.4): The hospital uses a systematic process to assess collected data.

Improve (PI.5): The hospital systematically improves its performance.

With a constant focus on quality, the JCAHO standards are easily attained. By instituting the above quality improvement methodologies, a structured standardized format can be developed to systematically assess and document the quality of services to the customer.

REFERENCES

1. College of American Pathologists: Commission of Inspection and Accreditation Inspection Checklist. Section 3A, 30: Urinalysis. College of American Pathologists, Skokie, IL, 1994.
2. Comprehensive Accreditation Manual for Hospitals: The Official Handbook, Improving Organization Performance. CAMH Update 4, November 1997.
3. Costaras, J: Urinalysis: It gets no respect. ADVANCE for Medical Laboratory Professionals, p.10, 11, August 11, 1997.
4. DiLorenzo, M, et al: Basic Laboratory Methods for Allied Health Professionals. University of Nebraska Medical Center, Division of Medical Technology, School of Allied Health Professions, Add-A-Competency Grant Project 1 D37 AHOO565-01, Funded by the United States Department of Health and Human Services, 1999.
5. Hodnett, J: Proficiency testing, we all do it—but what do the results mean?. Lab Med 30(5):316–323, 1999.
6. Holmes, R: Conquering performance improvement documentation for JCAHO. Medical Laboratory Observer 30(6):18,19,22,24, 1998.
7. Hrdlicka, D: Quality Improvement Made Simple. Advanced Management Information Technology—3, Add-A Competency, University of Nebraska Medical Center, Division of Medical Technology, 1998.
8. Hyduke, R: Quality Assurance, Urinalysis: Part 1A. Specimen Collections and Gross/Chemical Analysis, Virtual Hospital: Urinalysis for the Physical and Chemical Analysis: Quality Assurance, http://www.vh.org/Providers/CME/CLIA/UrineAnalysis/1.3Quality.htr.
9. National Committee for Clinical Laboratory Standards, NCCLS-Approved Guideline: GP16-A, Vol 15 No. 15,Urinalysis and Collection, Transportation, and Preservation of Urine Specimens: Approved Guideline, December, 1995.
10. Schweitzer, SC, Schumann, JL, and Schumann, GB: Quality assurance guidelines for the urinalysis laboratory. J Med Technol 3(11):567–572, 1986.
11. Strasinger, SK: Urinalysis and Body Fluids, ed 3. FA Davis, Philadelphia, 1994.
12. Trant, C, Broda, K, and Edwards, G: Department of Pathology Duke University Medical Center, Durham, NC, JCAHO Inspection: Preparing the Laboratory, AACC 50th Anniversary Meeting Workshop #2407, Chicago, Illinois, August 5, 1998.
13. Yablonsky, MA: Total quality management in the laboratory from under the microscope into practice. Lab Med 26(4):253–260, 1995.

STUDY QUESTIONS

1. Explain the difference between QC and QA.
2. When the CAP inspects the urinalysis laboratory, what piece of documentation is always required?
3. Name two times when a laboratory-designated person must document a review of a procedure manual.
4. Indicate whether each of the following would be considered a 1) preanalytical, 2) analytical, or 3) postanalytical factor by placing the appropriate number in the space:

_____ Reagent expiration date
_____ Rejection of a contaminated specimen
_____ Construction of a Levy-Jennings chart
_____ Telephoning a positive Clinitest result on a newborn

_____ Calibrating the centrifuge
_____ Collecting a timed urine specimen

5. Can a test be precise and not be accurate? Explain your answer.

6. Under what conditions must internal and external quality control tests be performed?

7. Would a control sample that has accidentally become diluted produce a trend or a shift in the Levy-Jennings plot?

8. List three steps that are taken when the results of reagent strip QC results are outside of the stated confidence limits.

9. When a new bottle of QC material is opened, what information is placed on the label?

10. When a control is run, what information is documented?

11. When a new bottle of reagent strips is opened, what two controls should be run?

12. List the four categories of laboratory tests designated by CLIA '88.

13. State which of the above categories is assigned to each of the following: reagent strip urinalysis, urine culture, complete urinalysis using the Clinitek 200, urine microscopic, and urine pregnancy test.

14. What three categories of laboratory testing require documented proficiency testing of personnel as mandated by CLIA '88?

15. What documentation of new employees must the laboratory perform?

16. How often does CLIA '88 require documentation of technical competency?

17. How does QA differ from TQM andCQI?

18. List six areas relating to patient outcomes that are included in the JCAHO standards.

19. Who are the laboratory's "customers" in CQI?

20. What is the primary goal of CQI?

21. State the purpose for developing each of the following: flowcharts, cause and effect diagrams, Pareto charts, and run charts.

22. Briefly explain the four steps of the PDCA method for quality improvement.

23. What is the purpose of the JCAHO 10-step process?

24. List the five essential elements for performance improvement as stated by JCAHO.

CASE STUDIES AND CLINICAL SITUATIONS

1. State a possible reason for an accreditation team to report a deficiency in the following situations:
   a. The urine microscopic reporting procedure has been recently revised.
   b. An unusually high number of urine specimens are being rejected because of improper collection.
   c. A key statement is missing from the Clinitest procedure.
   d. Open control bottles in the refrigerator are examined.

2. A physician consults a medical technologist to answer the following questions regarding CLIA '88:
   a. Can I perform urine microscopics?
   b. If I purchase an automated urinalysis strip reader and a chemistry analyzer:

      Will my CLIA status be affected?
      Will my office be required to perform proficiency testing?
      Will my office be subject to COLA inspections?

3. A hospital laboratory outreach coordinator is asked to develop a method to decrease the number of rejected specimens for urinalysis received from physicians' offices.
   a. What accepted process could the coordinator follow?
   b. Briefly outline the steps the coordinator should take to address this problem, including the use of visual documentation.

4. As the new supervisor of the urinalysis section, you encounter the following situations. Explain whether you would accept them or take corrective action.
   a. You are told that the supervisor always performs the CAP proficiency survey.
   b. QC is not performed daily on the Clinitest tablets.
   c. The urinalysis section is primarily staffed by personnel assigned to other departments for whom you have no personnel data.

CHAPTER 8

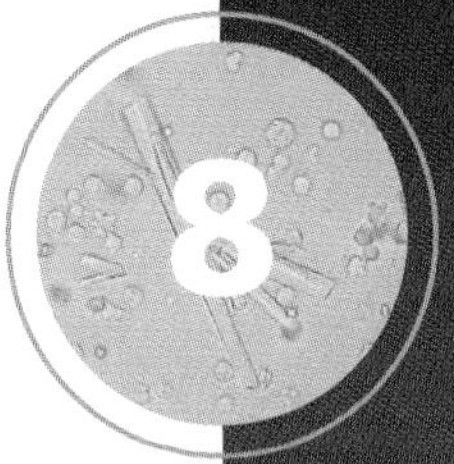
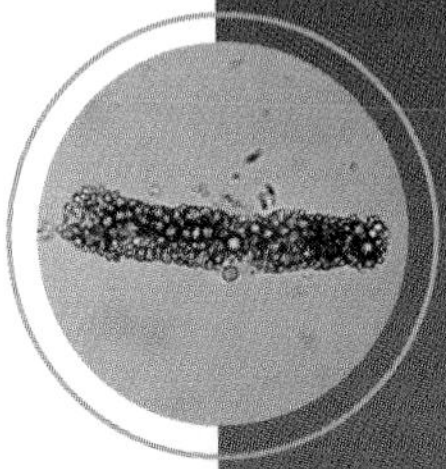
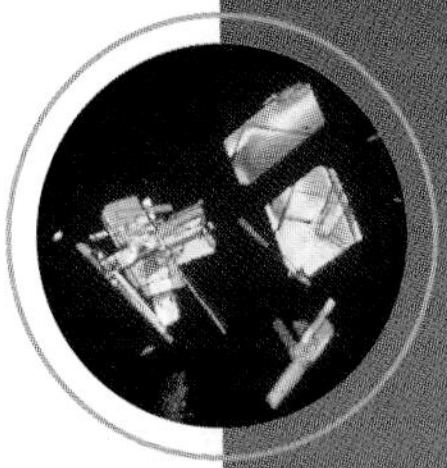
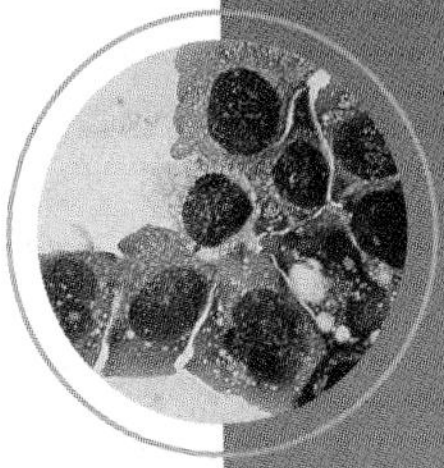
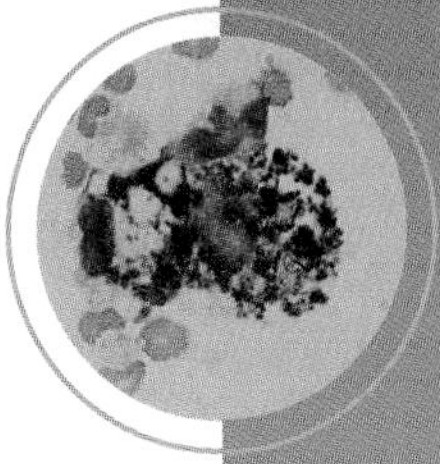

Renal Disease

LEARNING OBJECTIVES

Upon completion of this chapter, the reader will be able to:

1 Differentiate among renal diseases of glomerular, tubular, interstitial, and vascular origin.
2 Describe the processes by which immunologic damage is produced to the glomerular membrane.
3 Define glomerulonephritis.
4 Describe the characteristic clinical symptoms, etiology, and urinalysis findings in acute poststreptococcal and rapidly progressive glomerulonephritis, Goodpasture's syndrome, Wegener's granulomatosis, and Henoch-Schönlein purpura.
5 Name a significant urinary sediment constituent associated with all of the aforementioned disorders.
6 Name three renal disorders that also involve acute respiratory symptoms.
7 Differentiate between membranous and membranoproliferative glomerulonephritis.
8 Discuss the clinical course and significant laboratory results associated with immunoglobulin A nephropathy.
9 Relate laboratory results associated with the nephrotic syndrome to the disease process.
10 Compare and contrast the nephrotic syndrome and minimal change disease with regard to laboratory results and course of disease.
11 State two causes of acute tubular necrosis.
12 Name the urinary sediment constituent most diagnostic of renal tubular damage.
13 Define Fanconi's syndrome.
14 Compare and contrast the urinalysis results in patients with cystitis, pyelonephritis, and acute interstitial nephritis.
15 Differentiate among causes of laboratory results associated with prerenal, renal, and postrenal acute renal failure.
16 Discuss the formation of renal calculi, composition of renal calculi, and patient management techniques.

KEY TERMS

antiglomerular basement membrane antibody
cystitis
glomerulonephritis
lithiasis
nephrotic syndrome
pyelonephritis
tubulointerstitial disease

Disorders throughout the body can affect renal function and produce abnormalities in the urinalysis. Considering that the major function of the kidneys is filtration of the blood to remove waste products, it becomes evident that the kidneys are consistently exposed to potentially damaging substances.

Renal disease is often classified as being of glomerular, tubular, **interstitial**, or vascular origin based on the area of the kidney primarily affected. In this chapter, the most commonly encountered disorders will be covered in relation to the affected areas of the kidney, keeping in mind that some overlap will occur.

Glomerular Disorders

The majority of the disorders associated with the glomerulus are of immune origin, resulting from immunologic disorders throughout the body, including the kidney. **Immune complexes** formed as a result of immunologic reactions and increased serum immunoglobulins, such as immunoglobulin A (**IgA**), circulate in the bloodstream and are deposited on the glomerular membranes. Components of the immune system, including complement, neutrophils, lymphocytes, monocytes, and cytokines, are then attracted to the area, producing changes and damage to the membranes. Depending on the immune system mediators involved, damage may consist of cellular infiltration or proliferation and thickening of the glomerular basement membrane, which disrupt normal filtration by the glomerulus.

Nonimmunologic causes of glomerular damage include exposure to chemicals and toxins that also affect the tubules, disruption of the electrical membrane charges as occurs in the ***nephrotic syndrome***, deposition of amyloid material from systemic disorders that may involve chronic inflammation and acute-phase reactants, and the basement membrane thickening associated with diabetic nephropathy.

Glomerulonephritis

In general, ***glomerulonephritis*** refers to a sterile, inflammatory process that affects the glomerulus and is associated with the finding of blood, protein, and casts in the urine.[6] A variety of types of glomerulonephritis exist and also may progress from one form to another (i.e., acute glomerular nephritis (**AGN**) to chronic glomerulonephritis to the nephrotic syndrome and eventual renal failure).

ACUTE POSTSTREPTOCOCCAL GLOMERULONEPHRITIS

As its name implies, acute glomerulonephritis is a disease marked by the sudden onset of symptoms consistent with damage to the glomerular membrane. These may include fever; **edema**, most noticeably around the eyes; fatigue; hypertension; oliguria; and hematuria. Symptoms usually occur in children and young adults following respiratory infections caused by certain strains of group A streptococcus that contain M protein in the cell wall. During the course of the infection, these nephrogenic strains of streptococci form immune complexes with their corresponding circulating antibodies and become deposited on the glomerular membranes. The accompanying inflammatory reaction affects glomerular function.

In most cases, successful management of the secondary complications, hypertension, and electrolyte imbalance, until the immune complexes have been cleared from the blood and the inflammation subsides, will result in no permanent kidney damage. Similar symptoms also may be seen following pneumonia, endocarditis, and other severe infections.[8]

Primary urinalysis findings include marked hematuria, proteinuria, and oliguria, accompanied by red blood cell (RBC) casts, dysmorphic RBCs, hyaline and granular casts, and white blood cells (WBCs). As toxicity to the glomerular membrane subsides, the urinalysis results will return to normal, with the possible exception of microscopic hematuria that lasts until the membrane damage has been repaired. Blood urea nitrogen (**BUN**) may be elevated during the acute stages but, like the urinalysis, will return to normal. Demonstration of an elevated serum antistreptolysin O (**ASO**) titer provides evidence that the disease is of streptococcal origin.

RAPIDLY PROGRESSIVE (CRESCENTIC) GLOMERULONEPHRITIS

A more serious form of acute glomerular disease is called rapidly progressive (or crescentic) glomerulonephritis (**RPGN**) and has a much poorer prognosis, often terminating in renal failure. Symptoms are initiated by deposition of immune complexes in the glomerulus often as a complication of another form of glomerulonephritis or an immune systemic disorder such as **systemic lupus erythematosus**. Damage by macrophages to the capillary walls releases cells and plasma into Bowman's space, and the production of crescentic formations containing macrophages, fibroblasts, and polymerized fibrin causes permanent damage to the capillary tufts.

Initial laboratory results are similar to acute glomerulonephritis but become more abnormal as the disease progresses, including markedly elevated protein levels and very low glomerular filtration rates. Some forms may demonstrate increased fibrin degradation products, cryoglobulins, and the deposition of immunoglobulin A (IgA) immune complexes in the glomerulus.[4]

GOODPASTURE'S SYNDROME

Morphologic changes to the glomeruli resembling those in RPGN are seen in conjunction with the autoimmune disorder termed Goodpasture's syndrome. Appearance of a cytotoxic autoantibody against the glomerular and alveolar basement membranes can follow viral respiratory infections. Attachment of this autoantibody to the basement membrane followed by complement activation produces the capillary destruction. Referred to as ***antiglomerular basement membrane antibody***, the autoantibody can be detected in patient serum.

Initial pulmonary complaints are **hemoptysis** and **dyspnea** followed by the development of hematuria. Urinalysis results include proteinuria, hematuria, and the presence of RBC casts. Progression to chronic glomerulonephritis and end-stage renal failure is common.

Vasculitis

Several immune-mediated disorders affecting the systemic vascular system can result in glomerular involvement, producing symptoms and urinalysis results similar to those associated with acute glomerulonephritis. Damage may be the result of immune complex deposition, autoantibodies binding to vascular structures, and immune-mediate inflammation.[3] The vasculitis syndromes primarily associated with glomerular involvement are Wegener's granulomatosis and Henoch-Schönlein **purpura**.

Wegener's granulomatosis causes a **granuloma**-producing inflammation of the small blood vessels of primarily the kidney and respiratory system. Key to the diagnosis of Wegener's granulomatosis is the demonstration of antineutrophilic cytoplasmic antibody (**ANCA**) in the patient's serum.[9] Binding of these autoantibodies to the neutrophils located in the vascular walls may initiate the immune response and the resulting granuloma formation. Patients usually present first with pulmonary symptoms and later develop renal involvement including, hematuria, proteinuria, RBC casts, and elevated serum creatinine and BUN.

Henoch-Schönlein purpura is a disease occurring primarily in children following upper respiratory infections. As its name implies, initial symptoms include the appearance of raised, red patches on the skin. Respiratory and gastrointestinal symptoms including blood in the sputum and stools may be present. Renal involvement is the most serious complication of the disorder and may range from mild to heavy proteinuria and hematuria with RBC casts. Complete recovery with normal renal function is seen in more than 50 percent of patients. In other patients, progression to a more serious form of glomerulonephritis and renal failure may occur. Urinalysis and renal function assessment should be used to monitor patients following recovery from the original symptoms.

Immunogloblin A Nephropathy

Also known as Berger's disease, IgA **nephropathy**, in which immune complexes containing immunoglobulin A are deposited on the glomerular membrane, is the most common cause of glomerulonephritis. Patients have increased serum levels of IgA, which may be a result of a mucosal infection. The disorder is most frequently seen in children and young adults.

Patients usually present with an episode of macroscopic hematuria following an infection or strenuous exercise. Recovery from the macroscopic hematuria is spontaneous; however, asymptomatic microhematuria and elevated serum levels of IgA remain.[2] Except for periodic episodes of macroscopic hematuria, a patient with the disorder may remain essentially asymptomatic for 20 years or more; however, there is a gradual progression to chronic glomerulonephritis and end-stage renal disease.

Membranous Glomerulonephritis

The predominant characteristic of membranous glomerulonephritis is a pronounced thickening of the glomerular basement membrane resulting from the deposition of immunoglobulin G immune complexes. Disorders associated with the development of membranous glomerulonephritis include systemic lupus erythematosus, **Sjögren's syndrome**, secondary syphilis, hepatitis B, gold and mercury treatments, and malignancy. Many cases of unknown etiology have been reported. As a rule, the disease progresses slowly with possible remission; however, frequent development of nephrotic syndrome symptoms occurs.[13] There may also be a tendency toward **thrombosis**.

Laboratory findings include microscopic hematuria and elevated urine protein excretion that may reach concentrations similar to those in the nephrotic syndrome. Demonstration of one of the secondary disorders through blood tests can aid in the diagnosis.

Membranoproliferative Glomerulonephritis

Membranoproliferative glomerulonephritis (**MPGN**) is marked by two different alterations in the cellularity of the glomerulus and peripheral capillaries. Type I displays increased cellularity in the subendothelial cells of the mesangium (interstitial area of Bowman's capsule), causing thickening of the capillary walls, whereas type II displays extremely dense deposits in the glomerular basement membrane. Many of the patients are children, and the disease has a poor prognosis, with type I patients progressing to the nephrotic syndrome and type II patients experiencing symptoms of chronic glomerulonephritis. The laboratory findings are variable; however, hematuria, proteinuria, and decreased serum complement levels are usual findings. There appears to be an association with autoimmune disorders, infections, and malignancies.[5]

Chronic Glomerulonephritis

Depending on the amount and duration of the damage occurring to the glomerulus in the previously discussed glomerular disorders, progression to chronic glomerulonephritis and end-stage renal disease may occur. Gradually worsening symptoms include fatigue, anemia, hypertension, edema, and oliguria.

Examination of the urine reveals hematuria, proteinuria, glucosuria as a result of tubular dysfunction, and many varieties of casts, including broad casts. A markedly decreased glomerular filtration rate is present in conjunction with increased BUN and creatinine levels and electrolyte imbalance.

Nephrotic Syndrome

The nephrotic syndrome is marked by massive proteinuria (greater than 3.5 g/d), low levels of serum albumin, high levels of serum lipids, and pronounced edema.[6] Acute onset of the disorder can occur in instances of circulatory disruption producing systemic shock, which decreases the pressure and flow of blood to the kidney. Progression to the nephrotic syndrome also may occur as a complication of the previously discussed forms of glomerulonephritis.

Increased permeability of the glomerular membrane is attributed to damage to the membrane and changes in the electrical charges in the basal lamina and podocytes, producing a less tightly connected barrier. This facilitates the passage of high-molecular-weight proteins and lipids into the urine. Albumin is the primary protein depleted from the circulation. The ensuing hypoalbuminemia appears to stimulate the increased production of lipids by the liver. The lower oncotic pressure in the capillaries resulting from the depletion of plasma albumin increases the loss of fluid into the interstitial spaces, which, accompanied by sodium retention, produces the edema. Depletion of immunoglobulins and coagulation factors places patients at an increased risk of infection and coagulation disorders. Tubular damage, in addition to glomerular damage, occurs, and the nephrotic syndrome may progress to chronic renal failure.

Urinalysis observations include marked proteinuria; urinary fat droplets; oval fat bodies; renal tubular epithelial (RTE) cells; epithelial, fatty, and waxy casts; and microscopic hematuria. Absorption of the lipid-containing proteins by the RTE cells followed by cellular sloughing produces the characteristic oval fat bodies seen in the sediment examination.

Minimal Change Disease

As the name implies, minimal change disease (also known as lipid nephrosis) produces little cellular change in the glomerulus, although the podocytes appear to be less tightly fitting, allowing for the increased filtration of protein. Patients are usually children who present with edema, heavy proteinuria, transient hematuria, and normal BUN and creatinine results. Although the etiology is unknown at this time, allergic reactions, recent immunization, and possession of the human leukocyte antigen-B12 (HLA-B12) antigen have been associated. The disorder responds well to corticosteroids, and prognosis is generally good, with frequent complete remissions.[11]

Focal Segmental Glomerulosclerosis

In contrast to the previously discussed disorders, focal segmental **glomerulosclerosis (FSGS)** affects only certain numbers and areas of glomeruli, and the others remain normal. Symptoms may be similar to the nephrotic syndrome and minimal change disease owing to damaged podocytes. Immune deposits, primarily immunoglobulins M and C3, are a frequent finding and can be seen in undamaged glomeruli. FSGS is often seen in association with abuse of heroin and analgesics and with acquired immunodeficiency syndrome. Moderate to heavy proteinuria and microscopic hematuria are the most consistent urinalysis findings.

Laboratory testing and clinical information for the glomerular disorders are summarized in Tables 8–1 and 8–2.

Tubular Disorders

Disorders affecting the renal tubules include those in which tubular function is disrupted as a result of actual damage to the tubules and those in which a metabolic or hereditary disorder affects the intricate functions of the tubules.

Acute Tubular Necrosis

The primary disorder associated with damage to the renal tubules is acute tubular **necrosis (ATN)**. Damage to the RTE cells may be produced by decreased blood flow by causing lack of oxygen presentation to the tubules (**ischemia**), or the presence of toxic substances in the urinary filtrate.

Disorders causing ischemic ATN include shock, trauma, such as crushing injuries, and surgical procedures. Shock is a general term indicating a severe condition that decreases the flow of blood throughout the body. Examples of conditions that may cause shock are cardiac failures, sepsis involving toxogenic bacteria, anaphylaxis, massive hemorrhage, and contact with high-voltage electricity.

Exposure to a variety of nephrotoxic agents can damage and affect the function of the RTE cells. Substances include the aminoglycoside antibiotics, the antifungal agent amphotericin, cyclosporine, radiographic dye, organic solvents such as ethylene glycol, heavy metals, and mushroom poisoning. As discussed in Chapter 5, filtration of large amounts of hemoglobin and myoglobin also is nephrotoxic.

The disease course of ATN is variable. It may present as an acute complication of an ischemic event or more gradually during exposure to toxic agents. Correction of the ischemia and removal of toxic substances followed by effective management of the accompanying symptoms of acute renal failure frequently result in a complete recovery.

Urinalysis findings include mild proteinuria, microscopic hematuria, and most noticeably the presence of RTE cells and RTE cell casts containing tubular fragments consisting of three or more cells. As a result of the tubular damage, a variety of other casts may be present, including hyaline, granular, waxy, and broad.

Hereditary and Metabolic Tubular Disorders

Disorders affecting tubular function may be caused by systemic conditions that affect or override the tubular reabsorptive maximum (**Tm**) for particular substances normally reabsorbed by the tubules or by failure to inherit a gene or genes required for tubular reabsorption.

The disorder most frequently associated with tubular dysfunction is Fanconi's syndrome. The syndrome consists of a generalized failure of tubular reabsorption in the proximal convoluted tubule. Therefore, substances most noticeably affected include glucose, amino acids, phosphorous,

TABLE 8–1 **Summary of Laboratory Testing in Glomerular Disorders**

Disorder	Primary Urinalysis Result	Other Significant Tests
Acute glomerulonephritis	Macroscopic hematuria Proteinuria Red blood cell casts Granular casts	Antistreptolysin O titer Anti–group A streptococcal enzymes
Rapidly progressive glomerulonephritis	Macroscopic hematuria Proteinuria Red blood cell casts	Blood urea nitrogen Creatinine Creatinine clearance
Goodpasture's syndrome	Macroscopic hematuria Proteinuria Red blood cell casts	Antiglomerular basement membrane antibody
Wegener's granulomatosis	Macroscopic hematuria Proteinuria Red blood cell casts	Antineutrophilic cytoplasmic antibody
Henoch-Schönlein purpura	Macroscopic hematuria Proteinuria Red blood cell casts	Stool occult blood
IgA nephropathy (early stages)	Macroscopic or microscopic hematuria	Serum immunoglobulin A
IgA nephropathy (late stages)	See Chronic Glomerulonephritis	
Membranous glomerulonephritis	Microscopic hematuria Proteinuria	Antinuclear antibody Hepatitis B surface antigen Fluorescent treponemal antibody-absorption test (FTA-ABS)
Membranoproliferative glomerulonephritis	Hematuria Proteinuria	Serum complement levels
Chronic glomerulonephritis	Hematuria Proteinuria Glucosuria Cellular and granular casts Waxy and broad casts	Blood urea nitrogen Serum creatinine Creatinine clearance Electrolytes
Nephrotic syndrome	Heavy proteinuria Microscopic hematuria Renal tubular cells Oval fat bodies Fat droplets Fatty and waxy casts	Serum albumin Cholesterol Triglycerides
Minimal change disease	Heavy proteinuria Transient hematuria Fat droplets	Serum albumin Cholesterol Triglycerides
Focal segmental glomerulonephritis	Proteinuria Microscopic hematuria	Drugs of abuse HIV tests

sodium, potassium, bicarbonate, and water. Fanconi's syndrome may be inherited in association with cystinosis and Hartnup disease (see Chap. 9) or acquired through exposure to toxic agents, including heavy metals and outdated tetracycline, or as a complication of multiple myeloma and renal transplant.

Interstitial Disorders

Considering the close proximity between the renal tubules and the renal interstitium, disorders affecting the interstitium also affect the tubules, resulting in the commonly used term ***tubulointerstitial disease***. The majority of these disorders involve infections and inflammatory conditions.

The most common renal disease is urinary tract infection (**UTI**). Infection may involve the lower urinary tract (urethra and bladder) or the upper urinary tract (renal pelvis, tubules, and interstitium). Most frequently encountered is infection of the bladder (***cystitis***), which if untreated can then progress to a more serious upper UTI. Cystitis is seen more often in women and children who present with symptoms of urinary frequency and burning. Urinalysis reveals the presence of numerous WBCs and bacteria often accompanied by mild proteinuria and hematuria and an increased pH.

TABLE 8–2 **Summary of Clinical Information Associated with Glomerular Disorders**

Disorder	Etiology	Clinical Course
Acute glomerulonephritis	Deposition of immune complexes, formed in conjunction with group A *Streptococcus* infection, on the glomerular membranes	Rapid onset of hematuria and edema Permanent renal damage seldom occurs
Rapidly progressive glomerulonephritis	Deposition of immune complexes from systemic immune disorders on the glomerular membrane	Rapid onset with glomerular damage and possible progression to end-stage renal failure
Goodpasture's syndrome	Attachment of a cytotoxic antibody formed during viral respiratory infections to glomerular and alveolar basement membranes	Hemoptysis and dyspnea followed by hematuria Possible progression to end-stage renal failure
Wegener's granulomatosis	Antineutrophilic cytoplasmic autoantibody binds to neutrophils in vascular walls producing damage to small vessels in the lungs and glomerulus	Pulmonary symptoms including hemoptysis develop first followed by renal involvement and possible progression to end-stage renal failure
Henoch-Schönlein purpura	Occurs primarily in children following viral respiratory infections; a decrease in platelets disrupts vascular integrity	Initial appearance of purpura followed by blood in sputum and stools and eventual renal involvement Complete recovery is common, but may progress to renal failure
IgA nephropathy	Deposition of IgA on the glomerular membrane resulting from increased levels of serum IgA	Recurrent macroscopic hematuria following exercise with slow progression to chronic glomerulonephritis
Membranous glomerulonephritis	Thickening of the glomerular membrane following IgG immune complex deposition associated with systemic disorders	Slow progression to the nephrotic syndrome or possible remission
Membranoproliferative glomerulonephritis	Cellular proliferation affecting the capillary walls or the glomerular basement membrane, possibly immune mediated	Slow progression to chronic glomerulonephritis or nephrotic syndrome
Chronic glomerulonephritis	Marked decrease in renal function resulting from glomerular damage precipitated by other renal disorders	Noticeable decrease in renal function progressing to renal failure
Nephrotic syndrome	Disruption of the electrical charges that produce the tightly fitting podocyte barrier resulting in massive loss of protein and lipids	Acute onset following systemic shock Gradual progression from other glomerular disorders and then to renal failure
Minimal change disease	Disruption of the podocytes occuring primarily in children following allergic reactions and immunizations	Frequent complete remission following corticosteroid treatment
Focal segmental glomerulosclerosis	Disruption of podocytes in certain areas of glomeruli associated with heroin and analgesic abuse and acquired immunodeficiency syndrome	May resemble nephrotic syndrome or minimal change disease

Acute Pyelonephritis

Infection of the upper urinary tract including both the tubules and interstitium is termed ***pyelonephritis*** and can occur in both acute and chronic forms. Acute pyelonephritis most frequently occurs as a result of ascending movement of bacteria from a lower UTI into the renal tubules and interstitium. The ascending movement of bacteria from the bladder is enhanced with conditions that interfere with the downward flow of urine from the ureters to the bladder or the complete emptying of the bladder during urination. These include obstructions such as renal calculi, pregnancy, and reflux of urine from the bladder back into the ureters (**visicoureteral reflux**). With appropriate antibiotic therapy and removal of any underlying conditions, acute pyelonephritis can be resolved without permanent damage to the tubules.

Patients present with rapid onset of symptoms of urinary frequency and burning and lower back pain. A relatively high correlation between acute pylonephritis and bacteremia has been demonstrated, suggesting the need to perform blood cultures in addition to urine cultures.[12]

Urinalysis results are similar to those seen in cystitis, including numerous leukocytes and bacteria with mild proteinuria and hematuria. However, the additional finding of WBC casts, signifying infection within the tubules, is of primary diagnostic value for both acute and chronic pyelonephritis. Sediments also should be carefully observed for the presence of bacterial casts.

Chronic Pyelonephritis

As its name implies, chronic pyelonephritis is a more serious disorder that can result in permanent damage to the renal tubules and possible progression to chronic renal failure. Congenital urinary structural defects producing a reflux nephropathy are the most frequent cause of chronic pyelonephritis. The structural abnormalities may cause reflux between the bladder and ureters or within the renal pelvis, affecting emptying of the collecting ducts. Owing to its congenital origin, chronic pyelonephritis is often diagnosed in children and may not be suspected until tubular damage has become advanced.

Urinalysis results are similar to those seen in acute pyelonephritis, particularly in the early stages. As the disease progresses, a variety of granular, waxy, and broad casts accompanied by increased proteinuria and hematuria are present, and renal concentration is decreased.

Acute Interstitial Nephritis

Acute interstitial nephritis (**AIN**) is marked by inflammation of the renal interstitium followed by inflammation of the renal tubules. Patients present with a rapid onset of symptoms relating to renal dysfunction, including oliguria, edema, decreased renal concentrating ability, and a possible decrease in the glomerular filtration rate. Fever and the presence of a skin rash are frequent initial symptoms.

AIN is primarily associated with an allergic reaction to medications that occurs within the renal interstitium, possibly caused by binding of the medication to the interstitial protein. Symptoms tend to develop approximately 2 weeks following administration of medication. Medications commonly associated with AIN include penicillin, methicillin, ampicillin, cephalosporins, sulfonamides, nonsteroidal anti-inflammatory agents, and thiazide diuretics. Discontinuation of the offending medication and administration of steroids to control the inflammation frequently results in a return to normal renal function. However, supportive renal dialysis may be required to maintain patients until the inflammation subsides.

Urinalysis results include hematuria, possibly macroscopic, mild-to-moderate proteinuria, numerous WBCs, and WBC casts without the presence of bacteria. Performing differential leukocyte staining for the presence of increased eosinophils may be useful to confirm the diagnosis.[1]

Laboratory testing and clinical information for the tubulointerstitial disorders are summarized in Tables 8–3 and 8–4.

TABLE 8–3 **Summary of Laboratory Testing in Tubulointerstitial Disorders**

Disorder	Primary Urinalysis Results	Other Significant Tests
Acute tubular necrosis	Microscopic hematuria Proteinuria Renal tubular epithelial cells Renal tubular epithelial cell casts Hyaline, granular, waxy, broad casts	Hemoglobin Hematocrit Cardiac enzymes
Fanconi's syndrome	Glucosuria Possible cystine crystals	Serum and urine electrolytes Amino acid chromatography
Cystitis	Leukocyturia Bacteriuria Microscopic hematuria Mild proteinuria Increased pH	Urine culture
Acute pyelonephritis	Leukocyturia Bacteriuria White blood cell casts Bacterial casts Microscopic hematuria Proteinuria	Urine culture Blood cultures
Chronic pyelonephritis	Leukocyturia Bacteriuria White blood cell casts Bacterial casts Granular, waxy, broad casts Hematuria Proteinuria	Urine culture Blood cultures Blood urea nitrogen Creatinine Creatinine clearance
Acute interstitial nephritis	Hematuria Proteinuria Leukocyturia White blood cell casts	Urine eosinophils Blood urea nitrogen Creatinine Creatinine clearance

TABLE 8–4 **Summary of Clinical Information Associated with Tubulointerstitial Disorders**

Disorder	Etiology	Clinical Course
Acute tubular necrosis	Damage to the renal tubular cells caused by ischemia or toxic agents	Acute onset of renal dysfunction usually resolved when the underlying cause is corrected
Fanconi's syndrome	Inherited in association with cystinosis and Hartnup disease or acquired through exposure to toxic agents	Generalized defect in renal tubular reabsorption requiring supportive therapy
Cystitis	Ascending bacterial infection of the bladder	Acute onset of urinary frequency and burning resolved with antibiotics
Acute pyelonephritis	Infection of the renal tubules and interstitium related to interference of urine flow to the bladder, reflux of urine from the bladder, and untreated cystitis	Acute onset of urinary frequency, burning, and lower back pain resolved with antibiotics
Chronic pyelonephritis	Recurrent infection of the renal tubules and interstitium caused by structural abnormalities affecting the flow of urine	Frequently diagnosed in children, requires correction of the underlying structural defect Possible progression to renal failure
Acute interstitial nephritis	Allergic inflammation of the renal interstitium in response to certain medications	Acute onset of renal dysfunction often accompanied by a skin rash Resolves following discontinuation of medication and treatment with corticosteroids

Vascular Disorders

Renal function is affected by essentially any disorder of the circulatory system. Disorders include autoimmune disorders, vasculitis, and diabetes mellitus that affect the integrity of the renal blood vessels. In contrast, a sudden or chronic decrease in the pressure and amount of blood flow to the kidneys produces an overall renal ischemia and loss of functional renal tissue.

Renal Failure

Renal failure exists in both acute and chronic forms. As discussed in conjunction with many of the previous disorders, this may be a gradual progression from the original disorder to chronic renal failure or end-stage renal disease. The progression to end-stage renal disease is characterized by a marked decrease in the glomerular filtration rate (less than 25 mL/min.); steadily rising serum BUN and creatinine values (**azotemia**); electrolyte imbalance; lack of renal concentrating ability producing an isothenuric urine; proteinuria; renal glycosuria; and an abundance of granular, waxy, and broad casts, often referred to as a telescoped urine sediment.

Acute renal failure (**ARF**), in contrast to chronic renal failure, exhibits a sudden loss of renal function and is frequently reversible. Primary causes of ARF include a sudden decrease in blood flow to the kidney (prerenal), acute glomerular and tubular disease (renal), and renal calculi or tumor obstructions (postrenal). As can be seen from the variety of causes (Table 8–5), patients may present with many different symptoms relating to the particular disorder involved; however, a decreased glomerular filtration rate, oliguria, edema, and azotemia are general characteristics.

Similar to clinical symptoms, urinalysis findings are varied; however, because they relate to the primary cause of the ARF, they can be diagnostically valuable. For example, the presence of RTE cells and casts suggests ATN of prerenal origin; RBCs indicate glomerular injury; WBC casts with or without bacteria indicate interstitial infection or inflammation of renal origin; and postrenal obstruction may show normal and abnormal appearing urothelial cells possibly associated with malignancy.

Renal Lithiasis

Renal calculi (kidney stones) may form in the calyces and pelvis of the kidney, ureters, and bladder. In renal ***lithiasis***, the kidney stones vary in size from barely visible to large, staghorn calculi resembling the shape of the renal pelvis to smooth, round bladder stones with diameters of two or more inches. Small calculi may be passed in the urine, sub-

TABLE 8–5 **Causes of Acute Renal Failure**

Prerenal
Decreased blood pressure/cardiac output
Hemorrhage
Burns
Surgery
Septicemia
Renal
Acute glomerulonephritis
Acute tubular necrosis
Acute pyelonephritis
Acute interstitial nephritis
Postrenal
Renal calculi
Tumors
Crystallization of ingested substances

jecting the patient to severe pain radiating from the lower back to the legs. Larger stones cannot be passed and may not be detected until patients develop symptoms of urinary obstruction. **Lithotripsy**, a procedure using high-energy shock waves, can be used to break stones located in the upper urinary tract into pieces that can then be passed in the urine. Surgical removal also can be employed.

Conditions favoring the formation of renal calculi are similar to those favoring formation of urinary crystals, including pH, chemical concentration, and urinary stasis. Numerous correlation studies between the presence of crystalluria and the formation of renal calculi have been conducted with varying results. The finding of clumps of crystals in freshly voided urine suggests that conditions may be right for calculus formation. However, owing to the difference in conditions that affect the urine within the body and in a specimen container, little importance can be placed on the role of crystals in the prediction of calculi formation. Increased crystalluria has been noted during the summer months in persons known to form renal calculi.[7]

Analysis of the chemical composition of renal calculi plays an important role in patient management. Analysis can be performed chemically, but examination using x-ray crystallography provides a more comprehensive analysis.[10] Approximately 75 percent of the renal calculi are composed of calcium oxalate or phosphate. Magnesium ammonium phosphate (stuvite), uric acid, and cystine are the other primary calculi constituents. Patient management techniques include maintaining the urine at a pH incompatible with crystallization of the particular chemicals, maintaining adequate hydration to lower chemical concentration, and suggesting possible dietary restrictions.

Urine specimens from patients suspected of passing or being in the process of passing renal calculi are frequently received in the laboratory. The presence of microscopic hematuria resulting from irritation to the tissues by the moving calculus is the primary urinalysis finding.

REFERENCES

1. Bennett, WM, Elzinga, LW, and Porter, GA: Tubulointerstitial disease and toxic nephropathy. In Brenner, BM, and Rector, FC: The Kidney: Physiology and Pathophysiology. WB Saunders, Philadelphia, 1991.
2. Bricker, NS, and Kirschenbaum, MA: The Kidney: Diagnosis and Management. John Wiley, New York, 1984.
3. Bylund, DJ, and McCallum, RM: Vasculitis. In Henry, JB (ed): Clinical Diagnosis and Management by Laboratory Methods. WB Saunders, Philadelphia, 1996.
4. Couser, WG: Rapidly progressive glomerulonephritis. In Jacobson, HR, et al: Principles and Practice of Nephrology. BC Decker, Philadelphia, 1991.
5. Donadio, JV: Membranoproliferative glomerulonephritis. In Jacobson, HR, et al: Principles and Practice of Nephrology. BC Decker, Philadelphia, 1991.
6. Forland, M (ed): Nephrology. Medical Examination Publishing, New York, 1983.
7. Hallson, PC, and Rose, GA: Seasonal variations in urinary crystals. Br J Urol 49(4):277–284, 1977.
8. Johnson, RJ: Nonpoststreptococcal postinfectious glomerulonephritis. In Jacobson, HR, et al: Principles and Practice of Nephrology. BC Decker, Philadelphia, 1991.
9. Kallenberg, CG, Mulder, AH, and Tervaert, JW: Antineutrophil cytoplasmic autoantibodies: A still-growing class of autoantibodies in inflammatory disorders. Am J Med 93(6):675–682, 1992.
10. Mandel, N: Urinary tract calculi. Lab Med 17(8):449–458, 1986.
11. Sherbotle, JR, and Hayes, JR: Idiopathic nephrotic syndrome: Minimal change disease and focal segmental glomerulosclerosis. In Jacobson, HR, et al: Principles and Practice of Nephrology. BC Decker, Philadelphia, 1991.
12. Smith, WR, et al: Bacteremia in young urban women admitted with pyelonephritis. Am J Med Sci 313(1):50–57, 1997.
13. Wasserstein, AG: Membranous glomerulonephritis. In Jacobson, HR, et al: Principles and Practice of Nephrology. BC Decker, Philadelphia, 1991.

CASE STUDIES AND CLINICAL SITUATIONS

1. A 14-year-old boy who has recently recovered from a sore throat develops edema and hematuria. Significant laboratory results include a BUN of 30 mg/dL (normal 8 to 23 mg/dL) and an ASO titer of 833 Todd units (normal less than 166). Results of a urinalysis are as follows:

COLOR: Red	KETONES: Negative
CLARITY: Cloudy	BLOOD: Large
SP. GRAVITY: 1.020	BILIRUBIN: Negative
pH: 5.0	UROBILINOGEN: Normal
PROTEIN: 3+	NITRITE: Negative
GLUCOSE: Negative	LEUKOCYTE: Trace

Microscopic:
100 RBCs/hpf—many dysmorphic forms
5–8 WBCs/hpf
0–2 granular casts/lpf
0–1 RBC casts/lpf

a. What disorder do these results and history indicate?
b. What specific characteristic was present in the organism causing the sore throat?
c. What is the significance of the dysmorphic RBCs?
d. Are the WBCs significant? Why or why not?
e. What is the expected prognosis of this patient?
f. If the above urinalysis results were seen in a 5-year-old boy who has developed a red, patchy rash following recovery from a sore throat, what disorder would be suspected?

2. B.J. is a seriously ill 40-year-old man with a history of several episodes of macroscopic hematuria in the past 20 years. The episodes were associated with exercise or stress. Until recently the macroscopic hematuria had spontaneously reverted to asymptomatic microscopic hematuria. Significant laboratory results include a BUN of 80 mg/dL (normal 8 to 23 mg/dL), serum creatinine of 4.5 mg/dL (normal 0.6 to 1.2 mg/dL), creatinine clearance of 20 mL/min (normal 107 to 139 mL/min), serum calcium of 8.0 mg/dL (normal 9.2 to 11.0 mg/dL), serum phosphorus of 6.0 mg/dL (normal 2.3 to 4.7 mg/dL), and an elevated level of serum IgA. Results of a routine urinalysis are as follows:

COLOR: Red	KETONES: Negative
CLARITY: Slightly cloudy	BLOOD: Large
SP. GRAVITY: 1.010	BILIRUBIN: Negative

PH: 6.5	UROBILINOGEN: Normal
PROTEIN: 300 mg/dL	NITRITE: Negative
GLUCOSE: 250 mg/dL	LEUKOCYTE: Trace

Microscopic:

>100 RBCs/hpf	2–4 hyaline casts/lpf	1–5 granular casts/lpf
8–10 WBCs/hpf	0–2 waxy casts/lpf	0–2 broad waxy casts/lpf

a. What specific disease do the patient's laboratory results and history suggest?
b. Which laboratory result is most helpful in diagnosing this disease?
c. What additional diagnosis does his current condition suggest?
d. What is the significance of the positive result for urine glucose?
e. Is the specific gravity significant? Why or why not?
f. What is the significance of the waxy casts?

3. A 45-year-old woman recovering from injuries received in an automobile accident that resulted in her being taken to the emergency room with severe hypotension develops massive edema. Significant laboratory results include a BUN of 30 mg/dL (normal 8 to 23 mg/dL), cholesterol of 400 mg/dL (normal 150 to 240 mg/dL), triglycerides of 840 mg/dL (normal 10 to 190 mg/dL), serum protein of 4.5 mg/dL (normal 6.0 to 7.8 mg/dL), albumin of 2.0 mg/dL (normal 3.2 to 4.5 mg/dL), and a total urine protein of 3.8 g/d (normal 100 mg/d). Urinalysis results are as follows:

COLOR: Yellow	KETONES: Negative
CLARITY: Cloudy	BLOOD: Moderate
SP. GRAVITY: 1.015	BILIRUBIN: Negative
PH: 6.0	UROBILINOGEN: Normal
PROTEIN: 4+	NITRITE: Negative
GLUCOSE: Negative	LEUKOCYTE: Negative

Microscopic:

15–20 RBCs/hpf	0–2 granular casts/lpf	Moderate free fat droplets
0–5 WBCs/hpf	0–2 fatty casts/lpf	Moderate cholesterol crystals
0–2 oval fat bodies/hpf		

a. What renal disorder do these results suggest?
b. How does the patient's history relate to this disorder?
c. What physiologic mechanism accounts for the massive proteinuria?
d. What is the relationship of the proteinuria to the edema?
e. What mechanism produces the oval fat bodies?
f. State two additional procedures that could be performed to verify the presence of the oval fat bodies and the fatty casts.

4. A routinely active 4-year-old boy becomes increasingly less active after receiving several preschool immunizations. His pediatrician observes noticeable puffiness around the eyes. A blood test shows normal BUN and creatinine results and markedly decreased total protein and albumin values. Urinalysis results are as follows:

COLOR: Yellow	KETONES: Negative
CLARITY: Hazy	BLOOD: Small
SP. GRAVITY: 1.018	BILIRUBIN: Negative
PH: 6.5	UROBILINOGEN: Normal
PROTEIN: 4+	NITRITE: Negative
GLUCOSE: Negative	LEUKOCYTE: Negative

Microscopic:

10–15 RBCs/hpf	0–1 hyaline casts/lpf
0–4 WBCs/hpf	0–2 granular casts/lpf
Moderate fat droplets	0–1 oval fat bodies/hpf

a. What disorder do the patient history, physical appearance, and laboratory results suggest?
b. What other renal disorder produces similar urinalysis results?
c. What is the expected prognosis for this patient?

5. A 32-year-old construction worker experiences respiratory difficulty followed by the appearance of blood-streaked sputum. He delays visiting a physician until symptoms of extreme fatigue and red urine are present. A chest radiograph shows pulmonary infiltration and sputum culture is negative for pathogens. Blood test results indicate anemia, increased BUN and creatinine, and the presence of antiglomerular basement membrane antibody. Urinalysis results are as follows:

COLOR: Red	KETONES: Negative
CLARITY: Cloudy	BLOOD: Large
SP. GRAVITY: 1.015	BILIRUBIN: Negative
PH: 6.0	UROBILINOGEN: Normal
PROTEIN: 3+	NITRITE: Negative
GLUCOSE: Negative	LEUKOCYTE: Trace

Microscopic:

100 RBCs/hpf	0–3 hyaline casts/lpf
10–15 WBCs/hpf	0–3 granular casts/lpf
	0–2 RBCs casts/lpf

a. What disorder do the laboratory results suggest?
b. How is this disorder affecting the glomerulus?
c. If the antiglomerular membrane antibody test was negative, what disorder might be considered?
d. What is the diagnostic test for this disorder?
e. By what mechanism does this disorder affect the glomerulus?

6. A 25-year-old pregnant woman comes to the outpatient clinic with symptoms of lower back pain, urinary frequency, and a burning sensation when voiding. Her pregnancy has been normal up to this time. She is given a sterile container and asked to collect a midstream clean-catch urine specimen. Routine urinalysis results are as follows:

COLOR: Pale yellow	KETONES: Negative
CLARITY: Hazy	BLOOD: Small
SP. GRAVITY: 1.005	BILIRUBIN: Negative
PH: 8.0	UROBILINOGEN: Normal
PROTEIN: Trace	NITRITE: Positive
GLUCOSE: Negative	LEUKOCYTE: 2+

Microscopic:

6–10 RBCs/hpf	Heavy bacteria
40–50 WBCs/hpf	Moderate squamous epithelial cells

a. What is the most probable diagnosis for this patient?
b. What is the correlation between the color and the specific gravity?
c. What is the significance of the blood and protein tests?
d. Is this specimen suitable for the appearance of glitter cells? Explain your answer.
e. What other population is at a high risk for developing this condition?
f. What disorder might develop if this disorder is not treated?

7. A 10-year-old patient with a history of recurrent UTIs is admitted to the hospital for diagnostic tests. Initial urinalysis results are as follows:

COLOR: Yellow	KETONE: Negative
CLARITY: Cloudy	BLOOD: Small
SP. GRAVITY: 1.025	BILIRUBIN: Negative
pH: 8.0	UROBILINOGEN: Normal
PROTEIN: 2+ (SSA): (2+)	NITRITE: Positive
GLUCOSE: Negative	LEUKOCYTE: 2+

Microscopic:

6–10 RBCs/hpf	0–2 WBC casts/lpf	Many bacteria
>100 WBCs/hpf with clumps	0–1 bacterial casts/lpf	

A repeat urinalysis a day later has the following results:

COLOR: Yellow	KETONES: Negative
CLARITY: Cloudy	BLOOD: Small
SP. GRAVITY: >1.035	BILIRUBIN: Negative
pH: 7.5	UROBILINOGEN: Normal
PROTEIN: 2+ (SSA): (4+)	NITRITE: Positive
GLUCOSE: Negative	LEUKOCYTE: 2+

Microscopic:

6–10 RBCs/hpf	0–2 WBC casts/lpf	Many bacteria
>100 WBCs/hpf	0–1 bacterial casts/lpf	Moderate birefringent, flat crystals

a. What diagnostic procedure was performed on the patient that could account for the differences in the two urinalysis results?
b. Considering the patient's age and history, what is the most probable diagnosis?
c. What microscopic constituent is most helpful to this diagnosis?
d. What is the most probable cause of this disorder?
e. How can the presence of the bacterial cast be confirmed?
f. What is the most probable source of the crystals present in the sediment?

g. Without surgical intervention, what is the patient's prognosis?

8. A 35-year-old patient being treated for a sinus infection with methicillin develops fever, a skin rash, and edema. Urinalysis results are as follows:

COLOR: Dark yellow	KETONES: Negative
CLARITY: Cloudy	BLOOD: Moderate
SP. GRAVITY: 1.012	BILIRUBIN: Negative
pH: 6.0	UROBILINOGEN: Normal
PROTEIN: 3+	NITRITE: Negative
GLUCOSE: Negative	LEUKOCYTE: 2+

Microscopic:

20–30 RBCs/hpf	1–2 WBC casts/lpf
>100 WBCs/hpf	1–2 granular casts/lpf

After receiving the urinalysis report, the physician orders a test for urinary eosinophils. The urinary eosinophil result is 10 percent.

a. Is the urinary eosinophil result normal or abnormal?
b. What is the probable diagnosis for this patient?
c. Discuss the significance of the increased WBCs and WBC casts in the absence of bacteria.
d. How can this condition be corrected?

9. Following surgery to correct a massive hemorrhage, a 55-year-old patient exhibits oliguria and edema. Blood test results indicate increasing azotemia and electrolyte imbalance. The glomerular filtration rate is 20 mL/min. Urinalysis results are as follows:

COLOR: Yellow	KETONES: Negative
CLARITY: Cloudy	BLOOD: Moderate
SP. GRAVITY: 1.010	BILIRUBIN: Negative
pH: 7.0	UROBILINOGEN: Normal
PROTEIN: 3+	NITRITE: Negative
GLUCOSE: 2+	LEUKOCYTE: Negative

Microscopic:

50–60 RBCs/hpf	2–3 granular casts/lpf
3–6 WBCs/hpf	2–3 RTE cell casts/lpf
3–4 RTE cells/hpf	0–1 waxy casts/lpf
	0–1 broad granular casts/lpf

a. What diagnosis do the patient's history and laboratory results suggest?
b. What is the most probable cause of the patient's disorder? Is this considered to be of prerenal, renal, or postrenal origin?
c. What is the significance of the specific gravity result?
d. What is the significance of the RTE cells?
e. State two possible reasons for the presence of the broad casts.

10. A 40-year-old man develops severe back and abdominal pain after dinner. The pain subsides during the night but recurs in the morning, and he visits his family physician. Results of a complete blood count and an amylase are normal. Results of a routine urinalysis are as follows:

COLOR: Dark yellow	KETONES: Negative
CLARITY: Hazy	BLOOD: Moderate

SP. GRAVITY: 1.030	BILIRUBIN: Negative
pH: 5.0	UROBILINOGEN: Normal
PROTEIN: Trace	NITRITE: Negative
GLUCOSE: Negative	LEUKOCYTES: Negative

Microscopic
15–20 RBCs/hpf—appear crenated
0–2 WBCs/hpf
Few squamous epithelial cells

a. What condition could these urinalysis results and the patient's symptoms represent?
b. What would account for the crenated RBCs?
c. Is there a correlation between the urine color and specific gravity and the patient's symptoms?
d. Based on the primary substance that causes this condition, what type of crystals might have been present?
e. What changes will the patient be advised to make in his lifestyle to prevent future occurrences?

11. State a disorder or disorders that relate to each of the following descriptions:

a. A patient with severe lower back pain and microscopic hematuria is scheduled for lithotripsy.
b. The patient exhibits pulmonary and renal symptoms and a positive ANCA test.
c. A patient who tested positive for human immunodeficiency virus exhibits mild symptoms resembling the nephrotic syndrome.
d. A 40-year-old patient diagnosed with systemic lupus erythematosus develops macroscopic hematuria, proteinuria, and the presence of RBC casts in the urine sediment.
e. A 50-year-old patient diagnosed with systemic lupus erythematosus exhibits symptoms of gradually declining renal function and increasing proteinuria.
f. A patient who has taken outdated tetracycline develops glycosuria and a generalized aminoaciduria.
g. A patient known to form renal calculi develops oliguria, edema, and azotemia.

CHAPTER 9

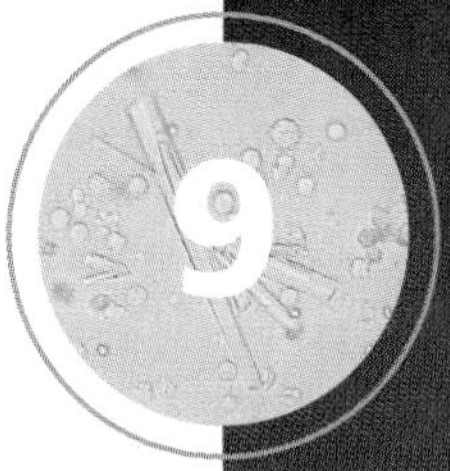

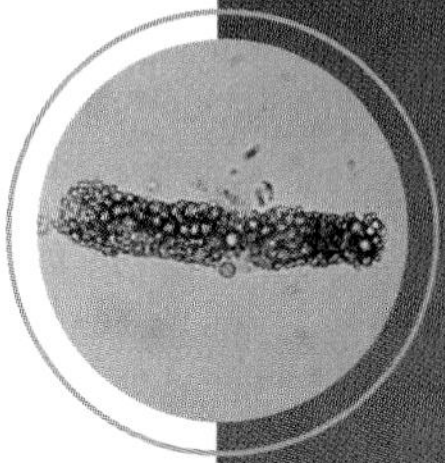

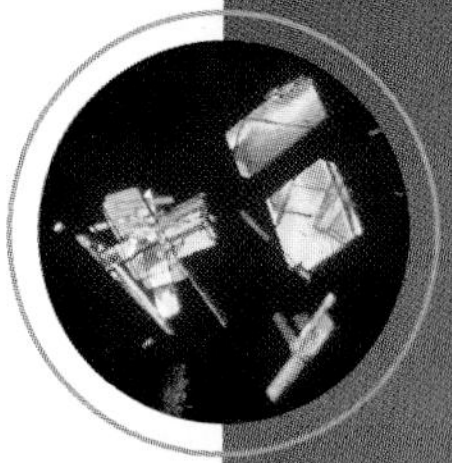

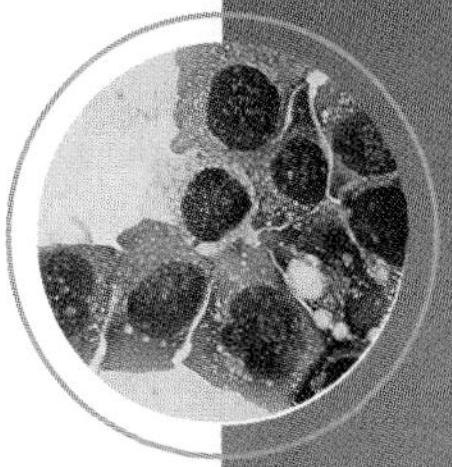

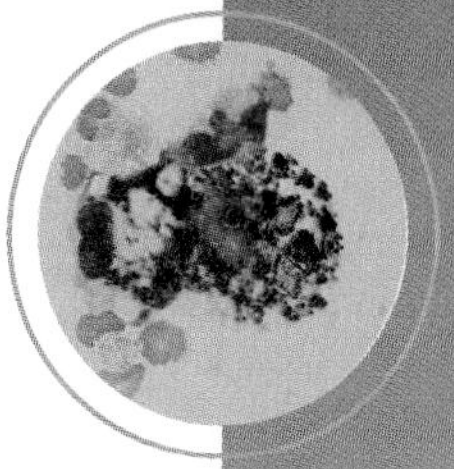

Urine Screening for Metabolic Disorders

LEARNING OBJECTIVES

Upon completion of this chapter, the reader will be able to:

1 Explain the abnormal accumulation of metabolites in the urine in terms of overflow and renal disorders.
2 Name the metabolic defect in phenylketonuria, and describe the clinical manifestations it produces.
3 Discuss the performance of the Guthrie and ferric chloride tests and their roles in the detection and management of phenylketonuria.
4 State three causes of tyrosyluria and the recommended screening test for its presence.
5 Name the abnormal urinary substance present in alkaptonuria, and tell how its presence may be suspected.
6 Discuss the appearance and significance of urine that contains melanin.
7 Describe a basic laboratory observation that has relevance in maple syrup urine disease.
8 Discuss the significance of ketonuria in a newborn.
9 Differentiate between the presence of urinary indican owing to intestinal disorders and Hartnup disease.
10 State the significance of increased urinary 5-hydroxyindoleacetic acid.
11 Differentiate between cystinuria and cystinosis, including the differences that are found during analysis of the urine and the disease processes.
12 Name the chemical screening test for cystine.
13 Describe the components in the heme synthesis pathway, including the primary fluids used for their analysis.
14 Briefly discuss the major porphyrias with regard to cause and clinical significance.
15 Differentiate between the Ehrlich reaction and fluorescent testing with regard to the testing of porphyrin components.
16 Describe the appearance of urine that contains increased porphyrins.
17 Define mucopolysaccharides, and name three syndromes in which they are involved.
18 List three screening tests for the detection of urinary mucopolysaccharides.
19 State the significance of increased uric acid crystals in newborns' urine.
20 Explain the reason for performing tests for urinary-reducing substances on all newborns.

KEY TERMS

alkaptonuria
cystinosis
cystinuria
galactosuria
homocystinuria
inborn error of metabolism
indicanuria
Lesch-Nyhan disease
maple syrup urine disease
melanuria
melituria
mucopolysaccharidoses
organic acidemias
phenylketonuria
porphyrinuria
tyrosinuria

As has been discussed in previous chapters, many of the abnormal results obtained in the routine urinalysis are related to metabolic rather than renal disease. Urine as an end product of body metabolism may contain additional abnormal substances not tested for by the routine urinalysis. Often, these substances can be detected by additional screening tests that can also be performed in the urinalysis laboratory. Positive screening tests can then be followed up with more sophisticated procedures performed in other sections of the laboratory.

The need to perform additional tests may be detected by the observations of alert laboratory personnel during the performance of the routine analysis or from observations of abnormal specimen color and odor by nursing staff and patients (Table 9–1). In other instances, clinical symptoms and family histories are the deciding factors. Several metabolic screening tests are routinely performed on all newborns.[3]

Overflow Versus Renal Disorders

The appearance of abnormal metabolic substances in the urine can be caused by a variety of disorders that can generally be grouped into two categories, termed the overflow type and renal type. Overflow disorders result from the disruption of a normal metabolic pathway that causes increased plasma concentrations of the nonmetabolized substances. These chemicals either override the reabsorption ability of the renal tubules or are not normally reabsorbed from the filtrate because they are only present in minute amounts. Abnormal accumulations of the renal type are caused by malfunctions in the tubular reabsorption mechanism as discussed in Chapter 8.

The most frequently encountered abnormalities are associated with metabolic disturbances that produce urinary overflow of substances involved in protein and carbohydrate metabolism. This is understandable when one considers the vast number of enzymes used in the metabolic pathways of proteins and carbohydrates and the fact that their function is essential for complete metabolism. Disruption of enzyme function can be caused by failure to inherit the gene to produce a particular enzyme, referred to as an ***inborn error of metabolism***,[7] or by organ malfunction from disease or toxic reactions. The most frequently encountered abnormal urinary metabolites are summarized in Table 9–2 and their appearance is classified according to functional defect. This table also includes those substances and conditions that are covered in this chapter.

TABLE 9–1 **Abnormal Metabolic Constituents or Conditions Detected in the Routine Urinalysis**

Color	Odor	Crystals
Homogentisic acid	Phenylketonuria	Cystine
Melanin	Maple syrup urine disease	Leucine
Indican	Isovaleric acidemia	Tyrosine
Porphyrins	Cystinuria	Lesch-Nyhan disease
	Cystinosis	
	Homocystinuria	

TABLE 9–2 **Major Disorders of Protein and Carbohydrate Metabolism Associated with Abnormal Urinary Constituents Classified as to Functional Defect**

Overflow		
Inherited	**Metabolic**	**Renal**
Phenylketonuria	Tyrosinemia	Hartnup disease
Tyrosinemia	Melanuria	Cystinuria
Alkaptonuria	Indicanuria	
Maple syrup urine disease	5-Hydroxyindoleacetic acid	
Organic acidemias	Porphyria	
Cystinosis		
Porphyria		
Mucopolysaccharidoses		
Melituria (galactosuria)		
Lesch-Nyhan disease		

Amino Acid Disorders

The amino acid disorders with urinary screening tests include ***phenylketonuria*** (PKU), ***tyrosinuria***, ***alkaptonuria***, ***melanuria***, ***maple syrup urine disease***, ***organic acidemias***, ***indicanuria***, ***cystinuria***, and ***cystinosis***.

PHENYLALANINE-TYROSINE DISORDERS

Many of the most frequently requested special urinalysis procedures are associated with the phenylalanine-tyrosine metabolic pathway. Major inherited disorders include PKU, tyrosyluria, and alkaptonuria. Metabolic defects cause production of excessive amounts of melanin. The relationship of these varied disorders is illustrated in Figure 9–1.

Phenylketonuria

The most well known of the **aminoacidurias**, PKU is estimated to occur in 1 of every 10,000 to 20,000 births and, if undetected, results in severe mental retardation. It was first identified in Norway by Ivan Følling in 1934, when a mother with other mentally retarded children reported a peculiar mousy odor to her child's urine. Analysis of the urine showed increased amounts of the keto acids, including phenylpyruvate. As shown in Figure 9–1, this will occur when the normal conversion of phenylalanine to tyrosine is disrupted. Interruption of the pathway also produces children with fair complexions even in dark-skinned families, owing to the decreased production of tyrosine and its pigmentation metabolite melanin.

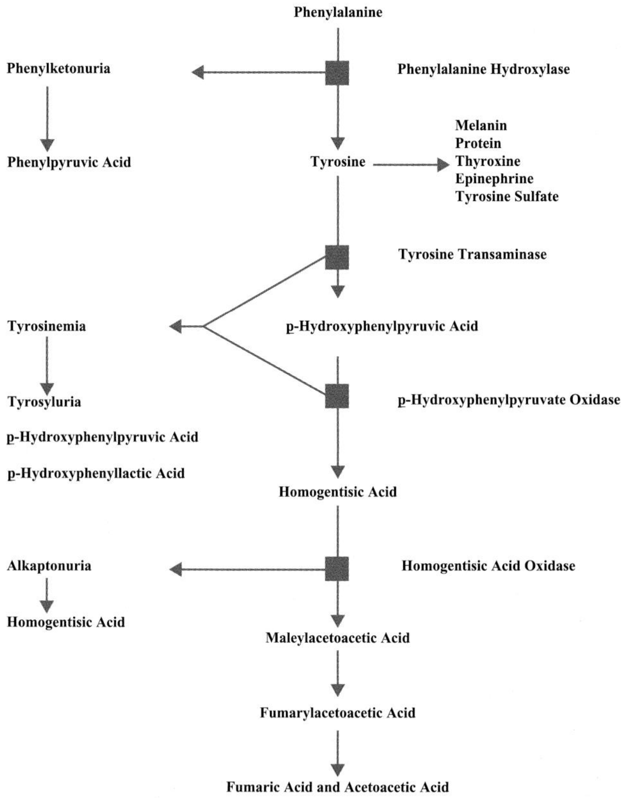

FIGURE 9–1 Phenylalanine and tyrosine metabolism. (Adapted from Frimpton,[6] and Kretchmer and Etzwiler.[15])

PKU is caused by failure to inherit the gene to produce the enzyme phenylalanine hydroxylase. The gene is inherited as an autosomal recessive trait with no noticeable characteristics or defects exhibited by heterozygous carriers. Fortunately, screening tests are available for early detection of the abnormality, and all states have laws that require the screening of newborns.[26] Once discovered, dietary changes that eliminate phenylalanine, a major constituent of milk, from the infant's diet can prevent the excessive buildup of serum phenylalanine and can thereby avoid damage to the child's mental capabilities. As the child matures, alternate pathways of phenylalanine metabolism develop, and dietary restrictions can be eased. Many products that contain large amounts of phenylalanine, such as aspartame, now have warnings for people with phenylketonuria.

The initial screening for PKU does not come under the auspices of the urinalysis laboratory, because increased blood levels of phenylalanine must, of course, occur prior to the urinary excretion of phenylpyruvic acid, which may take from 2 to 6 weeks. Blood samples must be obtained before the newborn is discharged from the hospital. The increasing tendency to release newborns from the hospital as early as 24 hours after birth has caused concern about the ability to detect increased phenylalanine levels at that early stage. Studies have shown that in many cases phenylalanine can be detected as early as 4 hours after birth and, if the cutoff level for normal results is lowered from 4 mg/dL to 2 mg/dL, the presence of PKU should be detected. Tests may need to be repeated during an early visit to the pediatrician.[5] More girls than boys escape detection of PKU during early tests because of slower rises in blood phenylalanine levels.[6]

Urine testing can be used as a follow-up procedure in questionable diagnostic cases, as a screening test to ensure proper dietary control in previously diagnosed cases, and, more recently, as a means of monitoring the dietary intake of pregnant women known to lack phenylalanine hydroxylase.

The most well-known blood test for PKU is the bacterial inhibition test developed by Guthrie.[9] In this procedure, blood from a heelstick is absorbed into filter paper circles. The circle must be completely saturated with a single layer of blood. The blood-impregnated disks are then placed on culture media streaked with the organism *Bacillus subtilis*. If increased phenylalanine levels are present in the blood, phenylalanine will counteract the action of beta-2-thienylalanine, an inhibitor of *B. subtilis* that is present in the media, and growth will be observed around the paper disks. Notice that in Figure 9–2 the bacterial

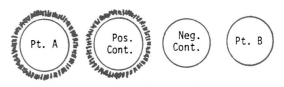

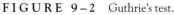

FIGURE 9–2 Guthrie's test.

PROCEDURE

Ferric Chloride Tube Test

1 Place 1 mL of urine in a tube.
2 Slowly add five drops of 10% ferric chloride.
3 Observe color.

growth around the disk from patient A corresponds to the positive control, indicating an increased level of phenylalanine. Modifications of the Guthrie test also will detect maple syrup urine disease, ***homocystinuria***, tyrosinemia, histidinemia, valinemia, and galactosemia.[23] Chemical and immunologic tests for many other substances including thyroid hormones, trypsin, and biotinidase can also be performed from dried blood collected by heel stick.[3] Additional methods are available for measuring serum levels of phenylalanine, including an automated technique that measures the fluorescence of phenylalanine when it is heated in the presence of Ninhydrin and L-leucyl-L-alanine or glycyl-L-leucine.[13]

Urine tests for phenylpyruvic acid are based upon the ferric chloride reaction performed by tube test. As will be seen in other discussions in this chapter, the ferric chloride test is a nonspecific reaction and will react with many other amino acids and commonly ingested medications (see Table 9–4 later in the chapter). Some brands of disposable diapers also produce false-positive reactions for PKU when tested with ferric chloride.[14] The addition of ferric chloride to urine containing phenylpyruvic acid produces a permanent blue-green color.

Tyrosyluria

The accumulation of excess tyrosine in the plasma (tyrosinemia) producing urinary overflow may be due to several causes and is not well categorized. As can be seen in Table 9–2, disorders of tyrosine metabolism may result from either inherited or metabolic defects. Also, because two reactions are directly involved in the metabolism of tyrosine, the urine may contain excess tyrosine or its degradation products *p*-hydroxyphenylpyruvic acid and *p*-hydroxyphenyllactic acid.

Most frequently seen is a transitory tyrosinemia in premature infants, which is caused by underdevelopment of the liver function necessary to complete the tyrosine metabolism. This condition seldom results in permanent damage, but it may be confused with PKU when urinary screening tests are performed, because the ferric chloride test will produce a green color. This reaction can be distinguished from the PKU reaction in the ferric chloride tube test because the green color fades rapidly when tyrosine is present.

Acquired severe liver disease also will produce tyrosyluria resembling that of the transitory newborn variety and, of course, is a more serious condition. In both instances, rarely seen tyrosine and leucine crystals may be observed during microscopic examination of the urine sediment.

Hereditary disorders in which enzymes required in the metabolic pathway are not produced present a serious and usually fatal condition that results in both liver and renal disease and in the appearance of a generalized aminoaciduria.

PROCEDURE

Nitroso-Napthol Test

1 Place five drops of urine in a tube.
2 Add 1 mL of 2.63N nitric acid.
3 Add one drop of 21.5% sodium nitrite.
4 Add 0.1 mL 1-nitroso-2-napthol.
5 Mix.
6 Wait 5 minutes.
7 Observe color.

The recommended urinary screening test for tyrosine and its metabolites is the nitroso-naphthol test. Like the ferric chloride test, the nitroso-naphthol test is nonspecific and, as shown in Table 9–4, will react with compounds other than tyrosine and its metabolites. However, the presence of an orange-red color shows a positive reaction and indicates that further testing is needed.

Alkaptonuria

Alkaptonuria was one of the six original inborn errors of metabolism described by Garrod in 1902. The name alkaptonuria was derived from the observation that urine from patients with this condition darkened after becoming alkaline from standing at room temperature. Therefore, the term "alkali lover," or alkaptonuria, was adopted. This metabolic defect is actually the third major one in the phenylalanine-tyrosine pathway and occurs from failure to inherit the gene to produce the enzyme homogentisic acid oxidase. Without this enzyme, the phenylalanine-tyrosine pathway cannot proceed to completion, and homogentisic acid accumulates in the blood, tissues, and urine. This condition does not usually manifest itself clinically in early childhood but observations of brown-stained or black-stained cloth diapers and reddish-stained disposable diapers have been reported.[21] In later life, brown pigment becomes deposited in the body tissues (particularly noticeable in the ears). Deposits in the cartilage eventually lead to arthritis. A high percentage of persons with alkaptonuria develop liver and cardiac disorders.[23]

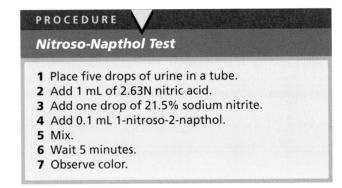

Homogentisic acid will react in several of the routinely used screening tests for metabolic disorders, including the ferric chloride test, in which a transient deep blue color is produced in the tube test. A yellow precipitate is produced in the Benedict's test or Clinitest, indicating the presence of a reducing substance. A more specific screening test for urinary homogentisic acid is to add alkali to freshly voided urine and to observe for darkening of the color; however, large amounts of ascorbic acid will interfere with this reaction.[24] The addition of silver nitrate and ammonium hydroxide also will produce a black urine. A spectrophotometric method to obtain quantitative measurements of both urine and plasma homogentisic acid is available, as are chromatography procedures.

PROCEDURE

Homogentisic Acid Test

1. Place 4 mL of 3% silver nitrate in a tube.
2. Add 0.5 mL of urine.
3. Mix.
4. Add 10% NH_4OH by drops.
5. Observe for black color.

Melanuria

The previous discussion has focused on the major phenylalanine-tyrosine metabolic pathway illustrated in Figure 9–1; however, as is the case with many amino acids, a second metabolic pathway also exists for tyrosine. This pathway is responsible for the production of melanin, thyroxine, epinephrine, protein, and tyrosine-sulfate. Of these substances, the major concern of the urinalysis laboratory is melanin, the pigment responsible for the dark color of hair, skin, and eyes. Deficient production of melanin results in **albinism**.

Like homogentisic acid, increased urinary melanin will produce a darkening of urine. The darkening appears after the urine is exposed to air. Elevation of urinary melanin is a serious finding that indicates the overproliferation of the normal melanin-producing cells (melanocytes), producing a malignant melanoma. These tumors secrete a colorless precursor of melanin, 5,6-dihydroxyindole, which oxidizes to melanogen and then to melanin, producing the characteristic dark urine. Differentiation between the presence of melanin and homogentisic acid must certainly be made.

Melanin will react with ferric chloride, sodium nitroprusside (nitroferricyanide), and Ehrlich's reagent. In the ferric chloride tube test, a gray or black precipitate will form in the presence of melanin and is easily differentiated from the reactions produced by other amino acid products. The sodium nitroprusside test provides an additional screening test for melanin. A red color is produced by the reaction of melanin and sodium nitroprusside. Interference due to a red color from acetone and creatinine can be avoided by adding glacial acetic acid, which will cause melanin to revert to a green-black color, whereas acetone turns purple, and creatinine becomes amber.[2]

Summary of Urine Screening Tests for Disorders of the Phenylalanine-Tyrosine Pathway

Phenylketonuria

Ferric chloride tube test

Tyrosyluria

Ferric chloride tube test
Nitroso-naphthol test

Alkaptonuria

Ferric chloride tube test
Benedict's test or Clinitest
Alkalization of fresh urine

Melanuria

Ferric chloride tube test
Sodium nitroprusside test
Ehrlich's test

BRANCHED-CHAIN AMINO ACID DISORDERS

The branched-chain amino acids differ from other amino acids by having a methyl group that branches from the main aliphatic carbon chain. Two major groups of disorders are associated with errors in the metabolism of the branched-chain amino acids. In one group, accumulation of one or more of the early amino acid degradation products occurs as is seen in maple syrup urine disease. Disorders in the other group are termed organic acidemias and result in accumulation of organic acids produced further down in the amino acid metabolic pathway.

A significant laboratory finding in branched-chain amino acid disorders is the presence of ketonuria in a newborn.

Maple Syrup Urine Disease

Although maple syrup urine disease is rare, a brief discussion is included in this chapter because the urinalysis laboratory can provide valuable information for the essential early detection of this disease.

Maple syrup urine disease is caused by an inborn error of metabolism, inherited as an autosomal recessive trait. The amino acids involved are leucine, isoleucine, and valine. The metabolic pathway begins normally, with the transamination of the three amino acids in the liver to the keto acids (α-ketoisovaleric, α-ketoisocaproic, and α-keto-β-methylvaleric). Failure to inherit the gene for the enzyme necessary to produce oxidative decarboxylation of these keto acids results in their accumulation in the blood and urine.[6]

Newborns with maple syrup urine disease begin to exhibit clinical symptoms associated with failure to thrive after approximately 1 week. The presence of the disease may be suspected from these clinical symptoms; however, many other conditions have similar symptoms. Personnel in the urinalysis laboratory or in the nursery may detect the disease through the observation of a urine specimen that produces a strong odor resembling maple syrup, which is caused by the rapid accumulation of keto acids in the urine. Even though a report of urine odor is not a part of the routine urinalysis, notifying the physician about this unusual finding can prevent the development of severe mental retardation and even death. Studies have shown that if maple syrup urine disease is detected by the 11th day, dietary regulation and careful monitoring of urinary keto acid concentrations can control the disorder.[4]

The screening test most frequently performed for keto acids is the 2,4-dinitrophenylhydrazine (**DNPH**) reaction. The DNPH test can also be used for home monitoring of

PROCEDURE

2,4-Dinitrophenylhydrazine (DNPH) Test

1 Place 1 mL of urine in a tube.
2 Add 10 drops of 0.2% 2,4-DNPH in 2N HCl.
3 Wait 10 minutes.
4 Observe for yellow or white precipitate.

diagnosed patients. Adding DNPH to urine that contains keto acids will produce a yellow turbidity or precipitate. Large doses of ampicillin will interfere with the DNPH reaction. Like many other urinary screening tests, the DNPH reaction is not specific for maple syrup urine disease, inasmuch as keto acids are present in other disorders, including PKU. In addition, all specimens with a positive reagent strip test result for ketones will produce a positive DNPH result. However, treatment can be started on the basis of odor, clinical symptoms, and a positive DNPH test while confirmatory procedures using amino acid chromatography are being performed.

Organic Acidemias

Generalized symptoms of the organic acidemias include early severe illness, often with vomiting accompanied by metabolic acidosis; hypoglycemia; ketonuria; and increased serum ammonia.[8] The three most frequently encountered disorders are isovaleric, propionic, and methylmalonic acidemia.

Isovaleric acidemia may be suspected when urine specimens, and sometimes even the patient, possess a characteristic odor of "sweaty feet." This is caused by the accumulation of isovalerylglycine due to a deficiency of isovaleryl coenzyme A in the leucine pathway. There is no screening test for isovalerylglycine, and its presence is identified using chromatography.

Propionic and methylmalonic acidemias result from errors in the metabolic pathway converting isoleucine, valine, threonine, and methionine to succinyl coenzyme A. Propionic acid is the immediate precursor to methylmalonic acid in this pathway.

A screening test is available for methylmalonic aciduria. The procedure uses *p*-nitroaniline to produce an emerald green color in the presence of methylmalonic acid.[24]

TRYPTOPHAN DISORDERS

The major concern of the urinalysis laboratory in the metabolism of tryptophan is the increased urinary excretion of the metabolites indican and 5-hydroxyindoleacetic acid (5-HIAA). Figure 9–3 shows a simplified diagram of the metabolic pathways by which these substances are produced. Other metabolic pathways of tryptophan are not included because they do not relate directly to the urinalysis laboratory.

Indicanuria

Under normal conditions, most of the tryptophan that enters the intestine is either reabsorbed for use by the body in the production of protein or is converted to indole by the

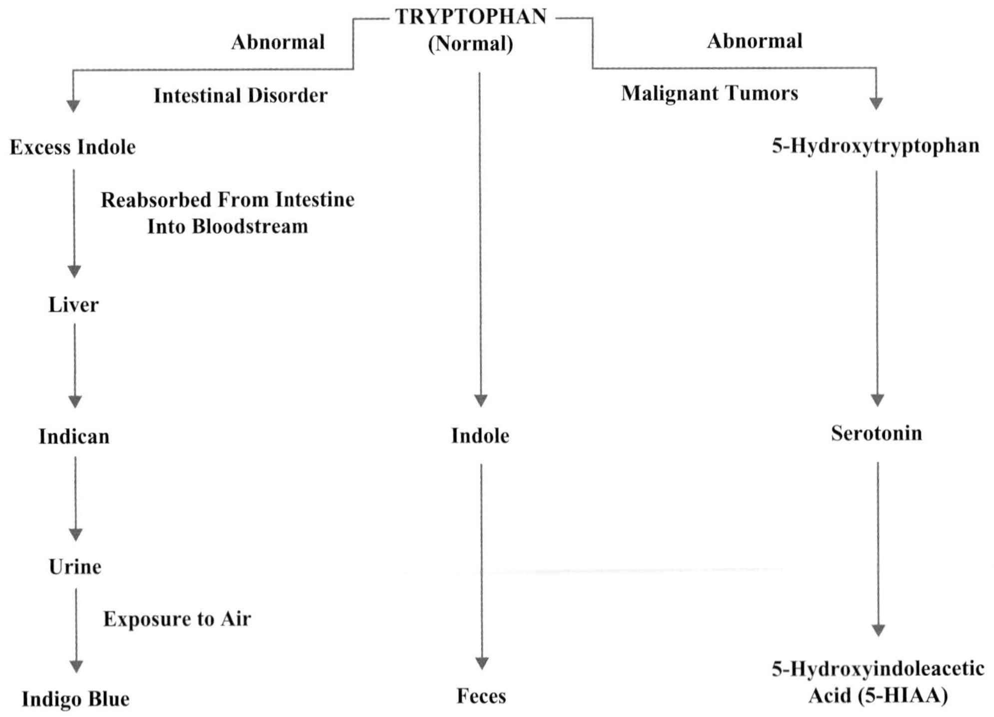

FIGURE 9–3 Tryptophan metabolism. (Adapted from Meister.[17])

PROCEDURE

p-*Nitroaniline Test*

1. Place one drop of urine in a tube.
2. Add 15 drops of 0.1% *p*-nitroaniline in 0.16 M HCl.
3. Add five drops of 0.5% sodium nitrite.
4. Mix.
5. Add 1 mL of 1 M sodium acetate buffer at pH 4.3.
6. Boil for 1 minute.
7. Add five drops of 8N NaOH.
8. Observe for emerald green color.

intestinal bacteria and excreted in the feces. However, in certain intestinal disorders (including obstruction; the presence of abnormal bacteria; malabsorption syndromes; and **Hartnup disease**, a rare inherited disorder) increased amounts of tryptophan are converted to indole. The excess indole is then reabsorbed from the intestine into the bloodstream and circulated to the liver, where it is converted to indican and then excreted in the urine. Indican excreted in the urine is colorless until oxidized to the dye indigo blue by exposure to air. Early diagnosis of Hartnup disease is sometimes made when mothers report a blue staining of their infant's diapers, referred to as the "blue diaper syndrome." Urinary indican will react with acidic ferric chloride to form a deep blue or violet color that can subsequently be extracted into chloroform.

Except in cases of Hartnup disease, correction of the underlying intestinal disorder will return urinary indican levels to normal. The inherited defect in Hartnup disease affects not only the intestinal reabsorption of tryptophan but also the renal tubular reabsorption of other amino acids, resulting in a generalized aminoaciduria (Fanconi's syndrome). The defective renal transport of amino acids does not appear to affect other renal tubular functions. Therefore, with proper dietary supplements, including niacin, persons with Hartnup disease have a good prognosis.[11]

5-Hydroxyindoleacetic Acid

As shown in Figure 9–3, a second metabolic pathway of tryptophan is for the production of serotonin used in the stimulation of smooth muscles. Serotonin is produced from tryptophan by the argentaffin cells in the intestine and is carried through the body primarily by the platelets. Normally, the body uses most of the serotonin, and only small amounts of its degradation product 5-HIAA are available for excretion in the urine. However, when carcinoid tumors involving the argentaffin (enterochromaffin) cells develop, excess amounts of serotonin are produced, resulting in the elevation of urinary 5-HIAA levels.

The addition of nitrous acid and 1-nitroso-2-naphthol to urine that contains 5-HIAA causes the appearance of a purple to black color, depending on the amount of 5-HIAA present. The normal daily excretion of 5-HIAA is 2 to 8 mg, and argentaffin cell tumors will produce from 160 to 628 mg per 24 hours.[22] Therefore, the test is usually performed on a random or first morning specimen because there can be little chance of false-negative results. If a 24-hour sample is used, it must be preserved with hydrochloric or boric acid. Patients must be given explicit dietary instructions prior to the collection of any sample to be tested for 5-HIAA, because serotonin is a major constituent of foods such as bananas, pineapples, and tomatoes. Medications, including phenothiazines and acetanilids, will also cause interference. Patients should be requested to withhold medications for 72 hours prior to specimen collection.

CYSTINE DISORDERS

There are two distinct disorders of cystine metabolism that exhibit renal manifestations. Confusion as to their relationship existed for many years following the discovery by Wollaston in 1810 of renal calculi consisting of cystine. It is now known that, although both disorders are inherited, one is a defect in the renal tubular transport of amino acids (cystinuria) and the other is an inborn error of metabolism (cystinosis). A noticeable odor of sulfur may be present in the urine in disorders of cystine metabolism.

Cystinuria

As the name implies, the condition is marked by elevated amounts of the amino acid cystine in the urine. The presence of increased urinary cystine is not due to a defect in the metabolism of cystine but, rather, to the inability of the renal tubules to reabsorb cystine filtered by the glomerulus. The demonstration that not only cystine but also lysine, arginine, and ornithine are not reabsorbed has ruled out the possibility of an error in metabolism even though the condition is inherited.[20] The disorder has two modes of inheritance: one in which reabsorption of all four amino acids—cystine, lysine, arginine, and ornithine—is affected, and the other in which only cystine and lysine are not reabsorbed. The primary clinical consideration in cystinuria is the tendency of persons with defective reabsorption of all four amino acids to form calculi. Approximately 65 percent of these people can be expected to produce calculi early in life.

Because cystine is much less soluble than the other three amino acids, laboratory screening determinations are based on the observation of cystine crystals in the sediment of concentrated or first morning specimens. Cystine is also the only amino acid found during the analysis of calculi from these patients. Elevations in the other three amino acids must be determined separately using chromatography procedures. A chemical screening test for urinary cystine can be performed using cyanide-nitroprusside. Reduction of cystine by sodium cyanide followed by the addition of nitroprusside will produce a red-purple color in a specimen that contains excess cystine. False-positive reactions will

PROCEDURE

Cyanide-Nitroprusside Test

1. Place 3 mL of urine in a tube.
2. Add 2 mL sodium cyanide.
3. Wait 10 minutes.
4. Add five drops 5% sodium nitroprusside.
5. Observe for red-purple color.

occur in the presence of ketones and homocystine, and additional tests may have to be performed.

Cystinosis

Regarded as a genuine inborn error of metabolism, cystinosis can occur in three variations, ranging from a severe fatal disorder developed in infancy to a benign form appearing in adulthood. The incomplete metabolism of cystine results in crystalline deposits of cystine in many areas of the body, including the cornea, bone marrow, lymph nodes, and internal organs. A major defect in the renal tubular reabsorption mechanism (Fanconi's syndrome) also occurs. Routine laboratory findings include polyuria, generalized aminoaciduria, positive test results for reducing substances, and lack of urinary concentration. In severe cases, there is a gradual progression to total renal failure. Renal transplants and the use of cystine-depleting medications to prevent the buildup of cystine in other tissues are extending lives.

Homocystinuria

Defects in the metabolism of homocystine can result in failure to thrive, cataracts, mental retardation, thromboembolic problems, and death. As mentioned previously, increased urinary homocystine gives a positive result with the cyanide-nitroprusside test. Therefore, an additional screening test for homocystinuria must be performed by following a positive cyanide-nitroprusside test result with a silver-nitroprusside test, in which only homocystine will react. The use of silver nitrate in place of sodium cyanide will reduce homocystine to its nitroprusside-reactive form but will not reduce cystine. Consequently, a positive reaction in the silver-nitroprusside test confirms the presence of homocystinuria.[24] Fresh urine should be used when testing for homocystine. The screening tests for cystine and homocystine have been converted to spectrophotometric procedures, which provide better detection of low levels.[27]

PROCEDURE

Silver Nitroprusside Test

1. Place 1 mL of urine in a tube.
2. Add two drops concentrated NH_4OH.
3. Add 0.5 mL 5% silver nitrate.
4. Wait 10 minutes.
5. Add five drops sodium nitroprusside.
6. Observe for red-purple color.

Porphyrin Disorders

Porphyrins are the intermediate compounds in the production of heme. The basic pathway for heme synthesis presented in Figure 9–4 shows the three primary porphyrins (uroporphyrin, coproporphyrin, and protoporphyrin) and the porphyrin precursors (α-aminolevulinic acid [**ALA**] and porphobilinogen). As can be seen, the synthesis of heme can be blocked at a number of stages. Blockage of a pathway reaction will result in the accumulation of the product formed just prior to the interruption. Detection and identification of this product in the urine, bile, feces, or blood can then aid in determining the cause of a specific disorder.

The solubility of the porphyrin compounds varies with their structure. ALA, porphobilinogen, and uroporphyrin are the most soluble and readily appear in the urine. Coproporphyrin is less soluble but is found in the urine, whereas protoporphyrin is not seen in the urine. Fecal analysis has usually been performed for the detection of cop-

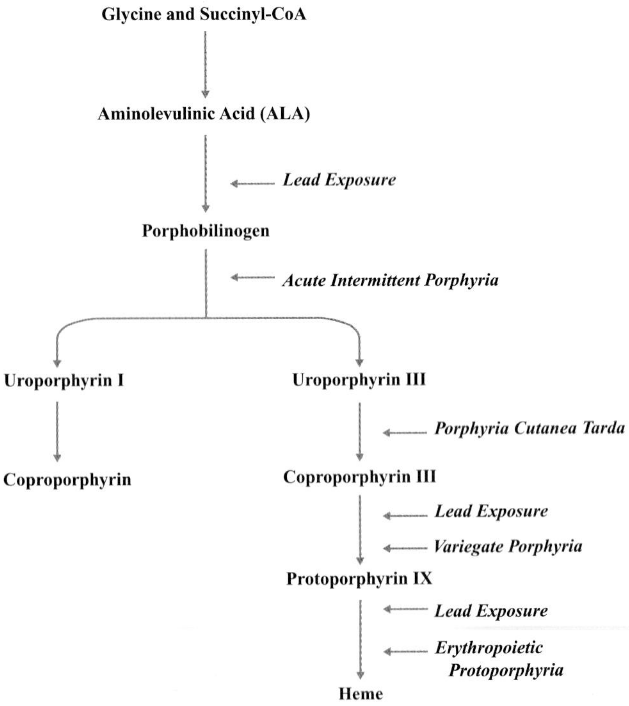

FIGURE 9–4 Pathway of heme formation, including stages affected by the major disorders of porphyrin metabolism. (Adapted from Miale.[18])

roporphyrin and protoporphyrin. However, to avoid false-positive interference, bile is a more acceptable specimen.[19] The Centers for Disease Control and Prevention recommends analysis of whole blood for the presence of free erythrocyte protoporphyrin (**FEP**) as a screening test for lead poisoning.

Disorders of porphyrin metabolism are collectively termed **porphyrias**. They can be inherited or acquired from erythrocytic and hepatic malfunctions or exposure to toxic agents. Common causes of acquired porphyrias include lead poisoning, excessive alcohol exposure, iron deficiency, and liver and renal disease. Inherited porphyrias are much rarer than acquired porphyrias. They are caused by failure to inherit the gene that produces an enzyme needed in the metabolic pathway. In Figure 9–4, the enzyme deficiency sites for some of the more common porphyrias are shown. The inherited porphyrias are frequently classified by their clinical symptoms, either neurologic/psychiatric or cutaneous photosensitivity or a combination of both (Table 9–3).

An indication of the possible presence of ***porphyrinuria*** is the observation of a red or port wine color to the urine. As seen with other inherited disorders, the presence of congenital porphyria is sometimes suspected from a red discoloration of an infant's diapers.

The two screening tests for porphyrinuria use the Ehrlich reaction and fluorescence under ultraviolet light in the 550 to 600 nm range. The Ehrlich reaction can be used only for the detection of ALA and porphobilinogen. Acetylacetone must be added to the specimen to convert the ALA to porphobilinogen prior to performing the Ehrlich test. The fluorescent technique must be used for the other porphyrins. The Ehrlich reaction, including the Watson-Schwartz test for differentiation between the presence of urobilinogen and porphobilinogen and the Hoesch test, were discussed in detail in Chapter 5. Testing for the presence of porphobilinogen is most useful when patients exhibit symptoms of an acute attack. Increased porphobilinogen is associated with acute intermittent porphyria. A negative test result will be obtained in the presence of lead poisoning unless ALA is first converted to porphobilinogen.

Fluorescent screening for the other porphyrins uses their extraction into a mixture of glacial acetic acid and ethyl acetate. The solvent layer is then examined. Negative reactions have a faint blue fluorescence. Positive reactions will fluoresce as violet, pink, or red, depending on the concentration of porphyrins. If the presence of interfering substances is suspected, the organic layer can be removed to a separate tube, and 0.5 mL of hydrochloric acid added to the tube. Only porphyrins will be extracted into the acid layer, which will then produce a bright orange-red fluorescence. The fluorescence method will not distinguish among uroporphyrin, coproporphyrin, and protoporphyrin, but it will rule out porphobilinogen and ALA. The identification of the specific porphyrins requires additional extraction techniques and the analysis of fecal and erythrocyte samples. Increased protoporphyrin is best measured in whole blood.

Mucopolysaccharide Disorders

Mucopolysaccharides, or glycosaminoglycans, are a group of large compounds located primarily in the connective tissue. They consist of a protein core with numerous polysaccharide branches. Inherited disorders in the metabolism of these compounds prevent the complete breakdown of the polysaccharide portion of the compounds, resulting in accumulation of the incompletely metabolized polysaccharide portions in the lysosomes of the connective tissue cells and their increased excretion in the urine. The products most frequently found in the urine are dermatan sulfate, keratan sulfate, and heparan sulfate, with the appearance of a particular substance being determined by the specific metabolic error that was inherited. Therefore, identification of the specific degradation product present may be necessary to establish a specific diagnosis.[16]

There are many types of ***mucopolysaccharidoses***, but the best known are Hurler's syndrome, Hunter's syndrome, and Sanfilippo's syndrome. In both Hurler's and Hunter's syndromes, the skeletal structure is abnormal and there is severe mental retardation; in Hurler's syndrome, mu-

TABLE 9–3 **Summary of Most Common Porphyrias**

Porphyria	Elevated Compound(s)	Clinical Symptoms	Laboratory Testing
Acute intermittent porphyria	ALA Porphobilinogen	Neurologic/psychiatric	Urine/Ehrlich's reaction
Porphyria cutanea tarda	Uroporphyrin	Photosensitivity	Urine fluorescence
Congenital erythropoietic porphyria	Uroporphyrin Coproporphyrin	Photosensitivity	Urine or feces fluorescence
Variegate porphyria	Coproporphyrin	Photosensitivity/neurologic	Bile or feces fluorescence
Erythropoietic protoporphyria	Protoporphyrin	Photosensitivity	Blood FEP Bile or feces fluorescence
Lead poisoning	ALA Protoporphyrin	Neurologic	Urine porphobilinogen/Ehrlich's reaction Blood FEP

PROCEDURE

Cetytrimethylammonium Bromide (CTAB) Test

1. Place 5 mL of urine in a tube.
2. Add 1 mL 5% CTAB in citrate buffer.
3. Read turbidity in 5 minutes.

PROCEDURE

Mucopolysaccharide (MPS) Paper Test

1. Place one drop of urine on dry MPS paper.
2. Dry.
3. Wash 5 minutes (in 1 mL acetic acid + 200 mL methanol diluted to a liter).
4. Dry.
5. Observe for blue spot.

copolysaccharides accumulate in the cornea of the eye. Both syndromes are usually fatal during childhood, whereas in Sanfilippo's syndrome, the only abnormality is mental retardation.[25]

Urinary screening tests for mucopolysaccharides are requested either as part of a routine battery of tests performed on all newborns or on infants who exhibit symptoms of mental retardation or failure to thrive. The most frequently used screening tests are the acid-albumin and cetyltrimethylammonium bromide (**CTAB**) turbidity tests and the metachromatic staining spot tests. In both the acid-albumin and the CTAB tests, a thick, white turbidity will form when these reagents are added to urine that contains mucopolysaccharides. Turbidity is usually graded on a scale of 0 to 4 after 30 minutes with acid-albumin and after 5 minutes with CTAB.[12] Metachromatic staining procedures use basic dyes to react with the acidic mucopolysaccharides. Papers can be prepared by dipping Whatman No. 1 filter paper into a 0.59 percent azure A dye in 2 percent acetic acid and letting it air dry.[1] Urine that contains mucopolysaccharides will produce a blue spot that cannot be washed away by a dilute acidified methanol solution.

Purine Disorders

A disorder of purine metabolism known as ***Lesch-Nyhan disease*** that is inherited as a sex-linked recessive results in massive excretion of urinary uric acid crystals. Failure to inherit the gene to produce the enzyme hypoxanthine guanine phosphoribosyltransferase is responsible for the accumulation of uric acid throughout the body. Patients suffer from severe motor defects, mental retardation, a tendency toward self-destruction, gout, and renal calculi. Development is usually normal for the first 6 to 8 months with the first symptom often being the observation of uric acid crystals resembling orange sand in diapers.[21] Laboratories should be alert for the presence of increased uric acid crystals in pediatric urine specimens.

Carbohydrate Disorders

The presence of increased urinary sugar (***melituria***) is most frequently due to an inherited disorder. In fact, **pentosuria** was one of Garrod's original six inborn errors of metabolism.[7] Fortunately, the majority of meliturias cause no disturbance to body metabolism.[10] However, as discussed in Chapter 5, pediatric urine should be routinely screened for the presence of reducing substances using the Benedict's or Clinitest copper reduction tests. The finding of a positive copper reduction test result combined with a negative reagent strip glucose oxidase test result is strongly suggestive of a disorder of carbohydrate metabolism. Of primary concern is the presence of ***galactosuria***, indicating the inability to properly metabolize galactose to glucose. The resulting galactosemia with toxic intermediate metabolic products results in infant failure to thrive, combined with liver disorders, the presence of cataracts, and severe mental retardation. Early detection of galactosuria followed by removal of lactose (the precursor of galactose) from the diet can prevent these symptoms.

Other causes of melituria include lactose, fructose, and pentose. **Lactosuria** may be seen during pregnancy and lactation. **Fructosuria** is associated with parenteral feeding and pentosuria with ingestion of large amounts of fruit. Whenever a nonglucose-reducing substance is encountered in pediatric urine, it should be further identified using chromatography. Urine screening tests for metabolic disasters are summarized in Table 9–4.

PROCEDURE

Lactose Screening Test

1. Mix 3 g lead acetate with 15 mL of urine.
2. Filter.
3. Add 2 mL of concentrated NH_4OH.
4. Boil and observe for a brick red precipitate.

PROCEDURE

Fructose Screening Test

1. Place 5 mL of urine in a tube.
2. Add 5 mL of 25% HCl.
3. Boil 5 minutes.
4. Add 5 mg resorcinol.
5. Boil 10 seconds.
6. Observe for a red precipitate.

TABLE 9–4 **Comparison of Urinary Screening Tests**

Test	Disorder	Observation
Color	Alkaptonuria	Black
	Melanuria	Black
	Indicanuria	Dark blue
	Porphyrinuria	Port wine
Odor	Phenylketonuria	Mousy
	Maple syrup urine disease	Maple syrup
	Isovaleric acidemia	Sweaty feet
	Cystinuria	Sulphur
	Cystinosis	Sulphur
	Homocystinuria	Sulphur
Crystals	Tyrosyluria	Sheaths of fine needles
	Cystinuria	Colorless hexagonal plates
	Lesch-Nyhan disease	Yellow-brown crystals
Ferric chloride tube test	Phenylketonuria	Blue-green
	Tyrosyluria	Transient green
	Alkaptonuria	Transient blue
	Melanuria	Gray-black
	Maple syrup urine disease	Green-gray
	Indicanuria	Violet-blue with chloroform
	5-HIAA	Blue-green
Nitroso-naphthol	Tyrosyluria	Red
	Maple syrup urine disease	Red
	5-HIAA	Violet with nitric acid
2,4-Dinitrophenylhydrazine	Phenylketonuria	Yellow
	Tyrosyluria	Yellow
	Maple syrup urine disease	Yellow
	Isovaleric acidemia	Yellow
	Propionic acidemia	Yellow
	Methylmalonic acidemia	Yellow
Acetest	Maple syrup urine disease	Purple
	Isovaleric acidemia	Purple
	Propionic acidemia	Purple
	Methylmalonic acidemia	Purple
	Melanuria	Red
p-Nitroaniline	Methylmalonic acidemia	Emerald green
Cyanide-nitroprusside	Cystinuria	Red-purple
	Cystinosis	Red-purple
	Homocystinuria	Red-purple
Silver nitroprusside	Homocystinuria	Red-purple
	Alkaptonuria	Black
Ehrlich's reaction	Porphyrinuria	Red
	Melanuria	Red
Cetytrimethylammonium bromide	Mucopolysaccharidoses	White turbidity
Mucopolysaccharide paper	Mucopolysaccharidoses	Blue spot
Clinitest	Melituria	Orange-red
	Cystinosis	Orange-red
	Alkaptonuria	Orange-red

REFERENCES

1. Bordon, M: Screening for metabolic disease. In Nyhan, WL: Abnormalities in Amino Acid Metabolism in Clinical Medicine. Appleton-Century-Crofts, Norwalk, CT, 1984.
2. Bradley, M, and Schumann, GB: Examination of urine. In Henry, JB (ed): Clinical Diagnosis and Management by Laboratory Methods. WB Saunders, Philadelphia, 1984.
3. Buist, NRM: Laboratory aspects of newborn screening for metabolic disorders. Lab Med 19(3):145–150, 1988.
4. Clow, CL, Reade, TH, and Scriver, CR: Outcome of early and long-term management of classical maple syrup urine disease. Pediatrics 68(6):856–862, 1981.
5. Doherty, LB, Rohr, FJ, and Levy, HL: Detection of phenylketonuria in the very early newborn specimen. Pediatrics 87(2):240–244, 1991.
6. Frimpton, GW: Aminoacidurias due to inherited disorders of metabolism. N Engl J Med 1289:835–901, 1973.
7. Garrod, AE: Inborn Errors of Metabolism. Henry Froude & Hodder & Stoughton, London, 1923.
8. Goodman, SI: Disorders of organic acid metabolism. In Emery, AEH,

and Rimoin, DL: Principles and Practice of Medical Genetics. Churchill Livingstone, New York, 1990.
9. Guthrie, R: Blood screening for phenylketonuria. JAMA 178(8):863, 1961.
10. Hiatt, HH: Pentosuria. In Stanbury, JB, Wyngaarden, JB, and Fredrickson, DS (eds): The Metabolic Basis of Inherited Diseases. McGraw-Hill, New York, 1983.
11. Jepson, JB: Hartnup's disease. In Stanbury, JB, Wyngaarden, JB, and Fredrickson, DS (eds): The Metabolic Basis of Inherited Diseases. McGraw-Hill, New York, 1983.
12. Kelly, S: Biochemical Methods in Medical Genetics. Charles C.Thomas, Springfield, IL, 1977.
13. Kirkman, H, et al: Fifteen year experience with screening for phenylketonuria with an automated fluorometric method. Am J Hum Genet 34(5):743–752, 1982.
14. Kishel, M, and Lighty, P: Some diaper brands give false-positive tests for PKU. N Engl J Med 300(4):200, 1979.
15. Kretchmer, N, and Etzwiler, DD: Disorders associated with the metabolism of phenylalanine and tyrosine. Pediatrics 21:445–475, 1958.
16. McKusick, VA, and Neufeld, EF: The mucopolysaccharide storage diseases. In Stanbury, JB, Wyngaarden, JB, and Fredrickson, DS (eds): The Metabolic Basis of Inherited Diseases. McGraw-Hill, New York, 1983.
17. Meister, A: Biochemistry of the Amino Acids. Academic Press, New York, 1965.
18. Miale, JB: Laboratory Medicine: Hematology. CV Mosby, St. Louis, 1982.
19. Nuttall, KL: Porphyrins and disorders of porphyrin metabolism. In Burtis, CA, and Ashwood, ER: Tietz Fundamentals of Clinical Chemistry. WB Saunders, Philadelphia, 1996.
20. Nyhan, WL: Abnormalities in Amino Acid Metabolism in Clinical Medicine. Appleton-Century-Crofts, Norwalk, CT, 1984.
21. Nyhan, WL, and Sakati, NO: Diagnostic Recognition of Genetic Disease. Lea & Febiger, Philadelphia, 1987.
22. Sjoerdsma, A, Weissbach, H, and Udenfriend, S: Simple test for diagnosis of metastatic carcinoid (argentaffinoma). JAMA 159(4):397, 1955.
23. Stanbury, JB: The Metabolic Basis of Inherited Diseases. McGraw-Hill, New York, 1983.
24. Thomas, GH, and Howell, RR: Selected Screening Tests for Metabolic Diseases. Yearbook Medical Publishers, Chicago, 1973.
25. Thompson, JS, and Thompson, MW: Genetics in Medicine. WB Saunders, Philadelphia, 1978.
26. Waber, L: Inborn errors of metabolism. Pediatr Ann 19(2):105–118, 1990.
27. Wu, JT, Wilson, LW, and Christensen, S: Conversion of a qualitative screening test to a quantitative measurement of urinary cystine and homocystine. Ann Clin Lab Sci 22(1):18–29, 1992.

STUDY QUESTIONS

1. State two reasons for the appearance of overflow metabolites in the urine.
2. Name two physical characteristics of urine that can alert medical personnel to the possibility of a metabolic disorder.
3. List four metabolic disorders associated with the phenylalanine-tyrosine metabolic pathway.
4. Why are laws present that require PKU testing of all newborns?
5. Why are the original PKU newborn tests performed on blood rather than urine?
6. Name the enzyme lacking in persons with PKU.
7. When performing the Guthrie test, does the presence of increased phenylalanine inhibit the growth of *B. subtilis*? Why or why not?
8. What is the purpose for testing urine from people with PKU with ferric chloride?
9. State three possible causes of tyrosyluria. Which is usually the least serious?
10. What is the significance of an orange-red color in the nitroso-naphthol test?
11. Why is increased urinary homogentisic acid called alkaptonuria?
12. Why does the presence of homogentisic acid produce a positive Clinitest result?
13. What is the significance of a urine that turns black following exposure to air and reacts with sodium nitroprusside and Ehrlich's reagent? Why is this of medical importance?
14. Describe the ferric chloride tube test in PKU, tyrosyluria, alkaptonuria, and melanuria.
15. How did maple syrup urine disease get its name?
16. What chemical test in the routine urinalysis is associated with a positive DNPH reaction?
17. Which organic acidemia produces urine with an odor of "sweaty feet"? Which reacts with *p*-nitroaniline?
18. Why are intestinal disorders associated with blue urine? How does the significance of a blue diaper differ from that of a blue urine specimen in an adult?
19. What is the significance of a urine that turns purple upon addition of nitrous acid and 1-nitroso-2-naphthol? How could this be a false-positive result?
20. Why is cystinosis considered an inborn error of metabolism and cystinuria is not?
21. Why are cystine crystals and not lysine crystals found in the urine in cystinuria?
22. How can cystinuria be differentiated from homocystinuria in the laboratory?
23. List three heme precursor substances that are tested for in urine, two in feces or bile, and one in blood.
24. Name an inherited porphyria with neurologic symptoms, one with photosensitivity, and one with both symptoms.
25. What is the most common cause of acquired porphyria?
26. Name three heme precursor substances elevated in lead poisoning.
27. How could you determine if porphobilinogen or uroporphyrin is the cause of a port wine–colored urine?

28. What is the signficance of a blue spot on paper containing azure A dye?

29. What is the characteristic urine abnormality in Lesch-Nyhan disease?

30. What is the primary concern when melituria is present in a newborn?

CASE STUDIES AND CLINICAL SITUATIONS

1. A premature infant develops jaundice. Laboratory tests are negative for hemolytic disease of the newborn, but the infant's bilirubin level continues to rise. Abnormal urinalysis results include a dark yellow color, positive Ictotest, and needle-shaped crystals seen on microscopic examination.

a. What is the most probable cause of the infant's jaundice?
b. How will urine from this infant react in the ferric chloride test?
c. Could these same urine findings be associated with an adult? Explain your answer.
d. What kind of crystals are present? Name another type of crystal with a spherical shape that is associated with this condition.
e. When blood is drawn from this infant, what precaution should be taken to ensure the integrity of the specimen?

2. A newborn develops severe vomiting and symptoms of metabolic acidosis. Urinalysis results are positive for ketones and negative for glucose and other reducing substances.

a. State a urinalysis screening test that would be positive in this patient.
b. If the urine had an odor of "sweaty feet," what metabolic disorder would be suspected?
c. If the newborn was producing dark brown urine with a sweet odor, what disorder would be suspected?
d. State an additional urinalysis screening test that might be ordered on the infant. If this test produces an emerald green color, what is the significance?
e. The urine produces a green-gray color when tested with ferric chloride. Is this an expected result? Why or why not?
f. For the most accurate diagnosis of the newborn's condition, what additional testing should be performed?

3. A 13-year-old boy is awakened with severe back and abdominal pain and is taken to the emergency room by his parents. A complete blood count is normal. Family history shows that both his father and uncle are chronic kidney stone formers. Results of a urinalysis are as follows:

COLOR: Yellow	KETONES: Negative
APPEARANCE: Hazy	BLOOD: Moderate
SP. GRAVITY: 1.025	BILIRUBIN: Negative
pH: 6.0	UROBILINOGEN: Normal
PROTEIN: Negative	NITRITE: Negative
GLUCOSE: Negative	LEUKOCYTE: Negative

Microscopic

>15–20 RBCs/hpf	Few squamous epithelial cells
0–3 WBCs/hpf	Many cystine crystals

a. What condition does the patient's symptoms represent?
b. What is the physiologic abnormality causing this condition?
c. If amino acid chromatography was performed on this specimen, what additional amino acids would you expect to find?
d. Why are they not present in the microscopic constituents?
e. What chemical test could be performed to confirm the identity of the cystine crystals?
f. What is the significance of the family history?

4. An 8-month-old boy is admitted to the pediatric unit with a general diagnosis of failure to thrive. The parents have observed slowness in the infant's development of motor skills. They also mention the occasional appearance of a substance resembling orange sand in the child's diapers. Urinalysis results are as follows:

COLOR: Yellow	KETONES: Negative
APPEARANCE: Slightly hazy	BLOOD: Negative
SP. GRAVITY: 1.024	BILIRUBIN: Negative
pH: 5.0	UROBILINOGEN: Normal
PROTEIN: Negative	NITRITE: Negative
GLUCOSE: Negative	LEUKOCYTE: Negative

Microscopic
Many uric acid crystals

a. Is the urine pH consistent with the appearance of uric acid crystals?
b. Is there any correlation between the urinalysis results and the substance observed in the child's diapers? Explain your answer.
c. What disorder do the patient's history and the urinalysis results indicate?
d. Is the fact that this is a male patient of any significance? Explain your answer.
e. Name the enzyme that is missing.

5. Shortly after arriving for the day shift in the urinalysis laboratory, a technician notices that an undiscarded urine has a black color. The previously completed report indicates the color to be yellow.

a. Is this observation significant? Explain your answer.
b. What two reactions might be seen with the ferric chloride test?
c. Which ferric chloride reaction would correlate with a positive Clinitest result?
d. The original urinalysis report showed the specimen to be positive for ketones. Is this significant? Why or why not?

6. Bobby Williams, age 8, is admitted through the emergency department with a ruptured appendix. Although surgery is successful, Bobby's recovery is slow, and the physicians are concerned about his health prior to the ruptured appendix. Bobby's mother states that he has always been noticeably underweight despite a balanced diet and strong appetite and that his younger brother exhibits similar characteristics. A note in his chart from the first postoperative day reports that the evening nurse noticed a purple coloration on the urinary catheter bag.
   a. Is the catheter bag color significant?
   b. What additional tests should be run?
   c. What condition can be suspected from this history?
   d. What is Bobby's prognosis?

7. A Watson-Schwartz test is performed on an anemic patient who is exhibiting signs of severe photosensitivity. The test result is negative.
   a. What metabolic disorder was suspected in this patient?
   b. Was sufficient testing performed to rule out this disorder? Why or why not?
   c. Can the Watson-Schwartz test be used to detect lead poisoning? Explain your answer.

8. The laboratory receives a request for a resorcinol test.
   a. What substance will be detected?
   b. What treatment might this patient be receiving?

CHAPTER 10

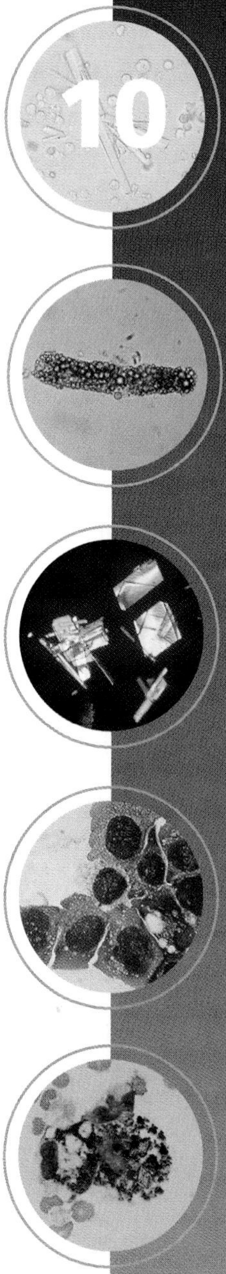

Cerebrospinal Fluid

LEARNING OBJECTIVES

Upon completion of this chapter, the reader will be able to:

1 State the three major functions of cerebrospinal fluid (CSF).
2 Distribute CSF specimen tubes numbered 1, 2, and 3 to their appropriate laboratory sections and correctly preserve them.
3 Describe the appearance of normal CSF.
4 Define xanthochromia and state its significance.
5 Differentiate between CSF specimens caused by intracranial hemorrhage and a traumatic tap.
6 Calculate CSF total, white blood cell and red blood cell counts when given the number of cells seen, amount of specimen dilution, and the squares counted in the Neubauer chamber.
7 Briefly explain the methods used to correct for WBCs and protein that are artificially introduced during a traumatic tap.
8 Describe the leukocyte content of the CSF in bacterial, viral, tubercular, and fungal meningitis.
9 Describe and give the significance of abnormal macrophages in the CSF.
10 Differentiate between the appearance of normal choroidal cells and malignant cells.
11 State the normal value for CSF total protein.
12 List three pathologic conditions that produce an elevated CSF protein.
13 Discuss the basic principles and advantages and disadvantages of the turbidimetric and the dye-binding methods of CSF protein analysis.
14 Determine whether increased CSF immunoglobulin is the result of damage to the blood-brain barrier or central nervous system production.
15 Discuss the significance of CSF electrophoresis findings in multiple sclerosis and the identification of CSF.
16 State the normal CSF glucose value.
17 Name the possible pathologic significance of a decreased CSF glucose.
18 Briefly discuss the diagnostic value of CSF lactate and glutamine determinations.
19 Name the microorganism associated with a positive India Ink preparation.
20 Briefly discuss the diagnostic value of the bacterial and cryptococcal antigen tests.
21 State the diagnostic value of the limulus lysate test.
22 Determine whether a suspected case of meningitis is most probably of bacterial, viral, fungal, or tubercular origin, when presented with pertinent laboratory data.
23 Describe the role of the Venereal Disease Research Laboratories test and fluorescent treponemal antibody-absorption test for syphilis in CSF testing.
24 Describe quality control procedures and safety precautions related to CSF procedures.

KEY TERMS

arachnoid villi
blood-brain barrier
choroid plexuses
meningitis
oligoclonal bands
pleocytosis
subarachnoid space
traumatic tap
xanthochromia

Formation and Physiology

First recognized by Cotugno in 1764, cerebrospinal fluid (**CSF**) is the third major fluid of the body.[16] The CSF provides a physiologic system to supply nutrients to the nervous tissue, to remove metabolic wastes, and to produce a mechanical barrier to cushion the brain and spinal cord against trauma. As shown in Figure 10–1, the brain and spinal cord are lined by the **meninges**, consisting of three layers: the dura mater, arachnoid mater, and pia mater. The CSF flows through the ***subarachnoid space*** located between the arachnoid mater and the pia mater. Approximately 20 mL of fluid is produced every hour in the ***choroid plexuses*** and reabsorbed by the ***arachnoid villi*** to maintain a total volume of 140 to 170 mL in adults and 10 to 60 mL in neonates.[23]

Production of CSF in the choroid plexuses is by filtration under hydrostatic pressure across the choroidal capillary wall and active transport secretion by the choroidal epithelial cells. Tightly fitting junctions between the endothelial cells of the capillaries and the choroid plexuses restrict entry of macromolecules such as protein, insoluble lipids, and substances bound to serum proteins. The chemical composition of the fluid does not resemble an ultrafiltrate of plasma owing to bidirectional active transport between the CSF, interstitial brain fluid, brain cells, and blood in the brain capillaries. The term ***blood-brain barrier*** is used to represent the control and filtration of blood components to the CSF and then to the brain.[10]

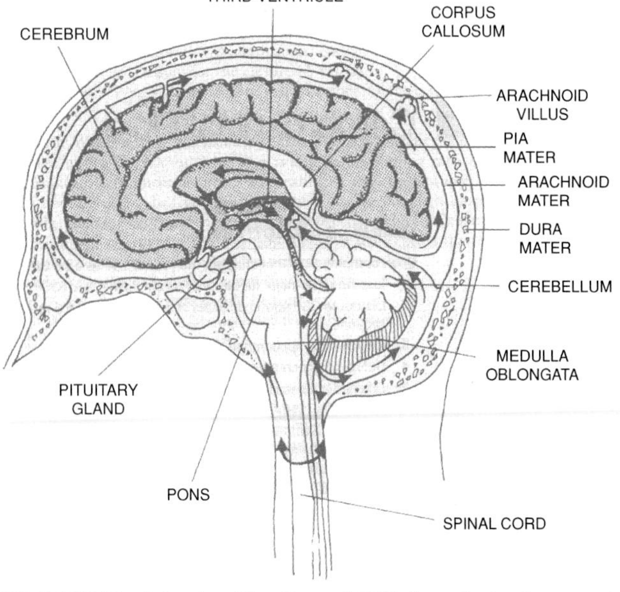

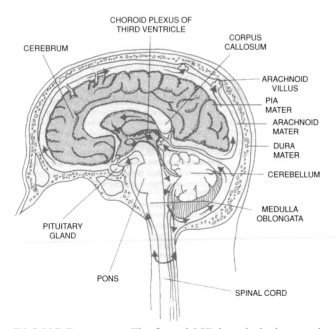

FIGURE 10–1 The flow of CSF through the brain and spinal column.

Specimen Collection and Handling

CSF is routinely collected by lumbar puncture between the third, fourth, or fifth lumbar vertebrae. Although this procedure is not complicated, it does require certain precautions, including measurement of the intracranial pressure and careful technique to prevent the introduction of infection or the damaging of neural tissue. Specimens are usually collected in three sterile tubes, which are labeled 1, 2, and 3 in the order in which they are withdrawn. Tube 1 is used for chemical and serologic tests; tube 2 is usually designated for the microbiology laboratory; and tube 3 is used for the cell count, because it is the least likely to contain cells introduced by the spinal tap procedure. If possible, a fourth tube may be drawn for the microbiology laboratory to provide better exclusion of skin contamination. Supernatant fluid that is left over after each section has performed its tests may be used for additional chemical or serologic tests. Excess fluid should not be discarded until there is no further use for it (Figure 10–2).

Considering the discomfort to the patient and the possible complications that can occur during specimen collection, laboratory personnel should handle CSF specimens carefully. Ideally, tests are performed on a STAT basis. If this is not possible, specimens are maintained in the following manner:

Hematology tubes are refrigerated.
Microbiology tubes remain at room temperature.
Chemistry and serology tubes are frozen.

Appearance

The initial appearance of the normally crystal clear CSF can provide valuable diagnostic information. Examination of the fluid occurs first at the bedside and is also included in the laboratory report. The major terminology used to describe CSF appearance includes crystal clear, cloudy or turbid, milky, xanthochromic, and hemolyzed/bloody (Figure

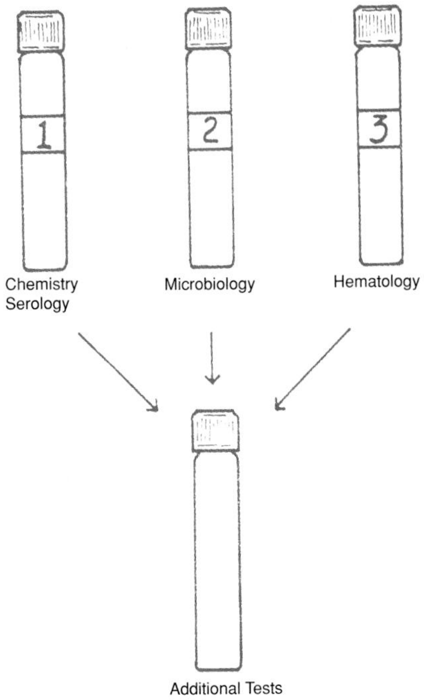

FIGURE 10–2 CSF specimen collection tubes.

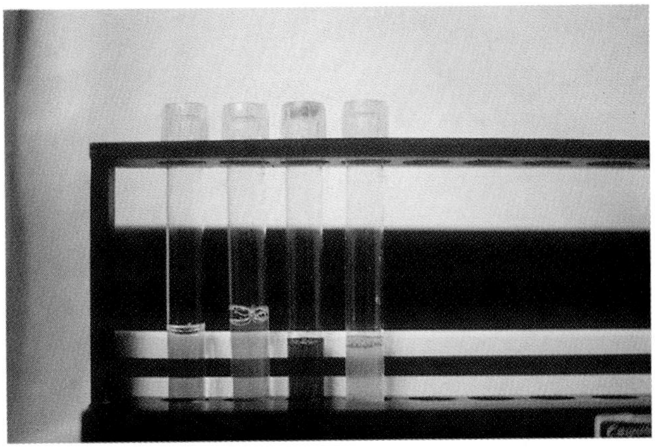

FIGURE 10–3 Tubes of CSF. Appearance left to right is normal, xanthochromic, hemolyzed, and cloudy.

10–3). A cloudy, turbid, or milky specimen can be the result of an increased protein or lipid concentration, but it also may be indicative of infection, with the cloudiness being caused by the presence of WBCs. All specimens should be treated with extreme care because they can be highly contagious; gloves must always be worn and face shields or splash guards should be used while preparing specimens for testing. Fluid for centrifugation must be in capped tubes.

Xanthochromia is a term used to describe CSF supernatant that is pink, orange, or yellow. A variety of factors can cause the appearance of xanthochromia, with the most common being the presence of RBC degradation products. Depending on the amount of blood and the length of time it has been present, the color will vary from pink (very slight amount of oxyhemoglobin) to orange (heavy hemolysis) to yellow (conversion of oxyhemoglobin to unconjugated bilirubin). Other causes of xanthochromia include elevated serum bilirubin, presence of the pigment carotene, markedly increased protein concentrations, and melanoma pigment. Xanthochromia that is due to immature liver function is also commonly seen in infants, particularly in those who are premature. The clinical significance of CSF appearance is summarized in Table 10–1.

TABLE 10–1 **Clinical Significance of Cerebrospinal Fluid Appearance**

Appearance	Cause	Major Significance
Crystal clear		Normal
Hazy, turbid, cloudy, milky	WBCs	Meningitis
	RBCs	Hemorrhage Traumatic tap
	Microorganisms	Meningitis
	Protein	Disorders that affect blood-brain barrier Production of IgG within the CNS
Oily	Radiographic contrast media	
Bloody	RBCs	Hemorrhage Traumatic tap
Xanthochromic	Hemoglobin	Old hemorrhage Lysed cells from traumatic tap
	Bilirubin	RBC degradation Elevated serum bilirubin level
	Carotene	Increased serum levels
	Protein	SEE ABOVE
	Melanin	Meningeal melanosarcoma
Clotted	Protein	SEE ABOVE
	Clotting factors	Introduced by traumatic tap
Pellicle	Protein	Disorders that affect blood-brain barrier
	Clotting factors	Tubercular meningitis

Traumatic Collection

Grossly bloody CSF can be an indication of intracranial hemorrhage, but it also may be due to the puncture of a blood vessel during the spinal tap procedure. Three visual examinations of the collected specimens can usually determine whether the blood is the result of hemorrhage or a ***traumatic tap***.

UNEVEN DISTRIBUTION OF BLOOD

Blood from a cerebral hemorrhage will be evenly distributed throughout the three CSF specimen tubes, whereas a traumatic tap will have the heaviest concentration of blood in tube 1, with gradually diminishing amounts in tubes 2 and 3. Streaks of blood also may be seen in specimens acquired following a traumatic procedure.

CLOT FORMATION

Fluid collected from a traumatic tap may form clots owing to the introduction of plasma fibrinogen into the specimen. Bloody CSF caused by intracranial hemorrhage will not contain enough fibrinogen to clot. Diseases in which damage to the blood-brain barrier allows increased filtration of protein and coagulation factors will also cause clot formation but do not usually produce a bloody fluid. These conditions include ***meningitis***, Froin's syndrome, and blockage of CSF circulation through the subarachnoid space. A classic weblike pellicle is associated with tubercular meningitis and is frequently seen after overnight refrigeration of the fluid.[27]

XANTHOCHROMIC SUPERNATANT

RBCs must usually remain in the CSF for approximately 2 hours before noticeable hemolysis begins; therefore, a xanthochromic supernatant would be the result of blood that has been present longer than that introduced by the traumatic tap. Care should be taken, however, to consider this examination in conjunction with those previously discussed, because a very recent hemorrhage would produce a clear supernatant, and introduction of serum protein from a traumatic tap could also cause the fluid to appear xanthochromic. To examine a bloody fluid for the presence of xanthochromia, the fluid should be centrifuged in a microhematocrit tube and the supernatant examined against a white background.

Additional testing for differentiation includes microscopic examination and the **D-dimer** test. The microscopic finding of macrophages containing ingested RBCs (**erythrophagocytosis**) or hemosiderin granules is indicative of intracranial hemorrhage. Detection of the fibrin degradation product, D-dimer, by latex agglutination immunoassay indicates the formation of fibrin at a hemorrhage site.

Cell Count

The cell count that is routinely performed on CSF specimens is the leukocyte (WBC) count. As discussed previously, the presence and significance of RBCs can usually be ascertained from the appearance of the specimen. Therefore, RBC counts are usually determined only when a traumatic tap has occurred and a correction for leukocytes or protein is needed. The RBC count can be calculated by performing a total cell count and a WBC count and subtracting the WBC count from the total count, if necessary. Any cell count should be performed immediately, because WBCs (particularly granulocytes) and RBCs will begin to lyse within 1 hour, with 40 percent of the leukocytes disintegrating after 2 hours.[6] Specimens that cannot be analyzed immediately should be refrigerated.

METHODOLOGY

Normal adult CSF contains 0 to 5 WBCs/μL. The number is higher in children, and as many as 30 mononuclear cells/μL can be considered normal in newborns.[32] Specimens that contain up to 200 WBCs or 400 RBCs/μL may appear clear, so it is necessary to examine all specimens microscopically.[12] An improved Neubauer counting chamber (Figure 10–4) is routinely used for performing CSF cell counts. Traditionally, electronic cell counters have not been used for performing CSF cell counts, owing to high background counts and poor reproducibility of low counts. However, newer instrumentation has greatly eliminated background interference and laboratories with documentation of linearity, background, and correlation studies can meet the requirements of accrediting agencies for automated body fluid cell counts.[36]

The standard Neubauer calculation formula used for blood cell counts is also applied to CSF cell counts to determine the number of cells per microliter.

$$\frac{\text{Number of cells counted} \times \text{dilution}}{\text{Number of squares counted} \times \text{volume of 1 square}} = \text{cells}/\mu\text{L}$$

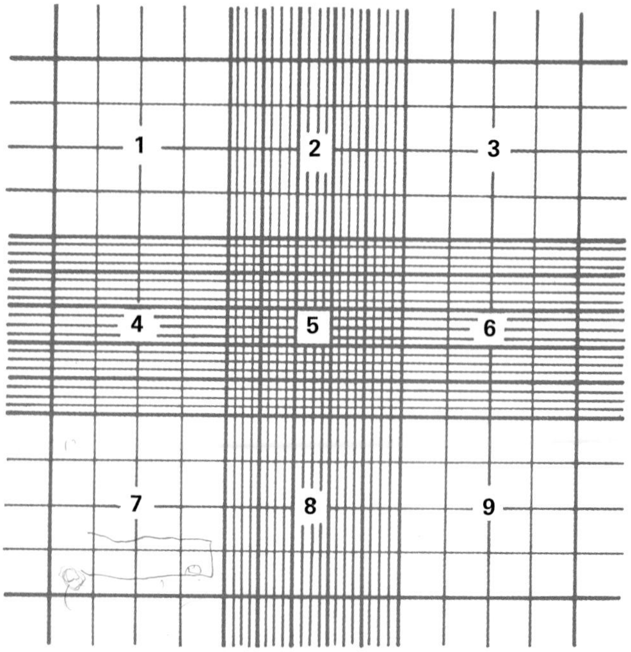

FIGURE 10–4 Neubauer counting chamber depicting the nine large, square counting areas.

This formula can be used for both diluted and undiluted specimens and offers flexibility in the number and size of the squares counted. Many varied calculations are available, including condensations of the formula to provide single factors by which to multiply the cell count. Keep in mind that the purpose of any calculation is to convert the number of cells counted in a specific amount of fluid to the number of cells that would be present in 1 μL of fluid. Therefore, a factor can be used only when the dilution and counting area are specific for that factor.

The methodology presented in this chapter eliminates the need to correct for the volume counted by counting the four large corner squares (0.4 μL) and the large center square (0.1 μL) on each side of the counting chamber.[35]

EXAMPLE:

$$\text{Number of cells counted} \times \text{dilution} \times \frac{1\ \mu\text{L}}{1\ \mu\text{L}\ (0.1 \times 10)\ \text{(volume counted)}} = \text{cells}/\mu\text{L}$$

TOTAL CELL COUNT

Clear specimens may be counted undiluted, provided no overlapping of cells is seen during the microscopic examination. When dilutions are required, calibrated automatic pipettes, not mouth pipetting, are used. A sample dilution method is as follows.[35]

Clarity	Dilution	Amount of Sample	Amount of Diluent
Slightly hazy	1:10	30 μL	270 μL
Hazy	1:20	30 μL	570 μL
Slightly cloudy	1:100	30 μL	2970 μL
Slightly bloody	1:200	30 μL	5970 μL
Cloudy			
Bloody	1:10,000	0.1 mL of a 1:100 dilution	9.9 mL
Turbid			

Dilutions for total cell counts are made with normal saline, mixed by inversion, and loaded into the hemocytometer with a Pasteur pipette. Cells are counted in the four corner squares and the center square on both sides of the hemocytometer. As shown in the preceding example, the number of cells counted multiplied by the dilution factor equals the number of cells per microliter.

WHITE BLOOD CELL COUNT

Lysis of RBCs must be obtained prior to performing the WBC count on either diluted or undiluted specimens. Specimens requiring dilution can be diluted in the manner described previously, substituting 3 percent acetic acid to lyse the RBCs. Addition of methylene blue to the diluting fluid will stain the WBCs providing better differentiation.

To prepare a clear specimen that does not require dilution for counting, place four drops of mixed specimen in a clean tube. Rinse a Pasteur pipette with glacial acetic acid, draining thoroughly, and draw the four drops of CSF into the rinsed pipette. Allow the pipette to sit for 1 minute, mix the solution in the pipette, discard the first drop, and load the hemocytometer. As in the total cell count, WBCs are counted in the four corner squares, and the center square on both sides of the hemocytometer and the number is multiplied by the dilution factor to obtain the number of WBCs per microliter. If a different number of squares is counted, the standard Neubauer formula should be used to obtain the number of cells per microliter.

CORRECTIONS FOR CONTAMINATION

Calculations are possible to correct for WBCs and protein artificially introduced into the CSF as the result of a traumatic tap. Determination of the CSF RBC count and the blood RBC and WBC counts is necessary to perform the correction. By determining the ratio of WBCs to RBCs in the peripheral blood and comparing this ratio with the number of contaminating RBCs, the number of artificially added WBCs can be calculated using the following formula:

$$\text{WBC (added)} = \frac{\text{WBC (blood)} \times \text{RBC (CSF)}}{\text{RBC (blood)}}$$

An approximate CSF WBC count can then be obtained by subtracting the "added" WBCs from the actual count. When peripheral blood RBC and WBC counts are in the normal range, many laboratories choose to simply subtract 1 WBC for every 700 RBCs present in the CSF.[32] Studies have shown a high percentage of error in the correction of fluids containing a large number of RBCs, indicating correction may be of little value under these circumstances.[28]

QUALITY CONTROL OF CEREBROSPINAL FLUID AND OTHER BODY FLUID CELL COUNTS

In-house controls can be prepared on a daily basis and performed on each shift to ensure the reliability of reagents and technique. This can be done by preparing dilutions of a selected patient sample and comparing manual results with those obtained on an automated cell counter. Results of the manual counts should agree with the automated counts by plus or minus 25 percent. The daily control specimen is refrigerated and manual counts are performed on each shift.[35] Spinalscopics Spinal Fluid Cell Count Controls (Quantimetrix, Redondo Beach, CA), which provides two levels of RBCs and WBCs, are available for purchase.

On a biweekly basis all diluents should be checked for contamination by examining in a counting chamber under 40× magnification. Contaminated diluents should be discarded and new solutions prepared.

On a monthly basis the speed of the cytocentrifuge should be checked with a tachometer and the timing should be checked with a stopwatch.

If nondisposable counting chambers are used, they must be soaked in a bactericidal solution for at least 15 minutes and then thoroughly rinsed with water and cleaned with isopropyl alcohol.

Differential Count on a Cerebrospinal Fluid Specimen

Identifying the type or types of cells present in the CSF is a valuable diagnostic aid. The differential count should be performed on a stained smear and not from the cells in the counting chamber. Poor visualization of the cells as they appear in the counting chamber has led to the laboratory practice of reporting only the percentage of mononuculear and polynuclear cells present, and this can result in the overlooking of abnormal cells with considerable diagnostic importance. To ensure that the maximum number of cells are available for examination, the specimen should be concentrated prior to the preparation of the smear.

Methods available for specimen concentration include sedimentation, filtration, centrifugation, and cytocentrifugation. Automated body fluid microscopy also is available on the IRIS Model 500 (International Remote Imaging Systems, Chatsworth, CA.). Sedimentation and filtration are not routinely used in the clinical laboratory, although they do produce less cellular distortion. Most laboratories that do not have a cytocentrifuge concentrate specimens with routine centrifugation. The specimen is centrifuged for 5 to 10 minutes; supernatant fluid is removed and saved for additional tests; and slides made from the suspended sediment are allowed to air dry and are stained with Wright's stain. When performing the differential count, 100 cells should be counted, classified, and reported in terms of percentage. If the cell count is low and finding 100 cells is not possible, report only the numbers of the cell types seen.

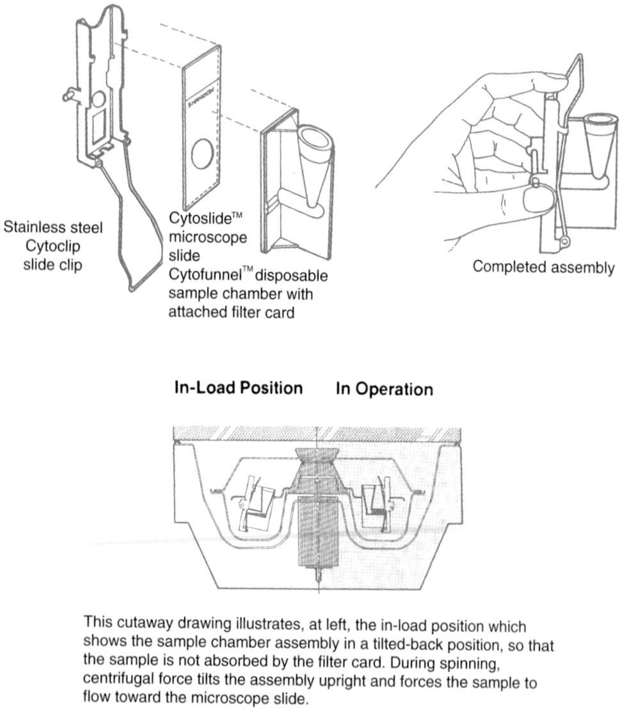
Stainless steel Cytoclip slide clip
Cytoslide™ microscope slide
Cytofunnel™ disposable sample chamber with attached filter card
Completed assembly
In-Load Position
In Operation
This cutaway drawing illustrates, at left, the in-load position which shows the sample chamber assembly in a tilted-back position, so that the sample is not absorbed by the filter card. During spinning, centrifugal force tilts the assembly upright and forces the sample to flow toward the microscope slide.

FIGURE 10–5 Cytospin 3 cytocentrifuge specimen processing assembly (Courtesy of Shandon, Inc., Pittsburgh, PA.)

CYTOCENTRIFUGATION

A diagramatic view of the principle of cytocentrifugation is shown in Figure 10–5. Fluid is added to the conical chamber, and as the specimen is centrifuged, cells present in the fluid are forced into a monolayer within a 6-mm diameter circle on the slide. Fluid is absorbed by the filter paper blotter, producing a more concentrated area of cells. As little as 0.1 mL of CSF combined with one drop of 30 percent albumin produces an adequate cell yield when processed with the cytocentrifuge. Addition of albumin increases the cell yield and decreases the cellular distortion frequently seen on cytocentrifuged specimens. Positively charged coated slides to attract cells (Shandon, Inc, Pittsburgh, PA) are also available. Cellular distortion may include cytoplasmic vacuoles, nuclear clefting, prominent nucleoli, and cellular clumping resembling malignancy. Cells from both the center and periphery of the slide should be examined because cellular characteristics may vary between areas of the slide.

A daily control slide for bacteria should also be prepared using 0.2 mL saline and two drops of 30 percent albumin. The slide is stained and examined if bacteria are seen on a patient's slide.[35]

In Table 10–2, a cytocentrifuge recovery chart is provided for comparison with chamber counts. The chamber count should be repeated if too many cells are seen on the slide, and a new slide should be prepared if not enough cells are seen on the slide.[35]

CEREBROSPINAL FLUID CELLULAR CONSTITUENTS

The cells found in normal CSF are primarily lymphocytes and monocytes (Figures 10–6 and 10–7). Adults usually have a predominance of lymphocytes to monocytes (70:30), whereas monocytes are more prevalent in children.[21] Improved concentration methods are also showing occasional neutrophils in normal CSF.[19] The presence of increased numbers of these normal cells (termed ***pleocytosis***) is considered abnormal, as is the finding of immature leukocytes, eosinophils, plasma cells, macrophages, increased tissue cells, and malignant cells.

When pleocytosis involving neutrophils, lymphocytes, or monocytes is present, the CSF differential count is most frequently associated with its role in providing diagnostic information about the type of microorganism that is causing an infection of the meninges (meningitis). A high CSF

TABLE 10–2 **Cytocentrifuge Recovery Chart[35]**

Number of White Blood Cells Counted in Chamber	Number of Cells Counted on Cytocentrifuge Slide
0	0–40
1–5	20–100
6–10	60–150
11–20	150–250
20	250

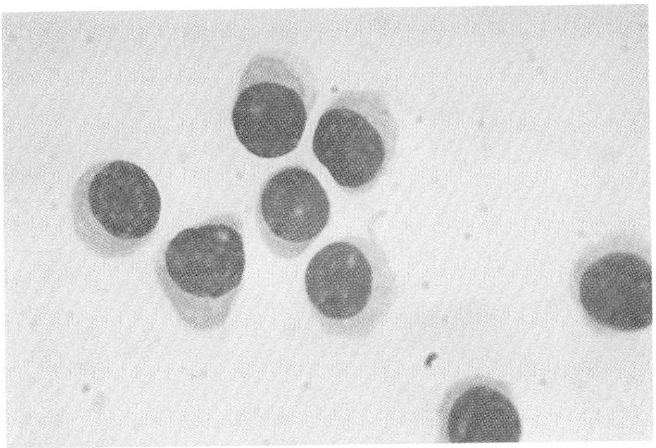

FIGURE 10–6 Normal lymphocytes. Some cytocentrifuge distortion of cytoplasm (×1000).

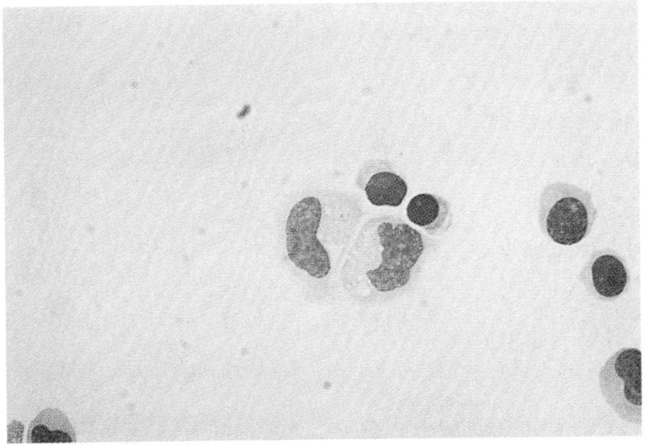

FIGURE 10–7 Normal lymphocytes and monocytes (×500).

WBC count of which the majority of the cells are neutrophils is considered indicative of bacterial meningitis. Likewise, a moderately elevated CSF WBC count with a high percentage of lymphocytes and monocytes suggests meningitis of viral, tubercular, fungal, or parasitic origin.

As seen in Table 10–3, many pathologic conditions other than meningitis can be associated with the finding of abnormal cells in the CSF. Therefore, because laboratory personnel become so accustomed to finding neutrophils, lymphocytes, and monocytes, they should be careful not to overlook other types of cells. Cell forms differing from those found in blood include macrophages, choroid plexus and ependymal cells, spindle-shaped cells, and malignant cells.

Increased neutrophils (Figure 10–8) also are seen in the early stages (1 to 2 days) of viral, fungal, tubercular, and parasitic meningitis. Neutrophils associated with bacterial meningitis may contain phagocytized bacteria (Figure 10–9). Although of little clinical significance, neutrophils may be increased following central nervous system **(CNS)** hemorrhage, repeated lumbar punctures, and injection of medications or radiographic dye.

A mixture of lymphocytes and monocytes is common in cases of viral, tubercular, and fungal meningitis (Figure

TABLE 10–3 **Predominant Cells Seen in Cerebrospinal Fluid**

Type of Cell	Major Clinical Significance	Microscopic Findings
Lymphocytes	Normal Viral, tubercular, and fungal meningitis Multiple sclerosis	All stages of development may be found
Neutrophils	Bacterial meningitis Early cases of viral, tubercular, and fungal meningitis Cerebral hemorrhage	Granules may be less prominent than in blood[19] Cells disintegrate rapidly
Monocytes	Normal Viral, tubercular, and fungal meningitis Multiple sclerosis	Found mixed with lymphocytes
Macrophages	RBCs in spinal fluid Contrast media	May contain phagocytized RBCs appearing as empty vacuoles or ghost cells and hemosiderin granules
Blast forms	Acute leukemia	Lymphoblasts, myeloblasts, or monoblasts
Plasma cells	Multiple sclerosis Lymphocyte reactions	Traditional and classic forms seen
Ependymal, choroidal, and spindle-shaped cells	Diagnostic procedures	Seen in clusters with distinct nuclei and distinct cell walls
Malignant cells	Metastatic carcinomas Primary central nervous system (CNS) carcinoma	Seen in clusters with fusing of cell borders and nuclei

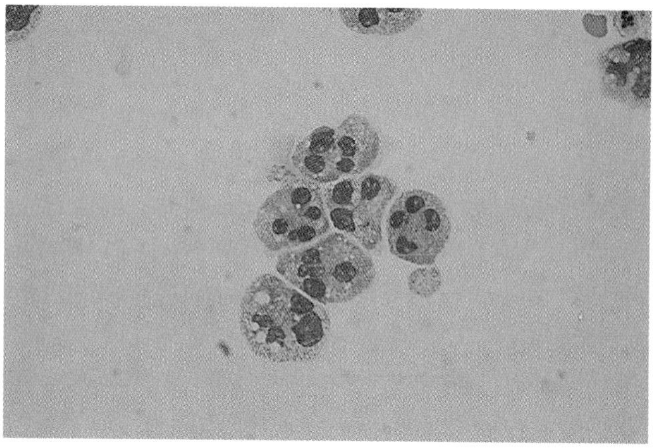

FIGURE 10–8 Neutrophils with cytoplasmic vacuoles resulting from cytocentrifugation (×500).

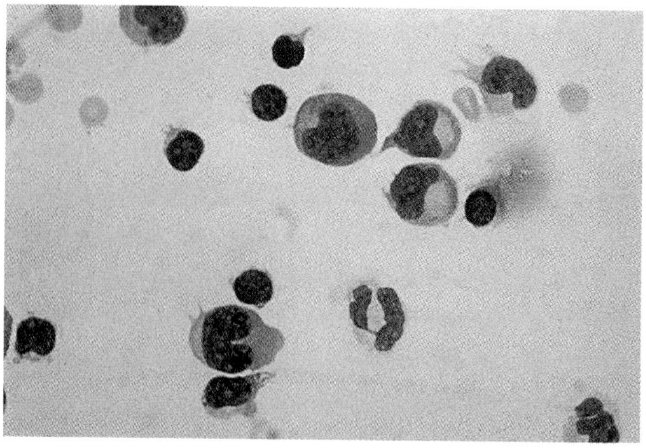

FIGURE 10–10 Broad spectrum of lymphocytes and monocytes in viral meningitis (×100).

10–10). Reactive lymphocytes containing increased dark blue cytoplasm and clumped chromatin are frequently present during viral infections in conjunction with normal cells. Increased lymphocytes are seen in cases of both asymptomatic human immunodeficiency virus (**HIV**) infection and acquired immunodeficiency syndrome (**AIDS**). A moderately elevated WBC count (less than 50 WBCs/μL) with increased normal and reactive lymphocytes and plasma cells may be indicative of multiple sclerosis or other degenerative neurologic disorders.[3]

Increased eosinophils are seen in the CSF in association with parasitic infections, fungal infections (primarily *Coccidioides immitis*), and introduction of foreign material, including medications and shunts into the CNS (Figure 10–11).

Macrophages appear within 2 to 4 hours after RBCs enter into the CSF and are frequently seen following repeated taps (Figure 10–12). The finding of increased macrophages containing RBCs is indicative of a previous hemorrhage (Figures 10–13 and 10–14). The macrophages may also contain hemosiderin granules and hematoidin crystals (Figures 10–15 through 10–17).

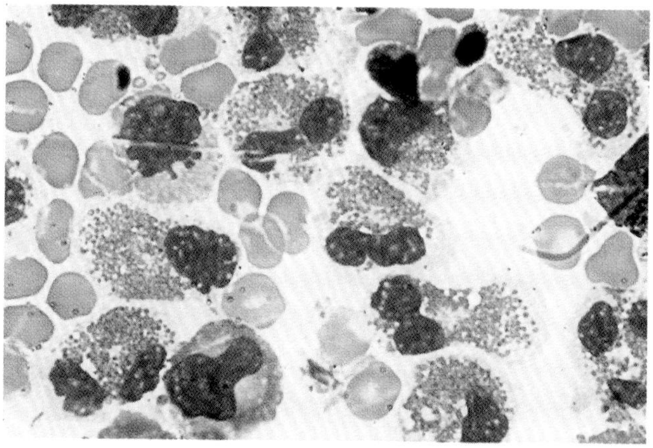

FIGURE 10–11 Eosinophils. Notice cytocentrifuge distortion (×1000).

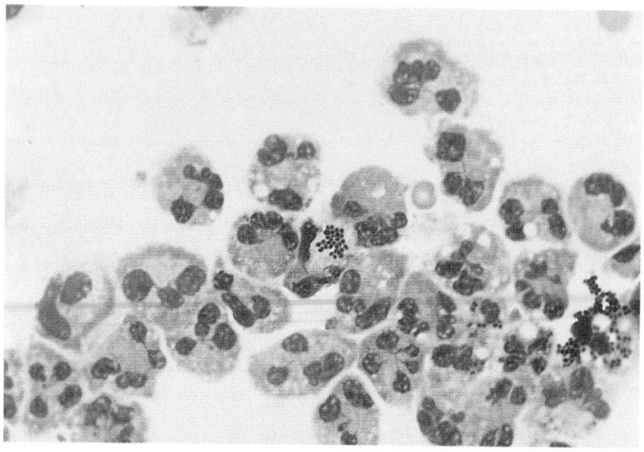

FIGURE 10–9 Neutrophils with intracellular bacteria (×1000).

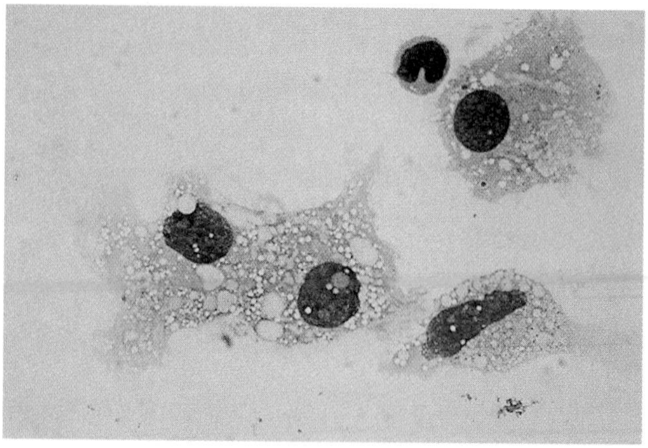

FIGURE 10–12 Macrophages. Notice the presence of large vacuoles (×500).

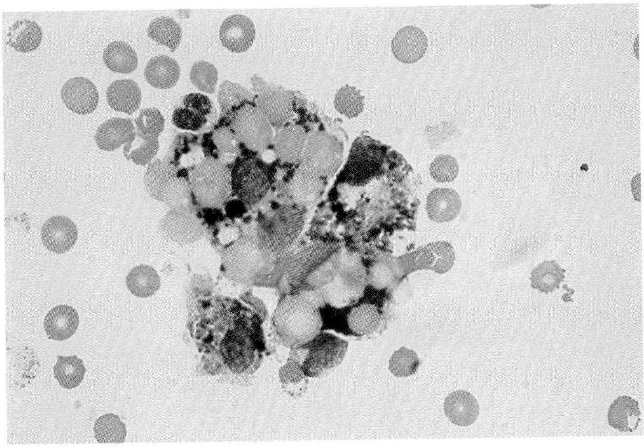

FIGURE 10–13 Macrophages showing erythrophagocytosis (×500).

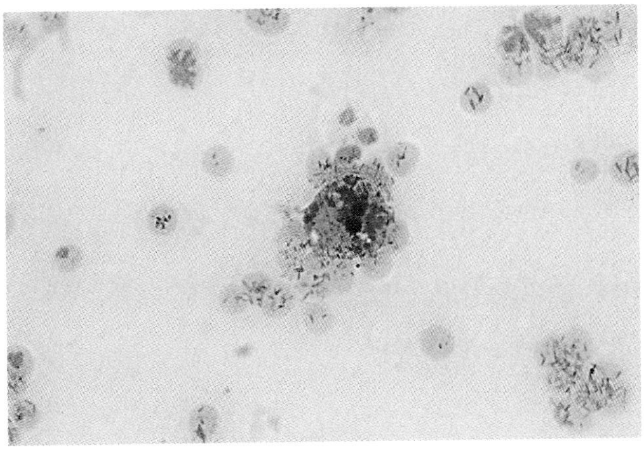

FIGURE 10–16 Macrophage containing hemosiderin stained with Prussian blue (×250).

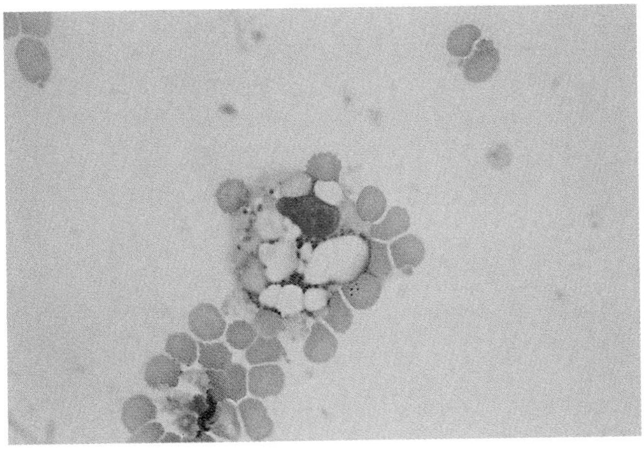

FIGURE 10–14 Macrophage with RBC remnants (×500).

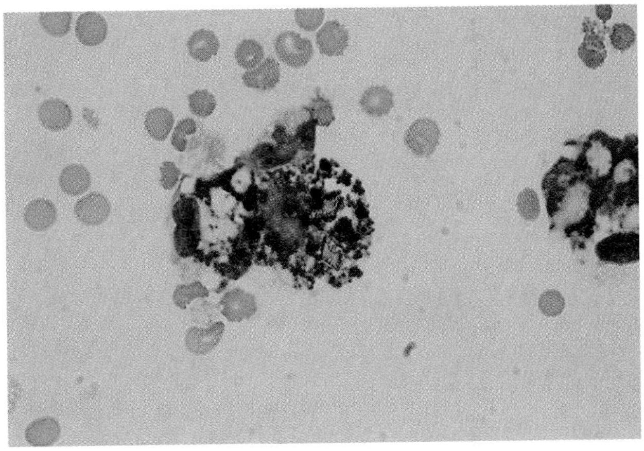

FIGURE 10–17 Macrophage containing hemosiderin and hematoidin crystals (×500).

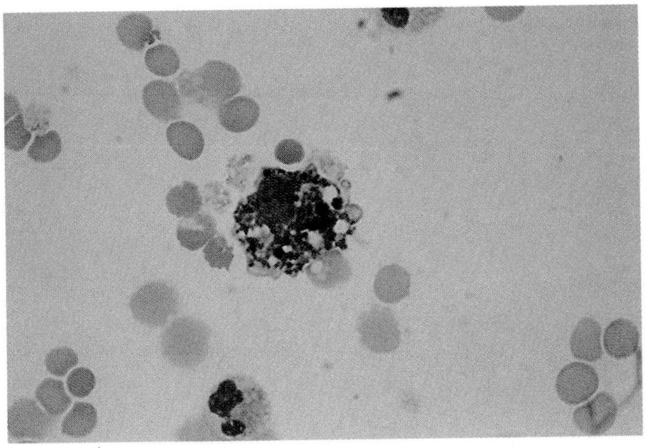

FIGURE 10–15 Macrophage with aggregated hemosiderin granules (×500).

Ependymal cells and choroid plexus cells (Figures 10–18 and 10–19) from the lining of the ventricles and spindle-shaped cells from the arachnoid lining (Figure 10–20) are not considered clinically significant. They are most frequently seen following diagnostic procedures such as pneumoencephalography and in fluid obtained from ventricular taps or during neurosurgery. These cells often appear as clusters and can be distinguished from malignant cells by their uniform appearance.

Nucleated RBCs are seen as a result of bone marrow contamination during the spinal tap (Figures 10–21 and 10–22). This is found in approximately 1 percent of specimens.[1] Capillary structures and endothelial cells may be seen following a traumatic tap (Figure 10–23).

Lymphoblasts, myeloblasts, and monoblasts (Figures 10–24 through 10–26) in the CSF are frequently seen as a complication of acute leukemias. Nucleoli are often more

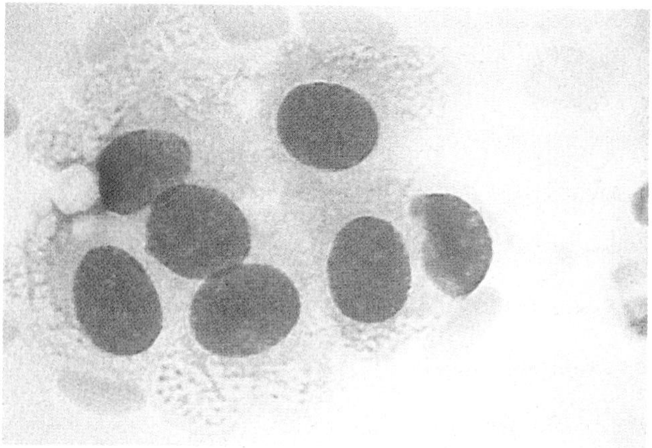

FIGURE 10-18 Ependymal cells (×1000).

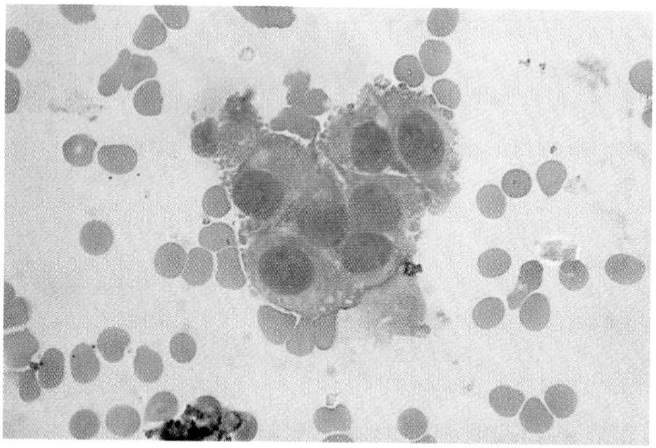

FIGURE 10-19 Choroid plexus cells showing distinct cell borders and nuclear uniformity (×500).

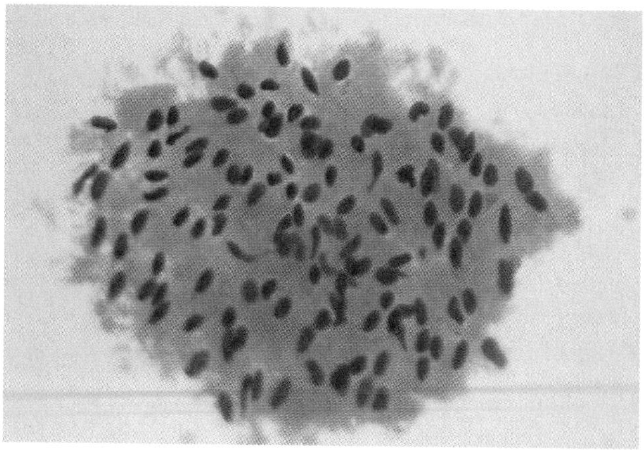

FIGURE 10-20 Cluster of spindle-shaped cells (×500).

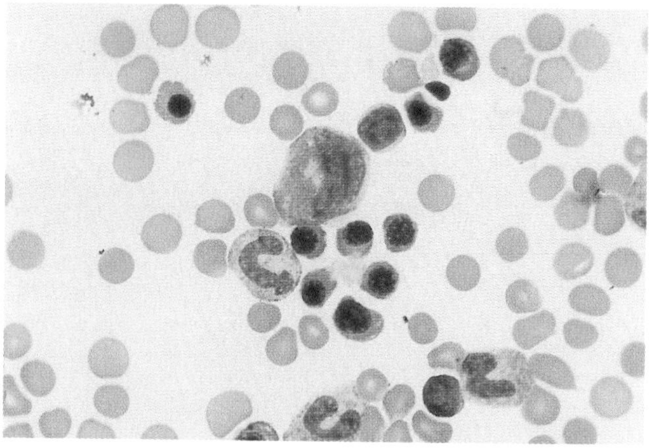

FIGURE 10-21 Nucleated RBCs seen with bone marrow contamination (×1000).

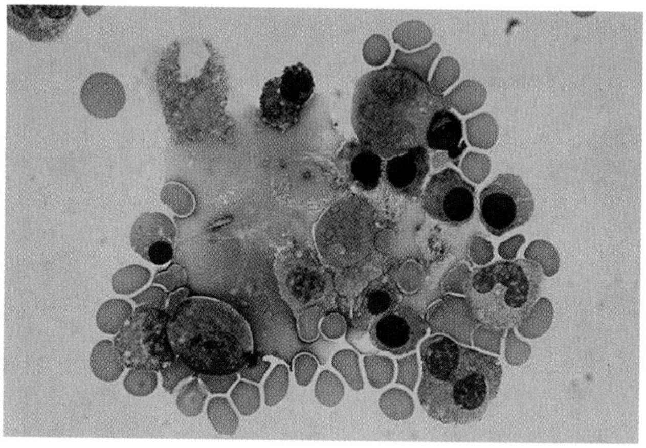

FIGURE 10-22 CSF bone marrow contamination (×500).

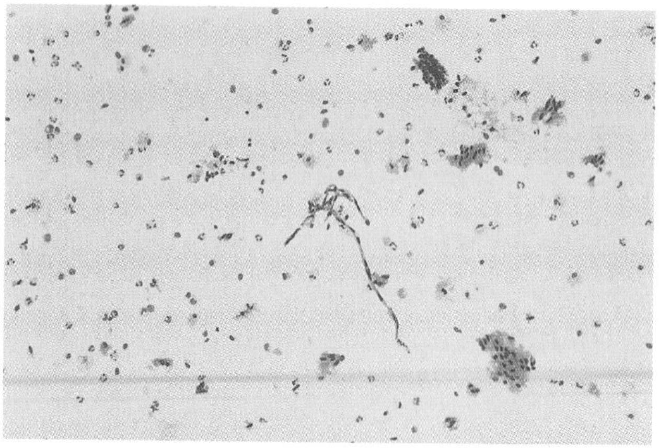

FIGURE 10-23 Capillary and RBCs seen with traumatic tap (×100).

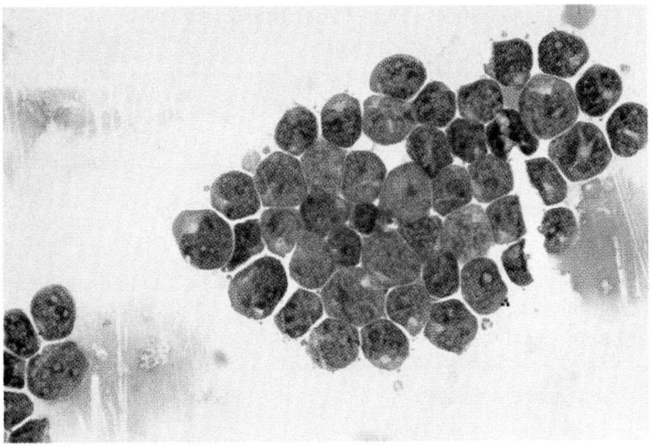

FIGURE 10-24 Lymphoblasts from acute lymphocytic leukemia (×500).

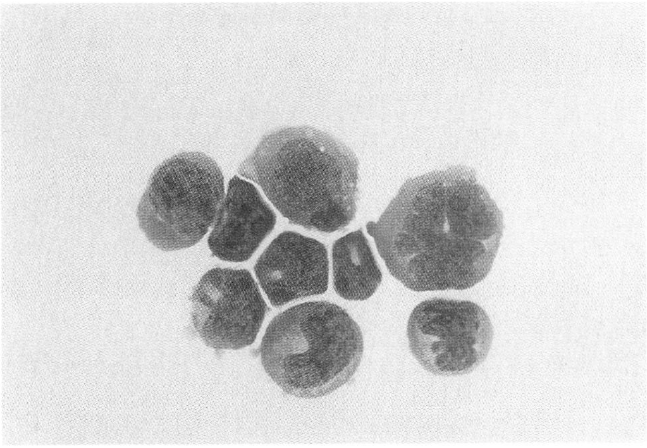

FIGURE 10-27 Noncleaved lymphoma cells (×1000).

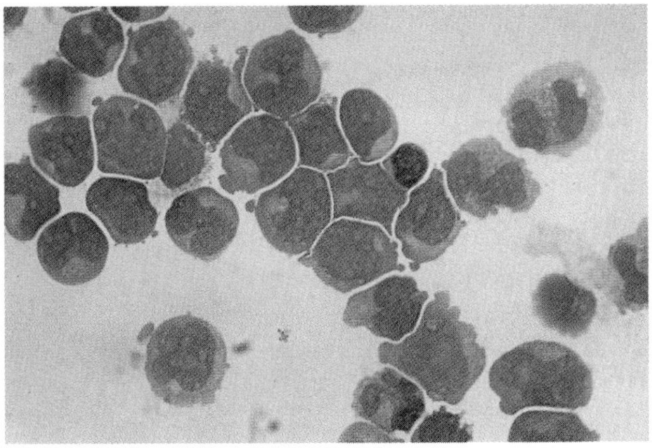

FIGURE 10-25 Myeloblasts from acute myelocytic leukemia (×500).

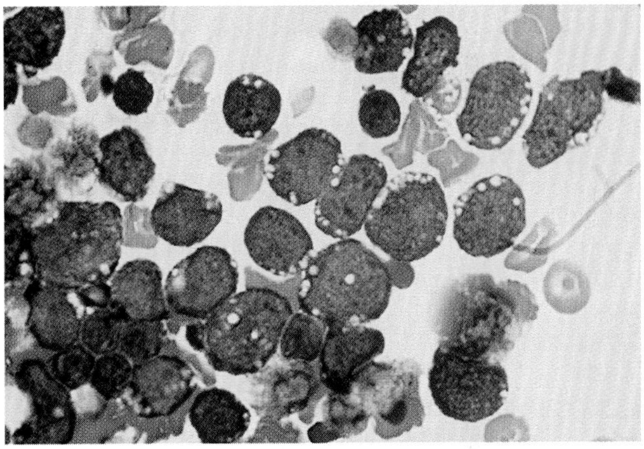

FIGURE 10-28 Burkitt's lymphoma. Notice characteristic vacuoles (×500).

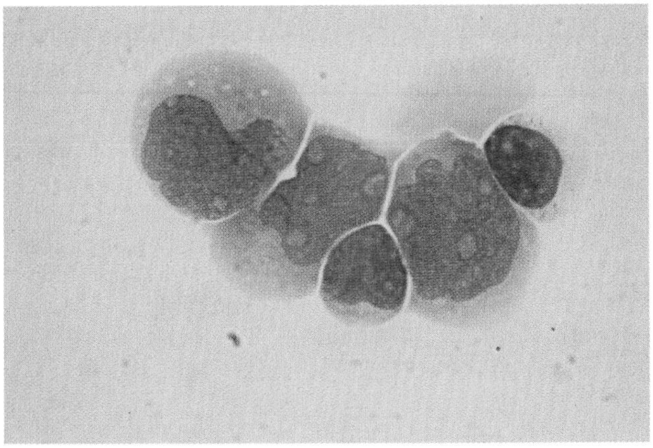

FIGURE 10-26 Monoblasts and two lymphocytes. Notice the prominent nucleoli (×1000).

prominent than in blood smears. Both cleaved and noncleaved lymphoma cells are also seen in the CSF (Figures 10–27 and 10–28).

Metastatic carcinoma cells are primarily from lung, breast, renal, and gastrointestinal malignancies and melanoma (Figure 10–29). Cells from primary CNS tumors include the astrocytomas and medulloblastomas, frequently occurring in children (Figure 10–30). They usually appear in clusters and must be distinguished from normal clusters of ependymal, choroid plexus, and leukemia cells. Fusing of cell walls and nuclear irregularities and hyperchromatic nucleoli are seen in clusters of malignant cells. Slides containing abnormal cells must be referred to pathology.

Chemistry Tests

Because CSF is formed by filtration of the plasma, one would expect to find the same low-molecular-weight chemicals in the CSF that are found in the plasma. This is essen-

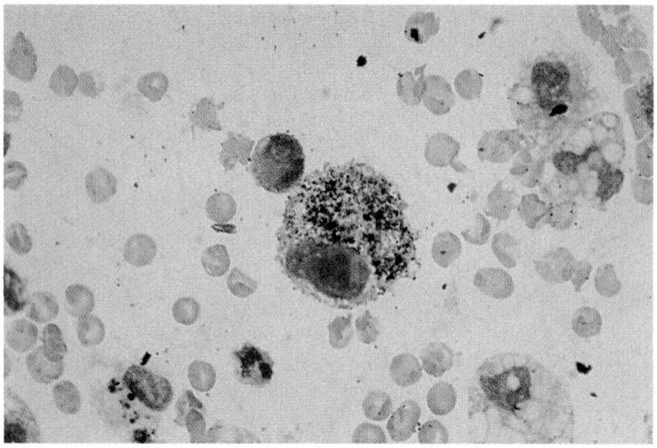

FIGURE 10–29 Malignant melanoma cell containing dustlike granules that are much finer than hemosiderin granules (×500).

tially true; however, because the filtration process is selective and the chemical composition is controlled by the blood-brain barrier, normal values for CSF chemicals are not the same as the plasma values. Abnormal values result from alterations in the permeability of the blood-brain barrier or increased production or metabolism by the neural cells in response to a pathologic condition, and they seldom have the same diagnostic significance as plasma abnormalities. The clinically important CSF chemicals are few in number, although under certain conditions, it may be necessary to measure a larger variety. Many CSF metabolites are currently under investigation to determine their possible diagnostic significance.

CEREBROSPINAL PROTEIN

The most frequently performed chemical test on CSF is the protein determination. Normal CSF contains a very small amount of protein. Normal values for total CSF protein are usually listed as 15 to 45 mg/dL, but are somewhat method dependent, and higher values are found in infants and older persons.[4] This value is reported in milligrams per deciliter and not grams per deciliter, as are plasma protein concentrations.

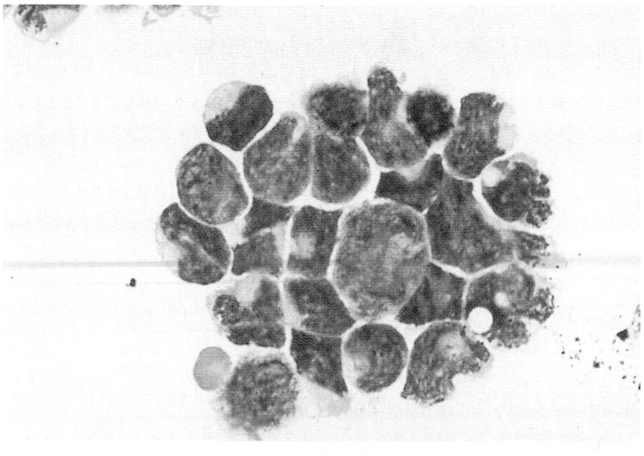

FIGURE 10–30 Medulloblastoma. Notice cellular clustering, nuclear irregularities, and rosette formation (×1000).

TABLE 10–4 **Cerebrospinal Fluid and Serum Protein Correlations**

	Cerebrospinal Fluid (mg/dL)	Serum (mg/dL)	Ratio
Prealbumin	1.7	23.8	14
Albumin	15.5	3600	236
Ceruloplasmin	0.1	36.6	366
Transferrin	1.4	204	142
Immunoglobulin G	1.2	987	802
Immunoglobulin A	0.13	175	1346

Adapted from Fishman.[10]

In general, the CSF contains protein fractions similar to those found in serum; however, as can be seen in Table 10–4, the ratio of CSF proteins to serum proteins varies among the fractions. As in serum, albumin comprises the majority of CSF protein. But in contrast to serum, prealbumin is the second most prevalent fraction in CSF. The alpha globulins include primarily haptoglobin and ceruloplasmin. Transferrin is the major beta globulin present; also, a separate carbohydrate-deficient transferrin fraction, referred to as "tau," is seen in CSF and not in serum. CSF gamma globulin is primarily immunoglobulin G (IgG), with only a small amount of IgA. IgM, fibrinogen, and beta lipoprotein are not found in normal CSF.[10]

Clinical Significance of Elevated Protein Values

Elevated total protein values are most frequently seen in pathologic conditions. Abnormally low values will be present when fluid is leaking from the CNS. The causes of elevated CSF protein include damage to the blood-brain barrier, production of immunoglobulins within the CNS, decreased clearance of normal protein from the fluid, and degeneration of neural tissue. Meningitis and hemorrhage conditions that damage the blood-brain barrier are the most common causes of elevated CSF protein. Many other neurologic disorders can elevate the CSF protein, and finding an abnormal result on a clear fluid with a low cell count is not unusual.

In the same manner as blood cells can be artificially introduced into a specimen by a traumatic tap, so can plasma protein. A correction calculation similar to that used in cell counts is available for protein measurements; however, if the correction is to be used, both the cell count and the protein determination must be done on the same tube.[12] When the blood hematocrit and serum protein values are normal, subtracting 1 mg/dL of protein for every 1200 RBCs counted is acceptable.[32]

$$\text{mg/dL protein added} = \frac{[\text{serum protein mg/dL} \times (1.00 - \text{Hct})] \times \text{CSF RBCs}/\mu\text{L} \ (\text{plasma volume})}{\text{blood RBCs}/\mu\text{L}}$$

Methodology

The two most routinely used techniques for measuring total CSF protein use the principles of turbidity production or dye-binding ability. Turbidimetric methods have been available for many years and rely on the precipitation of protein by either sulfosalicylic acid (SSA) or trichloroacetic acid. The reagent of choice is trichloroacetic acid because it will precipitate both albumin and globulin equally. Unless SSA is combined with sodium sulfate, albumin will contribute more to the turbidity than globulin. Standards should be prepared using a mixture of albumin and globulin and not just from albumin.

Dye-binding techniques offer the advantages of smaller sample size and less interference from external sources. The development of dye-binding procedures, which are almost as rapid and easy to perform as the turbidity methods, has greatly increased their acceptance in laboratories. This method uses the dye Coomassie brilliant blue G250 and the principle of "protein error of indicators" discussed in Chapter 5. Coomassie brilliant blue dye is used because it will bind to a variety of proteins rather than just to albumin. The color change of the pH-stabilized dye reagent from red to blue occurs when protein binds to the dye.[13] The concentration of protein present will determine the amount of blue color produced, thereby allowing a mathematic conversion of the intensity of the blue color present to the concentration of protein present (Beer's law).

Methods for the measurement of CSF protein are available for most automated chemistry analyzers.

Protein Fractions

Routine CSF protein procedures are designed to measure total protein concentration. However, diagnosis of neurologic disorders associated with abnormal CSF protein often requires measurement of the individual protein fractions. Protein that appears in the CSF as a result of damage to the integrity of the blood-brain barrier will contain fractions proportional to those in plasma, with albumin present in the highest concentration. Diseases, including multiple sclerosis, that stimulate the immunocompetent cells in the CNS will show a higher proportion of IgG.[34]

To accurately determine whether IgG is increased because it is being produced within the CNS or is elevated as the result of a defect in the blood-brain barrier, comparisons between serum and CSF levels of albumin and IgG must be made. Methods include the CSF/serum albumin index to evaluate the integrity of the blood-brain barrier and the CSF IgG index to measure IgG synthesis within the CNS.

The CSF to serum albumin index is calculated after determining the concentration of CSF albumin in milligrams per deciliter and the serum concentration in grams per deciliter. The formula used is as follows:

$$\text{CSF/serum albumin index} = \frac{\text{CSF albumin (mg/dL)}}{\text{Serum albumin (g/dL)}}$$

An index value less than 9 represents an intact blood-brain barrier. The index increases relative to the degree of damage to the barrier.

Calculation of an IgG index, which is actually a comparison of the CSF/serum albumin index with the CSF/serum IgG index, will compensate for any IgG entering the CSF via the blood-brain barrier.[17] It is performed by dividing the CSF/serum IgG index by the CSF/serum albumin index as follows:

$$\text{IgG index} = \frac{\text{CSF IgG (mg/dL)/serum IgG (g/dL)}}{\text{CSF albumin (mg/dL)/serum albumin (g/dL)}}$$

Normal IgG index values vary slightly among laboratories; however, in general values greater than 0.77 are indicative of IgG production within the CNS.

Techniques for the measurement of CSF albumin and globulin include electrophoresis, radial immunodiffusion, and nephelometry. Electrophoresis will provide an overall picture of all proteins present, and radial immunodiffusion and nephelometry measure individual fractions.

Electrophoresis

The primary purpose for performing CSF protein electrophoresis is for the detection of ***oligoclonal bands*** representing inflammation within the CNS. The bands are located in the gamma region of the protein electrophoresis, indicating Ig production. To ensure that the oligoclonal bands are present as the result of neurologic inflammation, simultaneous serum electrophoresis must be performed. Disorders, including leukemia, lymphoma, and viral infections, may produce serum banding, which can appear in the CSF as a result of blood-brain barrier leakage or traumatic introduction of blood into the CSF specimen. Banding representing both systemic and neurologic involvement is seen in the serum and CSF with HIV infection.[14]

The presence of two or more oligoclonal bands in the CSF that are not present in the serum can be a valuable tool in the diagnosis of multiple sclerosis, particularly when accompanied by an increased IgG index. Other neurologic disorders including encephalitis, neurosyphilis, Guillain-Barré syndrome, and neoplastic disorders also produce oligoclonal banding that may not be present in the serum. Therefore, the presence of oligoclonal banding must be considered in conjunction with clinical symptoms. Oligoclonal banding remains positive during remission of multiple sclerosis, but disappears in other disorders.[3]

Low protein levels in the CSF make concentration of the fluid prior to performing electrophoresis essential for most electrophoretic techniques. Agarose gel electrophoresis followed by Coomassie brilliant blue staining is most frequently performed in the clinical laboratory. Better resolution can be obtained using immunofixation electrophoresis (**IFE**) and isoelectric focusing (**IEF**) followed by silver staining. Specimen concentration is not required by the more sensitive IEF procedure.

Electrophoresis is also the method of choice when determining if a fluid is actually CSF. Identification can be made based on the appearance of the previously mentioned extra isoform of transferrin, tau, that is found only in CSF.[30]

Myelin Basic Protein

The presence of myelin basic protein (**MBP**) in the CSF is indicative of recent destruction of the myelin sheath that protects the axons of the neurons (**demyelination**). Measurement of the amount of MBP in the CSF can be used to monitor the course of multiple sclerosis.[15] It may also provide a valuable measure of the effectiveness of current and future treatments.[38]

CEREBROSPINAL FLUID GLUCOSE

Glucose enters the CSF by selective transport across the blood-brain barrier, which results in a normal value that is approximately 60 to 70 percent that of the plasma glucose. If the plasma glucose is 100 mg/dL, then a normal CSF glucose would be approximately 65 mg/dL. For an accurate evaluation of CSF glucose, a blood glucose test must be run for comparison. The blood glucose should be drawn about 2 hours prior to the spinal tap to allow time for equilibration between the blood and fluid. CSF glucose is analyzed using the same procedures employed for blood glucose. Specimens should be tested immediately because glycolysis occurs rapidly in the CSF.

The diagnostic significance of CSF glucose is confined to the finding of values that are decreased in relation to plasma values. Elevated CSF glucose values are always a result of plasma elevations. Low CSF glucose values can be of considerable diagnostic value in determining the causative agents in meningitis. The finding of a markedly decreased CSF glucose accompanied by an increased WBC count and a large percentage of neutrophils is indicative of bacterial meningitis. If the WBCs are lymphocytes instead of neutrophils, tubercular meningitis is suspected. Likewise, if a normal CSF glucose value is found with an increased number of lymphocytes, the diagnosis would favor viral meningitis. Classic laboratory patterns such as those just described may not be found in all cases of meningitis, but they can be helpful when they are present.

Decreased CSF glucose values are caused primarily by alterations in the mechanisms of glucose transport across the blood-brain barrier and by increased use of glucose by the brain cells. The common tendency to associate the decreased glucose totally with its use by microorganisms and leukocytes cannot account for the variations in glucose concentrations seen in different types of meningitis and the decreased levels seen in other disorders producing damage to the CNS.[24]

CEREBROSPINAL FLUID LACTATE

The determination of CSF lactate levels can be a valuable aid in the diagnosis and management of meningitis cases. In bacterial, tubercular, and fungal meningitis, the elevation of CSF lactate to levels greater than 25 mg/dL occurs much more consistently than does the depression of glucose and provides more reliable information when the initial diagnosis is difficult. Levels greater than 35 mg/dL are frequently seen with bacterial meningitis, whereas in viral meningitis lactate levels remain lower than 25 mg/dL. CSF lactate levels remain elevated during initial treatment but fall rapidly when treatment is successful, thus offering a sensitive method for evaluating the effectiveness of antibiotic therapy.

Destruction of tissue within the CNS owing to oxygen deprivation (**hypoxia**) causes the production of increased CSF lactic acid levels. Therefore, elevated CSF lactate is not limited to meningitis and can result from any condition that decreases the flow of oxygen to the tissues. CSF lactate levels are frequently used to monitor severe head injuries. RBCs contain high concentrations of lactate, and falsely elevated results may be obtained on xanthochromic or hemolyzed fluid.[19]

CEREBROSPINAL FLUID GLUTAMINE

Glutamine is produced in the CNS by the brain cells from ammonia and α-ketoglutarate. This process serves to remove the toxic metabolic waste product ammonia from the CNS. The normal concentration of glutamine in the CSF is 8 to 18 mg/dL.[18] Elevated levels are found in association with liver disorders that result in increased blood and CSF ammonia. Increased synthesis of glutamine is caused by the excess ammonia that is present in the CNS; therefore, the determination of CSF glutamine provides an indirect test for the presence of excess ammonia in the CSF. Several methods of assaying glutamine are available and are based on the measurement of ammonia liberated from the glutamine. This is preferred over the direct measurement of CSF ammonia because the concentration of glutamine remains more stable than that of the volatile ammonia in the collected specimen. The CSF glutamine level also correlates with clinical symptoms much better than does the blood ammonia.[18]

As the concentration of ammonia in the CSF increases, the supply of α-ketoglutarate becomes depleted; glutamine can no longer be produced to remove the toxic ammonia, and coma ensues. Some disturbance of consciousness is almost always seen when glutamine levels are more than 35 mg/dL.[10] Therefore, the CSF glutamine test is a frequently requested procedure for patients with coma of unknown origin. Approximately 75 percent of children with Reye's syndrome have elevated CSF glutamine levels.[11]

CEREBROSPINAL FLUID ENZYMES

Throughout the years, many enzymes in the CSF have been studied, but little clinical application of CSF enzyme tests has resulted. Measurement of lactate dehydrogenase (**LD**) and/or its isoenzymes LD1, LD2, LD3, LD4, and LD5 continues to be studied.

Measurement of the creatine kinase isoenzyme CK-BB in CSF after resuscitation from cardiac arrest has been shown to reliably predict recovery when levels are less than 17 mg/mL.[29]

Summary of Cerebrospinal Fluid Chemistry Tests

Protein

1. Normal concentration is 15–45 mg/dL.
2. Elevated values are most frequently seen in patients with meningitis, hemorrhage, and multiple sclerosis.

Glucose

1. Normal value is 60–70% of the plasma concentration.
2. Decreased levels are seen in patients with bacterial, tubercular, and fungal meningitis.

Lactate

1. Levels >35 mg/dL are seen in patients with bacterial meningitis.
2. Levels >25 mg/dL are found in patients with tubercular and fungal meningitis.
3. Lower levels are seen in patients with viral meningitis.

Glutamine

1. Normal concentration is 8–18 mg/dL.
2. Levels >35 mg/dL are associated with some disturbance of consciousness.

Creatine Kinase CK-BB Isoenzyme

1. Elevated levels in patients post cardiac arrest indicate a poor prognosis.

Microbiology Tests

The role of the microbiology laboratory in the analysis of CSF lies in the identification of the causative agent in meningitis. For positive identification, the microorganism must be recovered from the fluid by growing it on the appropriate culture medium. This can take anywhere from 24 hours in cases of bacterial meningitis to 6 weeks for tubercular meningitis. Consequently, in many instances, the CSF culture is actually a confirmatory rather than a diagnostic procedure. However, the microbiology laboratory does have several methods available to provide information for a preliminary diagnosis. These methods include the Gram stain, acid-fast stain, India Ink preparation, limulus lysate test, and latex agglutination tests. In Table 10–5, the laboratory tests used in the differential diagnosis of meningitis are compared.

GRAM STAIN

The Gram stain is routinely performed on CSF from all suspected cases of meningitis, although its value lies in the detection of bacterial and fungal organisms. All smears and cultures should be performed on concentrated specimens because often only a few organisms are present at the onset of the disease. The CSF should be centrifuged at 1500 g for 15 minutes, and slides and cultures should be prepared from the sediment.[25] Use of the cytocentrifuge will provide a highly concentrated specimen. Even when concentrated specimens are used, at least a 10 percent chance exists that Gram stains and cultures will be negative. Thus, blood cultures should be taken, because the causative organism will often be present in both the CSF and the blood.[19] A CSF Gram stain is one of the most difficult slides to interpret because the number of organisms present is usually small, and they can easily be overlooked, resulting in a false-negative report. Also, false-positive reports can occur if precipitated stain or debris is mistaken for microorganisms. Therefore, considerable care should be taken when interpreting a Gram stain. Organisms most frequently encountered include *Streptococcus pneumoniae* (gram-positive cocci), *Hemophilus influenzae* (pleomorphic gram-negative rods), *Escherichia coli* (gram-negative rods), and *Neisseria meningitidis* (gram-negative cocci). The gram-positive cocci, *Streptococcus agalactiae* and the gram-positive rods *Listeria monocytogenes* may be encountered in newborns.

TABLE 10–5 **Major Laboratory Results for the Differential Diagnosis of Meningitis**

Bacterial	Viral	Tubercular	Fungal
Elevated WBC count	Elevated WBC count	Elevated WBC count	Elevated WBC count
Neutrophils present	Lymphocytes present	Lymphocytes and monocytes present	Lymphocytes and monocytes present
Marked protein elevation	Moderate protein elevation	Moderate to marked protein elevation	Moderate to marked protein elevation
Markedly decreased glucose level	Normal glucose level	Decreased glucose level	Normal to decreased glucose level
Lactate level >35 mg/dL	Normal lactate level	Lactate level >25 mg/dL	Lactate level >25 mg/dL
Positive limulus lysate test result with gram-negative organisms		Pellicle formation	Positive India Ink with *Cryptococcus neoformans*
Positive Gram stain and bacterial antigen tests			Positive immunologic test for *C. neoformans*

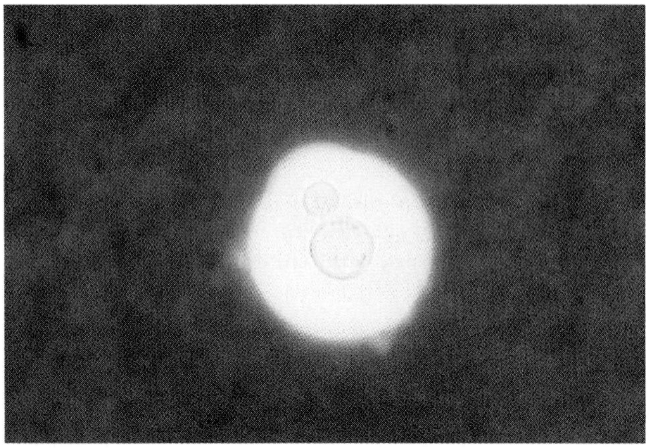

FIGURE 10–31 India Ink preparation of C. *neoformans*. Notice budding yeast form (×400). (Courtesy of Ann K. Fulenwider, MD.)

Acid-fast or fluorescent antibody stains are not routinely performed on specimens, unless tubercular meningitis is suspected. Considering the length of time required to culture mycobacteria, a positive report from this smear is extremely valuable.

Specimens from possible cases of fungal meningitis are Gram stained and often have an India Ink preparation performed on them. The India Ink preparation is performed to detect the presence of thickly encapsulated *Cryptococcus neoformans* (Figure 10–31). As one of the more frequently occurring complications of AIDS, cryptococcal meningitis is now commonly encountered in the clinical laboratory. Particular attention should be paid to the Gram stain for the classic starburst pattern produced by *Cryptococcus*, as this may be seen more often than a positive India Ink (Figure 10–32).[31]

Latex agglutination and enzyme-linked immunosorbent assay (**ELISA**) methods provide a rapid means for detecting and identifying microorganisms in CSF. Test kits are available to detect *Streptococcus* group B, *H. influenza type b*, *S. pneumoniae*, *N. meningitidis* A, B, C, Y, W135, and

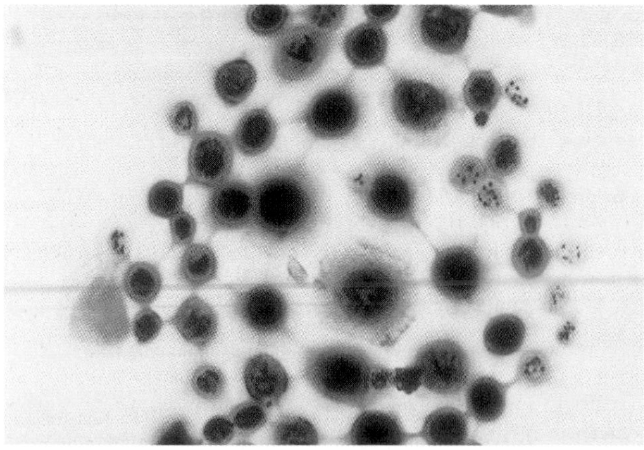

FIGURE 10–32 Gram stain of C. *neoformans* showing starburst pattern (×1000). (Courtesy of Ann K. Fulenwider, MD.)

E. coli K1 antigens. The bacterial antigen test (**BAT**) does not appear to be as sensitive to detection of *N. meningitidis* as it is to the other organisms.[5] The BAT should be used in combination with results from the hematology and clinical chemistry laboratories for diagnosing meningitis.[37] The Gram stain is still the recommended method for detection of organisms.[7]

Latex agglutination tests to detect the presence of C. *neoformans* antigen in serum and CSF provide a more sensitive method than the India Ink preparation. However, immunologic testing results should be confirmed by culture and demonstration of the organisms by India Ink, because false-positive reactions do occur. Interference by rheumatoid factor is the most common cause of false-positive reactions. Several commercial kits with pretreatment techniques are available and include incubation with dithiothreitol or pronase and boiling with ethylenediaminetetraacetic acid.[9,33] An enzyme immunoassay technique has been shown to produce fewer false-positive results.[20]

The limulus lysate test can be useful in the diagnosis of meningitis caused by gram-negative bacteria.[26] The reagent for this test is prepared from the blood cells of the horseshoe crab (*Limulus polyphemus*). These cells, termed amebocytes, contain a copper complex that gives them a blue color, thereby making the horseshoe crab a true "blue blood." Endotoxin found in the cell walls of gram-negative bacteria coagulates the amebocyte lysate within 1 hour if incubated at 37°C. The test is sensitive to minute amounts of endotoxin and will detect all gram-negative bacteria. The procedure must be performed using sterile technique to prevent false-positive results caused by contamination of specimens or tubes with endotoxin. Considerable amounts of endotoxin can be found in tap water.

Serologic Testing

In addition to the serologic procedures performed for identification of microorganisms, serologic testing of the CSF is performed to detect the presence of neurosyphilis. The use of penicillin in the early stages of syphilis has greatly reduced the number of cases of neurosyphilis. Consequently, the number of requests for serologic tests for syphilis on CSF is currently low. However, detection of the antibodies associated with syphilis in the CSF still remains a necessary diagnostic procedure.

Although many different serologic tests for syphilis are available when testing blood, the procedure recommended by the Centers for Disease Control and Prevention to diagnose neurosyphilis is the Venereal Disease Research Laboratories (VDRL) even though it is not as sensitive as the fluorescent treponemal antibody-absorption (FTA-ABS) test for syphilis. If the FTA-ABS is used, care must be taken to prevent contamination with blood, because the FTA-ABS remains positive in the serum of treated cases of syphilis.

The purpose of performing a test for syphilis on the CSF is to detect active cases of syphilis within the CNS. Therefore, the less sensitive VDRL procedure, the blood levels for which decrease in the later stages of syphilis, will be

PROCEDURE

Simulated Spinal Fluid Procedure

EQUIPMENT AND REAGENTS

1 Whole blood is collected the same day in EDTA. The "ideal" blood specimen for preparing SSF has a white count around 10 × 10^9 per liter, a low platelet count, and a normal-appearing differential with at least 20% lymphocytes. To prepare 50 mL of SSF, 5–7 mL of blood are needed.
2 Hanks' balanced salt solution (10×) without phenol red, sodium bicarbonate, calcium, or magnesium (Grand Island Biological Company, Grand Island, NY). Dilute 1:10 with deionized water.
3 30% bovine serum albumin.
4 Macrohematocrit tubes.
5 Capillary (Pasteur type) pipettes, both standard and 9-inch lengths.
6 Horizontal head centrifuge. A Beckman TJ6 model (Beckman Instruments, Inc, Palo Alto, CA) was used for this study.

STEPS

1 For each SSF sample, dispense 50-mL diluted balanced salt solution into a 125-mL Erlenmeyer flask. (The amount of balanced salt solution may be varied; 50 mL will make approximately 30 aliquots of SSF.)
2 Centrifuge the blood in the original collection tube at 300 g for 5 min. A gray-pink buffy coat layer should be visible at the interface between the plasma and the RBCs.
3 Aspirate off as much plasma as possible with a capillary pipette. Do not disturb the top (buffy coat) layer. Discard the plasma.
4 With a 9-inch capillary pipette and a circular motion, aspirate off the remaining plasma and the entire buffy coat layer. A small amount of the RBC layer will be aspirated into the pipette at the same time. This is acceptable.
5 Fill a macrohematocrit tube with this buffy coat mixture. Do not mix blood specimens from more than one source in one tube (they may agglutinate).
6 Centrifuge the macrohematocrit tube at 900 g for 10 min.
7 Pipette off as much of the plasma as possible and discard it. If a definite white layer (platelets) is visible above the gray buffy coat, carefully remove as much of it as possible without disturbing the gray layer.
8 Using a clean 9-inch capillary pipette, aspirate off the buffy coat (and as little of the red cell layer as possible) and add it to the flask containing diluted balanced salt solution. Rinse the pipette several times.

PROCEDURE

Simulated Spinal Fluid Procedure (continued)

9 Mix well and check the concentration of RBCs and WBCs by examining the SSF in a hemocytometer.
10 Adjust the concentration of cells as needed; add more balanced salt solution to decrease the number of RBCs and WBCs. The number of RBCs may be increased by adding more cells from the red cell layer. Since the entire buffy coat has been used, increasing the number of WBCs is not possible.
11 Add one drop (approximately 0.05 mL) of 30% bovine serum albumin to each 50 mL of SSF for each 30 mg/dL total protein desired.
12 Mix well and dispense aliquots of approximately 1.5 mL SSF into appropriate tightly stoppered containers.

From Lofsness and Jensen,[22] with permission

more specific for infection of the CNS.[8] The rapid plasma reagin (**RPR**) test is not recommended for use on CSF, because it is less sensitive and specific than the VDRL. To prevent unnecessary testing of the CSF in suspected cases of neurosyphilis, a positive serum test should be obtained using the FTA-ABS. Fluid can be frozen until serum results are available.[2]

Teaching Cerebrospinal Fluid Analysis

Many of the problems that occur in the analysis of CSF are the result of inadequate training of the personnel performing the tests. This is understandable when one considers that not only is CSF difficult to collect, but also there is often very little fluid left for student practice after the required tests have been run. Preparation of simulated fluids by adding blood cells to saline has met with limited success owing to the instability of the cells in saline and the inability to perform routine chemical analyses for glucose and protein. More satisfactory results can be achieved using the simulated spinal fluid procedure presented in this chapter, which provides the teaching laboratory with a specimen suitable for all types of cell analyses and glucose and protein determinations. The advantages of this procedure over others include the absence of bicarbonate, which may cause bubbling with acidic diluting fluids; the absence of calcium, which prevents clot formation when blood is added; stability for 48 hours under refrigeration; no distortion of cellular morphology; and the presence of glucose and protein.[22]

REFERENCES

1. Abrams, J, and Schumacher, HR: Bone marrow in cerebrospinal fluid and possible confusion with malignancy. Arch Pathol Lab Med 110:366–369, 1986.
2. Albright, RE, et al: Issues in cerebrospinal fluid management. Am J Clin Pathol 95(3):397–401, 1991.
3. Bentz, JS: Laboratory investigation of multiple sclerosis. Lab Med 26(6):393–399, 1995.
4. Biou, D, et al: Cerebrospinal fluid protein concentrations in children: Age-related values in patients without disorders of the central nervous system. Clin Chem 46(3):399–403, 2000.
5. Buck, GE: Nonculture methods for detection and identification of microorganisms in clinical specimens. Pediatr Clin North Am 36(1):95–100, 1989.
6. Chow, G, and Schmidley, JW: Lysis of erythrocytes and leukocytes in traumatic lumbar punctures. Arch Neurol 41:1084–1085, 1984.
7. Coovadia, YM, and Soliva, Z: Three latex agglutination tests compared with Gram staining for the detection of bacteria in cerebrospinal fluid. S Afr Med J 71(7):442, 1987.
8. Davis, LE, and Schmitt, JW: Clinical significance of cerebrospinal fluid tests for neurosyphilis. Ann Neurol 25:50–53, 1989.
9. Eng, RHK, and Person, A: Serum cryptococcal antigen determination in the presence of rheumatoid factor. J Clin Microbiol 14: 700–702, 1981.
10. Fishman, RA: Cerebrospinal Fluid in Diseases of the Nervous System, ed. 2. WB Saunders, Philadelphia, 1992.
11. Glasgow, AM, and Dhiensiri, K: Improved assay for spinal fluid glutamine and values for children with Reye's syndrome. Clin Chem 20(6):642–644, 1974.
12. Glasser, L: Tapping the wealth of information in CSF. Diagn Med 4(1):23–33, 1981.
13. Godd, K: Protein estimation in spinal fluid using Coomassie blue reagent. Med Lab Sci 38:61–63, 1981.
14. Grimaldi, LME, et al: Oligoclonal IgG bands in cerebrospinal fluid and serum during asymptomatic human immunodeficiency virus infection. Ann Neurol 24:277–279, 1988.
15. Gupta, MK, et al: Measurement of immunoreactive myelin basic protein in cerebrospinal fluid. Ann Neurol 23:274–276, 1988.
16. Hammock, M, and Milhorat, T: The cerebrospinal fluid: Current concepts of its formation. Ann Clin Lab Sci 6(1):22–28, 1976.
17. Hershey, LA, and Trotter, JL: The use and abuse of the cerebrospinal fluid IgG profile in the adult: A practical evaluation. Ann Neurol 8(4):426–434, 1980.
18. Hourani, BT, Hamlin, EM, and Reynolds, TB: Cerebrospinal fluid glutamine as a measure of hepatic encephalopathy. Arch Intern Med 127:1033–1036, 1971.
19. Kjeldsberg, CR, and Knight, JA: Body Fluids: Laboratory Examination of Amniotic, Cerebrospinal, Seminal, Serous and Synovial Fluids: A Textbook Atlas. ASCP, Chicago, 1993.
20. Knight, FR: New enzyme immunoassay for detecting cryptococcal antigen. J Clin Pathol 45(9):836–837, 1992.
21. Kolmel, HW: Atlas of Cerebrospinal Fluid Cells. Springer-Verlag, New York, 1976.
22. Lofsness, KG, and Jensen, TL: The preparation of simulated spinal fluid for teaching purposes. Am J Med Technol 49(7):493–496, 1983.
23. McComb, JG: Recent research into the nature of cerebrospinal fluid formation and absorption. J Neurosurg 59:369–383, 1983.
24. Menkes, J: The causes of low spinal fluid sugar in bacterial meningitis: Another look Pediatrics 44(1):1–3, 1969.
25. Murray, PR, and Hampton, CM: Recovery of pathogenic bacteria from cerebrospinal fluid. J Clin Microbiol 12:554–557, 1980.
26. Nachum, R, and Neely, M: Clinical diagnostic usefulness of the limulus amebocyte lysate assay. Lab Med 13(2):112–117, 1982.
27. Nagda, KK: Procoagulant activity of cerebrospinal fluid in health and disease. Indian J Med Res 74:107–110, 1981.
28. Novak, RW: Lack of validity of standard corrections for white blood cell counts of blood contaminated cerebrospinal fluid in infants. Am J Clin Pathol 82:95–97, 1984.
29. Roine, RO, et al: Neurological outcome after out-of-hospital cardiac arrest. Predictions by cerebrospinal fluid enzyme analysis. Arch Neurol 46:753–756, 1989.
30. Rouah, E, Rogers, BB, and Buffone, GJ: Transferrin analysis by immunofixation as an aid in the diagnosis of cerebrospinal fluid otorrhea. Arch Pathol Lab Med 111:756–757, 1987.
31. Sato, Y, et al: Rapid diagnosis of cryptococcal meningitis by microscopic examination of centrifuged cerebrospinal fluid sediment. J Neurol Sci 164(1):72–75, 1999.
32. Smith, GP, and Kjeldsberg, CR: Cerebrospinal, synovial, and serous body fluids, ed. 19. In Henry, JB (ed): Clinical Diagnosis and Management by Laboratory Methods. WB Saunders, Philadelphia, 1996.
33. Stockman, L, and Roberts, GD: Specificity of the latex test for cryptococcal antigen: A rapid simple method for eliminating interference. J Clin Microbiol 17(5):945–947, 1983.
34. Tourtellotte, WW: Cerebrospinal fluid in multiple sclerosis. In Vinken, PJ, and Bruyn, GW (eds): Handbook of Clinical Neurology. Elsevier, New York, 1970.
35. University of Virginia Health Sciences Center: Clinical Laboratory Procedure Manual. Charlottesville, VA, 1993.
36. Walter, J: Hematology and the analysis of body fluids. Advance for Medical Laboratory Professional 4:10–19, 1996.
37. Werner, V, and Kruger, RL: Value of the bacterial antigen test in the absence of CSF fluid leukocytosis. Lab Med 22(11):787–789, 1991.
38. Whitaker, JN: Myelin basic protein in cerebrospinal fluid and other body fluids. Mult Scler 4(1):16–21, 1998.

STUDY QUESTIONS

1. List three functions of the CSF.
2. State the function of the following structures with regard to the CSF: choroid plexuses, subarachnoid space, and arachnoid villi.
3. State a possible discrepancy associated with the following actions:
   a. CSF tube 1 is sent to the microbiology laboratory.
   b. CSF tube 2 is sent to the hematology laboratory.
   c. CSF tube 1 remains at room temperature for 4 hours.
   d. CSF tube 3 remains at room temperature for 4 hours.
4. How does pink xanthochromia differ clinically from yellow xanthochromia?
5. Indicate whether each of the following statements represents a hemorrhage or a traumatic tap by placing an "H" or a "T" in the blank.
   _____ Clot formation
   _____ Erythrophagocytosis
   _____ Positive D-dimer test
   _____ Clear supernatant
   _____ Even distribution of blood
6. What is the clinical significance of a weblike pellicle in the CSF?
7. Should a cell count be performed on a clear CSF? Why or why not?
8. Given the following information, calculate the total CSF cell count.
   Cells counted = 50
   Dilution = 1:10
   Large Neubauer squares counted = 10
9. What diluting fluid is used for a total CSF cell count? A CSF WBC count?
10. What is the purpose of the WBC and protein correction calculation?

11. How must the CSF be prepared prior to performing a cell differential count?

12. What is the purpose of adding albumin to the cytocentrifuge preparation?

13. Name the primary clinical concern when a pleocytosis of neutrophils or lymphocytes is present.

14. Name the type of cell(s) that predominate in each of the following conditions: multiple sclerosis, following pneumoencephalography, malfunctioning shunts, AIDS, and cerebral hemorrhage.

15. What is the significance of nucleated RBCs in the CSF?

16. How do clusters of choroid plexus and malignant cells differ in appearance?

17. Name four sources of malignant cells found in CSF.

18. Why does the chemical composition of the CSF differ from that of plasma?

19. True or False? The normal range of CSF protein is 15 to 45 g/dL.

20. What is the primary difference in the concentration of protein fractions between CSF and plasma?

21. Name four causes of elevated CSF protein levels.

22. Why is trichloroacetic acid recommended over SSA in turbidometric methods measuring CSF protein? Coomassie brilliant blue in dye-binding methods?

23. How does the clinical significance of the CSF/serum albumin index differ from that of the IgG index?

24. Why must electrophoresis to detect oligoclonal banding be performed on both CSF and serum? In the diagnosis of what disorder is this most important?

25. How can an unidentified fluid be determined to be CSF?

26. What is the significance of MBP in the CSF?

27. Why are serum and CSF samples for glucose analyzed simultaneously?

28. What is the cause of decreased CSF glucose levels in patients with bacterial meningitis?

29. Explain the relationship of increased blood and CSF ammonia to increased levels of CSF glutamine.

30. Prior to performing Gram staining and culture of CSF, what must be done to the fluid?

31. State a cause of a false-negative CSF Gram stain report and a cause of a false-positive report.

32. Why is the laboratory currently receiving increased requests for India Ink preparations?

33. Will the limulus lysate test detect the presence of *S. pneumoniae* or *E. coli*?

34. What is the most probable cause of a false-positive Cryptococcal antigen test?

35. What is the significance of a positive serum FTA-ABS with a negative CSF VDRL test? With a positive CSF VDRL test?

CASE STUDIES AND CLINICAL SITUATIONS

1. Three tubes of CSF containing evenly distributed visible blood are drawn from a 75-year-old disoriented patient and delivered to the laboratory. Initial test results are as follows:

   WBC COUNT: 250 μL PROTEIN: 150 mg/dL
   GLUCOSE: 70 mg/dL GRAM STAIN: No organisms seen
   DIFFERENTIAL: Neutrophils, 68%; monocytes, 3%; lymphocytes, 28%; eosinophils, 1%
   Many macrophages containing ingested RBCs

   a. What is the most probable condition indicated by these results? State two reasons for your answer.
   b. Are the elevated WBC count and protein of significance? Explain your answer.
   c. Are the percentages of the cells in the differential of any significance? Explain your answer.
   d. If this patient had recently experienced a cardiac arrest, what additional test performed on the CSF might be of value?
   e. If the blood was unevenly distributed and nucleated RBCs and capillary structures were seen instead of macrophages, what would this indicate?
   f. Combining the patient's condition and the information in "e," what additional chemical test might be requested?

2. A patient with AIDS is hospitalized with symptoms of high fever and rigidity of the neck. Routine laboratory tests on the CSF show a WBC count of 100/μL with a predominance of lymphocytes and monocytes, glucose of 55 mg/dL (plasma: 85 mg/dL), and a protein of 70 mg/dL. The Gram stain shows a questionable starburst pattern.
   a. What additional microscopic examination should be performed?
   b. If the test is positive, what is the patient's diagnosis?
   c. If the results of the test are questionable, what additional testing can be performed?
   d. What could cause a false positive reaction in this test?
   e. If the tests named in "a" and "c" are negative, the glucose level is 35 mg/dL and a pellicle is observed in the fluid, what additional testing should be performed?
   f. If CSF and serum IFE was performed on this patient, what unusual findings might be present?

3. A 35-year-old woman is admitted to the hospital with symptoms of intermittent blurred vision, weakness, and loss of sensation in her legs. A lumbar puncture is performed with the following results:

   APPEARANCE: Colorless, clear
   WBC COUNT: 35 cells/μL (90% lymphocytes)
   GLUCOSE: 60 mg/dL (plasma: 100 mg/dL)

PROTEIN: 50 mg/dL (serum: 7 g/dL)
ALBUMIN: 30 mg/dL (serum: 5 g/dL)
IgG GLOBULIN: 15 mg/dL (serum: 2 g/dL)

a. Name and perform the calculation to determine the integrity of the patient's blood-brain barrier.
b. Does the patient have an intact barrier?
c. Name and perform the calculation used to determine if IgG is being synthesized within the CNS.
d. What does this result indicate?
e. Considering the patient's clinical symptoms and the calculation results, what diagnosis is suggested?
f. If immunofixation electrophoresis is performed on the patient's serum and CSF, what findings would be expected?
g. What substance in the CSF can be measured to monitor this patient?

4. Mary Howard, age 5, is admitted to the pediatrics ward with a temperature of 105°F, lethargy, and cervical rigidity. A lumbar spinal tap is performed, and three tubes of cloudy CSF are delivered to the laboratory. Preliminary tests results are as follows:

APPEARANCE: White and cloudy
WBC COUNT: 6,000 cells/μL
DIFFERENTIAL: 90% neutrophils, 10% lymphocytes
PROTEIN: 150 mg/dL
GLUCOSE: 10 mg/dL
GRAM STAIN: No organisms seen

a. From these results, what preliminary diagnosis could the physician consider?
b. Is the Gram stain result of particular significance?
c. What additional rapid test could be performed to supplement the Gram stain?
d. Would a CSF lactate test be of any value for the diagnosis? Why or why not?

5. State possible technical errors that could result in the following discrepancies:

a. An unusual number of Gram stains reported as gram-positive cocci fail to be confirmed by positive cultures.
b. A physician complains that CSF differentials are being reported only as polynuclear and mononuclear cells.
c. Bacteria observed on the cytospin differential cannot be confirmed by Gram stain or culture.
d. The majority of CSF specimens sent to the laboratory from the neurology clinic have glucose readings less than 50 percent of the corresponding blood glucose results performed in the clinic.

CHAPTER 11

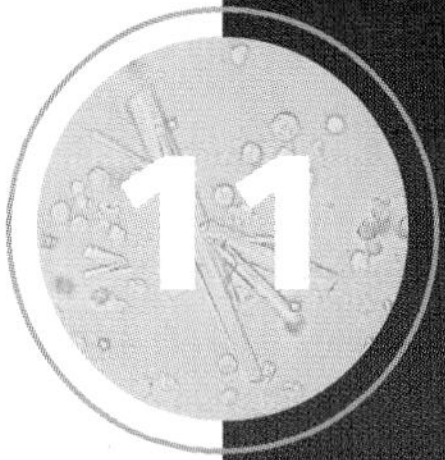

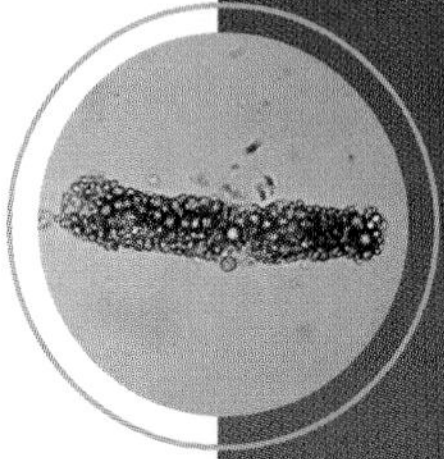

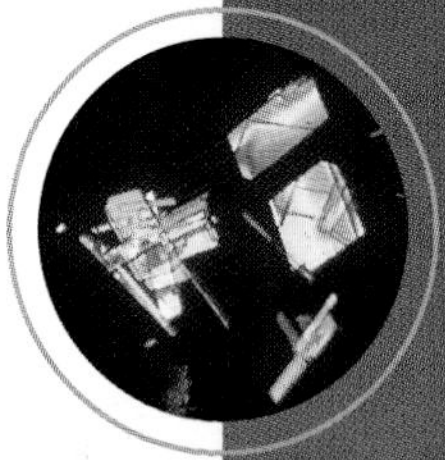

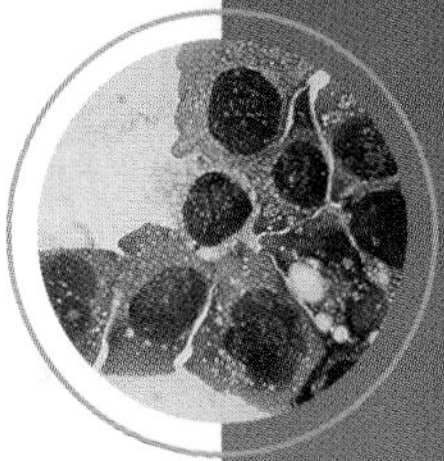

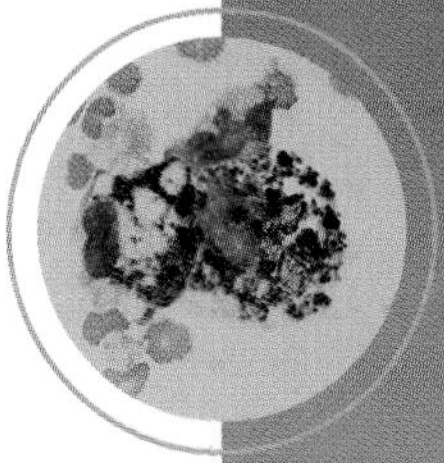

Semen

LEARNING OBJECTIVES

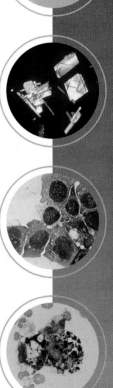

Upon completion of this chapter, the reader will be able to:

1. Describe the four components of semen with regard to source and function.
2. Describe the normal appearance of semen and three abnormalities in appearance.
3. State two possible causes of low semen volume.
4. Discuss the significance of semen liquefaction and viscosity.
5. Calculate a sperm concentration and count when provided with the number of sperm counted, the dilution, the area of the counting chamber used, and the ejaculate volume.
6. Define round cells, and explain their significance.
7. State the two parameters considered when evaluating sperm motility.
8. Describe the appearance of normal sperm, including structures and their functions.
9. Differentiate between routine and strict criteria for evaluation of sperm morphology.
10. Given an abnormal result in the routine semen analysis, determine additional tests that might be performed.
11. Describe the two routinely used methods for detection of antisperm antibodies.
12. List two methods for identifying a questionable fluid as semen.
13. State the World Health Organization normal values for routine and follow-up semen analysis.
14. Discuss the types and significance of sperm function tests.
15. Describe methods of quality control appropriate for the semen analysis.

KEY TERMS

andrology
infertility
semen
spermatids
spermatozoa

Advances in the field of ***andrology*** and assisted reproductive technology (**ART**) and increased concern over fertility, particularly by couples choosing to have children later in life, have resulted in increased emphasis on the analysis of ***semen***. Patients with abnormal results on the routine semen analysis performed in the clinical laboratory often are referred to specialized andrology laboratories for further testing to determine the need for in vitro fertilization (**IVF**). Clinical laboratory personnel also may be employed in andrology laboratories and perform both routine and specialized testing.

In addition to fertility testing, the clinical laboratory performs postvasectomy semen analysis and forensic analyses to determine the presence of semen.

Physiology

Semen is composed of four fractions that are contributed individually by the testes and epididymis, the seminal vessels, the prostate, and the bulbourethral glands (Figure 11–1). Each fraction differs in its composition, and the mixing of all four fractions during ejaculation is essential for the production of a normal semen specimen.

Spermatozoa are produced in the seminiferous tubules of the testes. They mature and are stored in the epididymis. Spermatozoa and fluid from the epididymis contribute about 5 percent of the semen volume. The seminal vessels produce the majority of the fluid (60 percent) present in the semen. The fluid contains a high content of fructose that the spermatozoa readily metabolize. Spermatozoa do not become motile until they are exposed to the fluid from the seminal vessels.

Approximately 20 to 30 percent of the semen volume is acidic fluid produced by the prostate gland. It contains high concentrations of acid phosphatase, citric acid, and zinc and proteolytic enzymes responsible for both the coagulation and **liquefaction** of the semen following ejaculation.

The bulbourethral glands contribute about 5 percent of the fluid volume in the form of a thick, alkaline mucus that helps to neutralize acidity from the prostate secretions and the vaginal acidity.

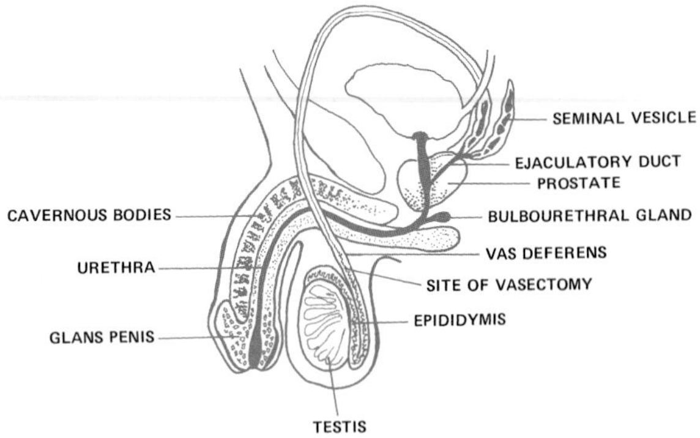

FIGURE 11–1 Diagram of the male genitalia.

Specimen Collection

The variety in the composition of the semen fractions makes proper collection of a complete specimen essential for accurate evaluation of male fertility. The majority of sperm are contained in the first portion of the ejaculate, making complete collection essential for accurate testing of both fertility and postvasectomy specimens. Patients should receive detailed instructions for specimen collection.

Specimens are collected following a period of sexual abstinence of at least 3 days and not longer than 5 days. Specimens collected following prolonged abstinence tend to have higher volumes and decreased motility.[12] When performing fertility testing, two or three samples are usually tested at 2-week intervals with two abnormal samples considered significant. The laboratory should provide warm sterile glass or plastic containers. Whenever possible, the specimen is collected in a room provided by the laboratory. However, if this is not appropriate, the specimen should be kept at room temperature and delivered to the laboratory within 1 hour of collection. Laboratory personnel must record the time of specimen collection and specimen receipt. A fresh semen specimen is clotted and should liquefy within 30 to 60 minutes after collection; therefore, the time of collection is essential for evaluation of semen liquefaction. Analysis of the specimen cannot begin until after liquefaction has occurred. Specimens awaiting analysis should be kept at 37°C. Specimens should be collected by masturbation. If this is not possible, only nonlubricant-containing polymeric silicone (Silastic) condoms should be used.

SPECIMEN HANDLING

All semen specimens are potential reservoirs for human immunodeficiency and hepatitis viruses, and Standard Precautions must be observed at all times during the analysis. Specimens are discarded as biohazardous waste.

Semen Analysis

The semen analysis for fertility evaluation consists of both macroscopic and microscopic examination. Parameters reported include appearance, volume, **viscosity**, pH, sperm concentration and count, motility, and morphology. Normal values are shown in Table 11–1.

TABLE 11–1 **Normal Values for Semen Analysis**[13]

Volume	2–5 mL
Viscosity	Pours in droplets
pH	7.2–8.0
Sperm concentration	20–160 million/mL
Sperm count	740 million/ejaculate
Motility	>50% within 1 h
Quality	>2.0
Morphology	>30% normal forms (strict criteria) >50% normal forms (routine criteria)
White blood cells	<1.0 million/mL

APPEARANCE

Normal semen has a gray-white color, appears translucent, and has a characteristic musty odor. Increased white turbidity indicates the presence of white blood cells and infection within the reproductive tract. Should the specimen require culturing, this is performed prior to continuing with the semen analysis. During the microscopic examination, WBCs must be differentiated from immature sperm (***spermatids***). The leukocyte esterase reagent strip test may be useful to screen for the presence of WBCs.[7] Varying degrees of red coloration are associated with the presence of red blood cells and are abnormal. Yellow coloration may be caused by urine contamination, specimen collection following prolonged abstinence, and medications. Urine is toxic to sperm, thereby affecting the evaluation of motility.

As stated previously, fresh semen specimens are clotted and should liquefy within 30 to 60 minutes. Failure of liquefaction to occur may be caused by a deficiency in prostatic enzymes and should be reported. Semen analysis cannot be performed until liquefaction has occurred and the specimen can be thoroughly mixed.

VOLUME

Normal semen volume ranges between 2 and 5 mL. It can be measured by pouring the specimen into a clean graduated cylinder calibrated in 0.1-mL increments. Increased volume may be seen following periods of extended abstinence. Decreased volume is more frequently associated with ***infertility*** and may indicate improper functioning of one of the semen-producing organs. Incomplete specimen collection must also be considered.

VISCOSITY

Specimen viscosity refers to the consistency of the fluid and may be related to specimen liquefaction. Incompletely liquefied specimens will be clumped and highly viscous. The normal semen specimen should be easily drawn into a pipette and form droplets that do not appear clumped or stringy when discharged from the pipette. Ratings of 0 (watery) to 4 (gel-like) can be assigned to the viscosity report.[10] Increased viscosity and incomplete liquefaction will impede sperm motility.

pH

The normal pH of semen is alkaline with a range of 7.2 to 8.0. Increased pH is indicative of infection within the reproductive tract. A decreased pH is associated with increased prostatic fluid. Semen for pH testing can be applied to the pH pad of a urinalysis reagent strip and the color compared with the manufacturer's chart. Dedicated pH testing paper also can be used.

SPERM CONCENTRATION/COUNT

Even though fertilization is accomplished by one spermatozoon, the actual number of sperm present in a semen specimen is a valid measurement of fertility. Normal values for sperm concentration are commonly listed as 20 to 160 million sperm per milliliter, with concentrations between 10 and 20 million per milliliter considered borderline. The total sperm count for the ejaculate can be calculated by multiplying the sperm concentration by the specimen volume. Total sperm counts greater than 40 million per ejaculate are considered normal (20 million per milliliter $\times$ 2 mL).

In the clinical laboratory, sperm concentration is usually performed using the Neubauer counting chamber. The sperm are counted in the same manner as cells in the cerebrospinal fluid cell count, that is, by diluting the specimen and counting the cells in the Neubauer chamber. The amount of the dilution and the number of squares counted vary among laboratories.

The most commonly used dilution is 1:20 prepared using a mechanical (positive-displacement) rather than a Thoma pipette.[13] Dilution of the semen is essential because it immobilizes the sperm prior to counting. The traditional diluting fluid contains sodium bicarbonate and formalin, which immobilize and preserve the cells; however, good results can also be achieved using tap water.

The Makler Counting Chamber (Sefi-Medical Instruments, Hafia, Israel) provides a method for counting undiluted specimens using a counting chamber with 1 mm^2 grid divided into 100 squares (0.12 $\times$ 0.1 mm^2) engraved in the cover plate. Sperm are immobilized by heating part of the specimen prior to charging the chamber. Sperm motility using the unheated portion of the specimen can also be evaluated in the chamber.[8]

Using the Neubauer hemocytometer, sperm are usually counted in the four corner and center squares of the large center square—similar to a manual RBC count (Figure 11–2). Both sides of the hemocytometer are loaded and

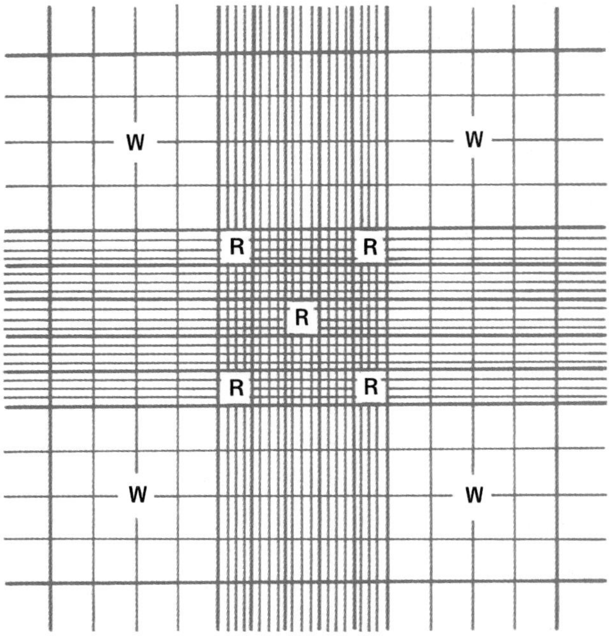

FIGURE 11–2 Areas of Neubauer counting chamber used for red and white blood cell counts. (W = typical white blood cell counting area and R = typical red blood cell counting area.)

counted, and the counts should agree within 10 percent. An average of the two counts is then used in the calculation. If the counts do not agree, both the dilution and the counts are repeated. Counts are performed using either phase or bright-field microscopy. The addition of stain, such as crystal violet, to the diluting fluid will aid in visualization when using bright-field microscopy.

Only fully developed sperm should be counted. Immature sperm and WBCs, often referred to as "round" cells, must not be included. However, their presence can be significant, and they may need to be identified and counted separately. Stain included in the diluting fluid aids in differentiation between immature sperm cells and leukocytes, and they can be counted in the same manner as mature sperm. Greater than 1 million leukocytes per milliliter is associated with inflammation of the reproductive organs.

Calculation of sperm concentration is dependent on the dilution used and the size and number of squares counted. When using the 1:20 dilution and counting the five squares (RBCs) in the large center square as described previously, the number of sperm can be multiplied by 1,000,000 (add 6 zeros) to equal the sperm concentration per milliliter. Notice that unlike blood cell counts, the sperm concentration is reported in milliliters rather than microliters. Calculation of sperm concentration can also be performed using the basic formula for cell counts covered in Chapter 10. Because this formula provides the number of cells per microliter, the figure must then be multiplied by 1000 to calculate the number of sperm per milliliter. The total sperm count is calculated by multiplying the number of sperm per milliliter by the specimen volume.

EXAMPLES:

1. Using a 1:20 dilution, an average of 60 sperm are counted in the five RBC counting squares. Calculate the sperm concentration per milliliter and the total sperm count in a specimen with a volume of 4 mL.

60 sperm counted × 1,000,000 = 60,000,000 sperm/mL
60,000,000 sperm/mL × 4 mL = 240,000,000 sperm/ejaculate

2. Using a 1:20 dilution, 600 sperm are counted in two WBC counting squares. Calculate the sperm concentration per milliliter and the total sperm count in a specimen with a volume of 2 mL.

$$\frac{600 \text{ sperm} \times 20 \text{ (dilution)}}{2 \text{ (squares counted)} \times 0.1\ \mu\text{L (volume counted)}} = 60{,}000 \text{ sperm } \mu\text{L}$$

60,000 sperm/μL × 1,000 = 60,000,000 sperm/mL
60,000,000/mL × 2 mL = 120,000,000 sperm/ejaculate

SPERM MOTILITY

The presence of sperm capable of forward, progressive movement is critical for fertility, because once presented to the cervix, the sperm must propel themselves through the cervical mucosa to the uterus, fallopian tubes, and ovum. Traditionally, clinical laboratory reporting of sperm motility has been a subjective evaluation performed by examining an undiluted specimen and determining the percentage of motile sperm and the quality of the motility.

TABLE 11–2 **Sperm Motility Grading**

Grade	Criteria
4.0	Rapid, straight-line motility
3.0	Slower speed, some lateral movement
2.0	Slow forward progression, noticeable lateral movement
1.0	No forward progression
0	No movement

Assessment of sperm motility should be performed on well mixed, liquefied semen within 1 hour of specimen collection. The practice of examining sperm motility at timed intervals over an extended period has been shown to serve no useful purpose.[11] To provide continuity in reporting, laboratories should place a consistent amount of semen under the same size coverslip, such as 10 μL under a 22 × 22 mm coverslip. The percentage of sperm showing actual forward movement can then be estimated after evaluating approximately 20 high-power fields. Motility is evaluated as to the speed and direction of the motility and graded on a scale of 0 to 4, with 4 indicating rapid, straight-line movement and 0 indicating no movement (Table 11–2). A minimum motility of 50 percent with a rating of 2.0 after 1 hour is considered normal.[12] The presence of a high percentage of immobile sperm and clumps of sperm requires further evaluation to determine sperm viability or the presence of sperm agglutinins.

In recent years, instrumentation capable of performing computer-assisted semen analysis (**CASA**) has been developed. CASA provides objective determination of both sperm velocity and trajectory (direction of motion). Sperm concentration is also included in the analysis. Currently CASA instrumentation is found primarily in laboratories that specialize in andrology and perform a high volume of semen analysis.

SPERM MORPHOLOGY

Just as the presence of a normal number of sperm that are nonmotile will produce infertility, the presence of sperm that are morphologically incapable of fertilization also will result in infertility.

Sperm morphology is evaluated with respect to both head and tail appearance. Abnormalities in head morphology are associated with poor ovum penetration, whereas tail abnormalities affect motility.

The normal sperm has an oval-shaped head approximately 5 μm long and 3 μm wide and a long, flagellar tail approximately 45 μm long (the only flagella in the human body). As shown in Figure 11–3, the head and tail are connected by the neck and the middle piece, which contains mitochondria that provide energy for flagellar tail motion. Critical to ovum penetration is the enzyme-containing **acrosomal cap** located at the tip of the head. The acrosomal cap should encompass approximately one-half of the head.[13]

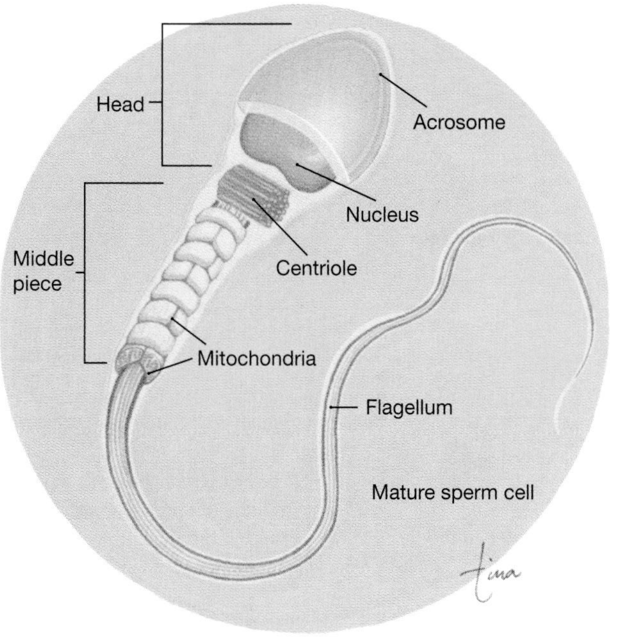

FIGURE 11–3 Normal spermatozoa structure. (From Scanlon, VC, and Sanders, T: Essentials of Anatomy and Physiology, ed. 3. FA Davis, Philadelphia, 1999, p. 439, with permission.)

Sperm morphology is evaluated from a thinly smeared, stained slide under oil immersion. Staining can be performed using Wright's, Giemsa, or Papanicolaou's stain and is a matter of laboratory preference. Air-dried slides are stable for 24 hours. At least 200 sperm should be evaluated and the percentage of abnormal sperm reported. Routinely identified abnormalities in head structure include double heads, giant and amorphous heads, pinheads, tapered heads, and constricted heads (Figures 11–4 and 11–5). Abnormal sperm tails are frequently double, coiled, or bent (Figure 11–6 and 11–7). Abnormalities in the neck and middle piece may cause the sperm head to bend backward.

Additional parameters in the evaluation of sperm morphology include measurement of head, neck, and tail size, the size of the acrosome, and the presence of vacuoles. Inclusion of these parameters is referred to as Kruger's strict criteria.[6] Performance of strict criteria evaluation requires the use of a stage micrometer or morphometry.[4] At present, evaluation of sperm morphology using strict criteria is not routinely performed in the clinical laboratory but is recommended by the World Health Organization (**WHO**).[13]

Normal values for sperm morphology depend on the method of evaluation used and vary from less than 50 percent abnormal forms when using routine criteria to less than 70 percent abnormal forms when using strict criteria.[13]

Differentiation and enumeration of round cells (immature sperm and neutrophils) can also be made during the morphology examination (Figure 11–8). By counting the number of spermatids or neutrophils seen in conjunction with 100 mature sperm, the amount per milliliter can be calculated using the formula:

$$C = \frac{N \times S}{100}$$

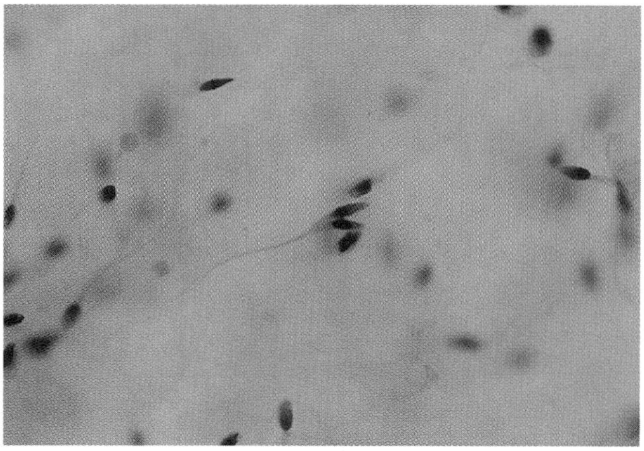

FIGURE 11–4 Spermatozoa with double head, hematoxylin-eosin (×1000).

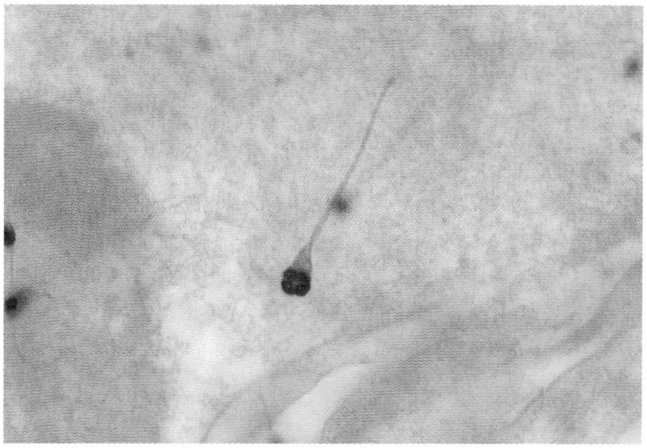

FIGURE 11–5 Spermatozoa with amorphous head, hematoxylin-eosin (×1000).

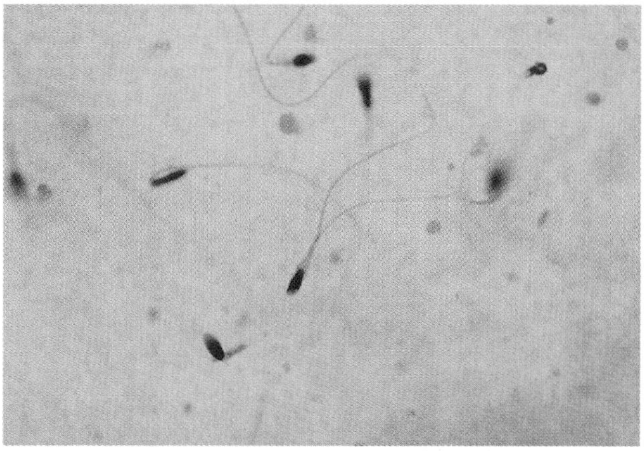

FIGURE 11–6 Spermatozoa with double tail, hematoxylin-eosin (×1000).

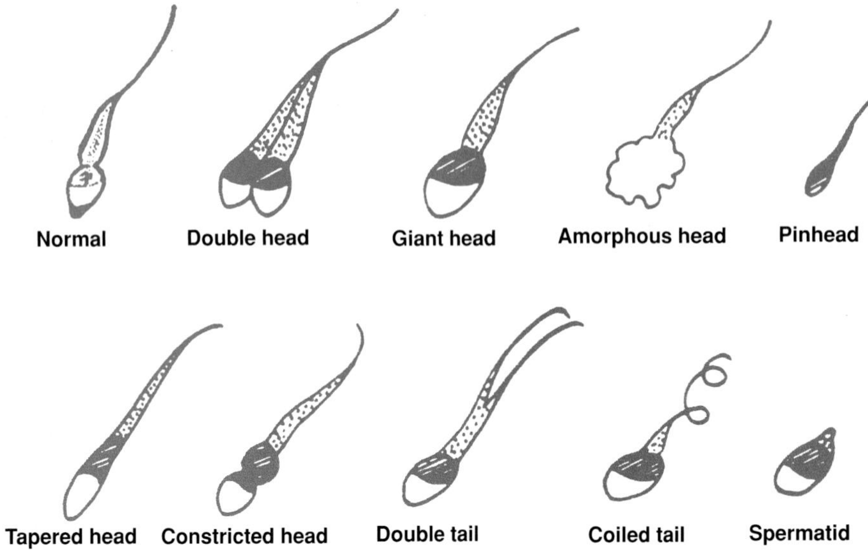

FIGURE 11–7 Abnormalities of sperm heads and tails are illustrated.

N equals the number of spermatids or neutrophils counted per 100 mature sperm, and S equals the sperm concentration in millions per milliliter. This method can be used when counting cannot be performed during the hemocytometer count and to verify counts performed by hemocytometer.

Additional Testing

Should abnormalities be discovered in any of these routine parameters, additional tests may be requested (Table 11–3). The most common are tests for sperm viability, seminal fluid fructose level, sperm agglutinins, and microbial infection.

SPERM VIABILITY

Decreased sperm viability may be suspected when a specimen has a normal sperm concentration with markedly decreased motility. Viability is evaluated by mixing the specimen with an eosin-nigrosin stain, preparing a smear, and counting the number of dead cells in 100 sperm. Living cells are not infiltrated by the dye and remain a bluish-white color, whereas dead cells stain red against the purple background (Figure 11–9). Normal viability requires 75 percent living cells and should correspond to the previously evaluated motility.

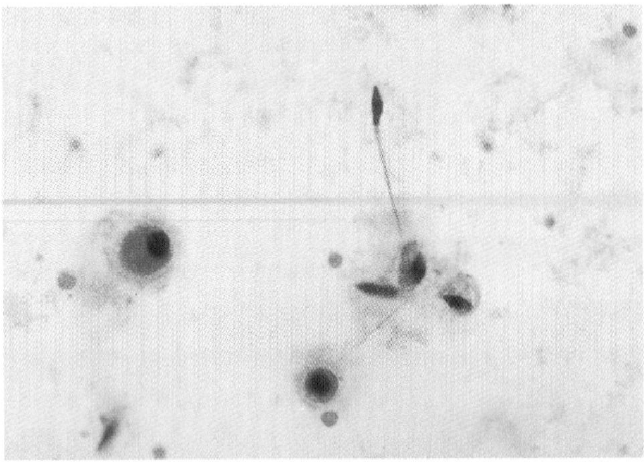

FIGURE 11–8 Immature spermatozoa, hematoxylin-eosin (×1000).

SEMINAL FLUID FRUCTOSE

Low sperm concentration may be caused by lack of the support medium produced in the seminal vesicles. This can be indicated by a low to absent fructose level in the semen. Specimens can be screened for the presence of fructose using the resorcinol test.

A normal quantitative level of fructose is equal to or greater than 13 µmol per ejaculate. Specimens for fructose levels should be tested within 2 hours or frozen to prevent fructolysis.

ANTISPERM ANTIBODIES

Antisperm antibodies can be present in both men and women. They may be detected in semen, cervical mucosa, or serum and are considered a possible cause of infertility. It

PROCEDURE

Seminal Fructose Screening Test[11]

1. Prepare reagent. (50 mg resorcinol in 33 mL concentrated HCl diluted to 100 mL with water).
2. Mix 1 mL semen with 9 mL reagent.
3. Boil.
4. Observe for orange-red color.

TABLE 11–3 **Additional Testing for Abnormal Semen Analysis**

Abnormal Result	Possible Abnormality	Test
Decreased motility with normal count	Viability	Eosin-nigrosin stain
Decreased count	Lack of seminal vesicle support medium	Fructose level
Decreased motility with clumping	Male antisperm antibodies	Mixed agglutination reaction and immunobead tests Sperm agglutination with male serum
Normal analysis with continued infertility	Female antisperm antibodies	Immunobead test Sperm agglutination with female serum

is not unusual for both partners to demonstrate antibodies, although male antisperm antibodies are more frequently encountered.

Under normal conditions, the blood-testes barrier separates sperm from the male immune system. When this barrier is disrupted, as can occur following surgery, **vasectomy** reversal (**vasovasostomy**), trauma, and infection, the antigens on the sperm produce an immune response that damages the sperm. The damaged sperm may then cause the production of antibodies in the female partner.[2]

The presence of antibodies in the male partner can be suspected when clumps of sperm are observed during a routine semen analysis. The presence of antisperm antibodies in the female partner will result in a normal semen analysis accompanied by continued infertility. The presence of antisperm antibodies in women may be demonstrated by mixing the semen with the female cervical mucosa or serum and observing for agglutination.

Two frequently used tests to detect the presence of antibody-coated sperm are the mixed agglutination reaction (**MAR**) test and the immunobead test. The MAR test is a screening procedure used primarily to detect the presence of IgG antibodies. The semen sample containing motile sperm is incubated with IgG antihuman globulin (**AHG**) and a suspension of latex particles or treated RBCs coated with IgG. The bivalent AHG will bind simultaneously to both the antibody on the sperm and the antibody on the latex particles or RBCs, forming microscopically visible clumps of sperm and particles or cells. Less than 10 percent of the motile sperm attached to the particles is considered normal.

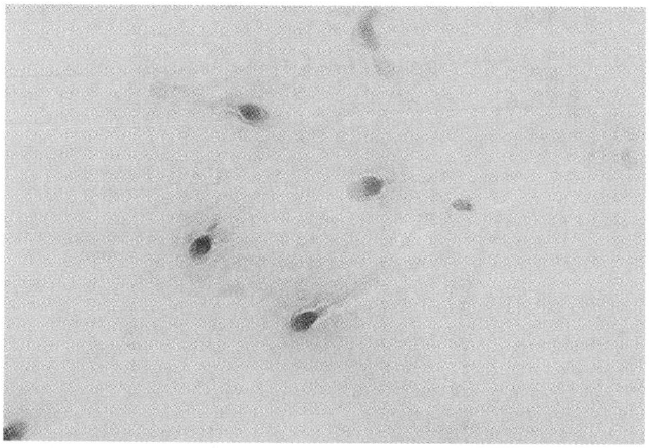

FIGURE 11–9 Nonviable spermatozoa demonstrated by the eosin-nigrosin stain (×1000).

The immunobead test is a more specific procedure in that it can be used to detect the presence of IgG, IgM, and IgA antibodies and will demonstrate what area of the sperm (head, neck, or tail) the autoantibodies are affecting. Head-directed antibodies can interfere with penetration into the cervical mucosa or ovum, whereas tail-directed antibodies affect movement through the cervical mucosa.[9] In the immunobead test, sperm are mixed with polyacrylamide beads known to be coated with either anti-IgG, anti-IgM, or anti-IgA. Microscopic examination of the sperm will show the beads attached to sperm at particular areas. Depending on the type of beads used, the test could be reported as "IgM tail antibodies," "IgG head antibodies," and so forth. The presence of beads on less than 20 percent of the sperm is considered normal.

MICROBIAL AND CHEMICAL TESTING

The presence of more than 1 million leukocytes per millimeter indicates infection within the reproductive system, frequently the prostate. Routine aerobic and anaerobic cultures and tests for *Chlamydia trachomatis*, *Mycoplasma hominis*, and *Ureaplasma urealyticum* are most frequently performed.

Additional chemical testing performed on semen may include determination of the levels of neutral α-glucosidase, zinc, citric acid, and acid phosphatase. Just as decreased fructose levels are associated with a lack of seminal fluid, decreased neutral α-glucosidase suggests a disorder of the epididymis. Decreased zinc, citrate, and acid phosphatase indicate a lack of prostatic fluid (Table 11–4).

TABLE 11–4 **Normal Semen Chemical Values**[13]

Neutral α-glucosidase	≥20 mμ/ejaculate
Zinc	≥2.4 μmol/ejaculate
Citric acid	≥52 μmol/ejaculate
Acid phosphatase	≥200 μ/ejaculate

On certain occasions, the laboratory may be called on to determine whether semen is actually present in a specimen. A primary example is in cases of alleged rape. Microscopically examining the specimen for the presence of sperm may be possible, with the best results being obtained by enhancing the specimen with xylene and examining under phase microscopy.[3] However, a more reliable procedure is to test the material chemically for acid phosphatase. Because seminal fluid is the only body fluid with a high concentration of acid phosphatase, the detection of this enzyme can confirm the presence of semen in a specimen. Further, information can often be obtained by performing ABO blood grouping and DNA analysis on the specimen.

POSTVASECTOMY SEMEN ANALYSIS

Postvasectomy semen analysis is a much less involved procedure when compared with the infertility analysis, inasmuch as the only concern is the presence or absence of spermatozoa. The length of time required for complete sterilization can vary greatly among patients and depends on both time and number of ejaculations. Therefore, finding viable sperm in a postvasectomy patient is not uncommon, and care should be taken not to overlook even a single sperm. Specimens are routinely tested at monthly intervals, beginning at 2 months postvasectomy and continuing until two consecutive monthly specimens show no spermatozoa.

Recommended testing includes examination of a wet preparation using phase microscopy for the presence of motile and nonmotile sperm. A negative wet preparation is followed by centrifugation of the specimen for 10 minutes and examination of the sediment.[11]

SPERM FUNCTION TESTS

Advances in assisted reproduction and IVF have resulted in a need for more sophisticated semen analysis to assess not only the characteristics of sperm but also the functional ability. The tests are most commonly performed in specialized andrology laboratories and include the hamster egg penetration assay, cervical mucus penetration test, hypo-osmotic swelling test, and the in vitro acrosome reaction (Table 11–5).[14]

TABLE 11–5 **Sperm Function Tests**

Test	Description
Hamster egg penetration	Sperm are incubated with species-nonspecific hamster eggs and penetration is observed microscopically
Cervical mucus penetration	Observation of sperm penetration ability of partner's midcycle cervical mucus
Hypo-osmotic swelling	Sperm exposed to low-sodium concentrations are evaluated for membrane integrity and sperm viability
In vitro acrosome reaction	Evaluation of the acrosome to produce enzymes essential for ovum penetration

SEMEN ANALYSIS QUALITY CONTROL

Traditionally, the semen routine analysis has been subject to very little quality control.[1] This has resulted from a lack of appropriate control materials and the subjectivity of the motility and morphology analyses. The analysis is rated as a high complexity test under the Clinical Laboratory Improvement Amendments '88, and testing personnel standards must be observed.

Increased interest in fertility testing has promoted the development of quality control materials and in-depth training programs. The standardized procedures developed by the World Health Organization have provided a basis for laboratory testing and reporting. The use of CASA has aided in reducing the subjectivity of the analysis. However, even computerized, the analysis has been shown to vary among operators.[5]

Laboratories can now participate in proficiency testing programs offered by the College of American Pathologists and the American Association of Bioanalysts (**AAB**) that include sperm concentration, viability, and morphology. Commercial quality control materials and training aids are available and should be incorporated into laboratory protocols.

REFERENCES

1. Baker, DJ, et al: Semen evaluations in the clinical laboratory. Lab Med 25(8):509–514, 1994.
2. Cearlock, DM: Autoimmune antispermatozoa antibodies in men: Clinical detection and role in infertility. Clin Lab Sci 2(3):165–168, 1989.
3. Fraysier, HD: A rapid screening technique for the detection of spermatozoa. J Forensic Sci 32(2):527–528, 1987.
4. Harr, R: Characterization of spermatozoa by planar morphometry. Clin Lab Sci 10(4):190–196, 1997.
5. Krause, W, and Viethen, G: Quality assessment of computer-assisted semen analysis (CASA) in the andrology laboratory. Andrologia 31(3):125–129, 1999.
6. Kruger, T, et al: Predictive value of sperm morphology in IVF. Fertil Steril 112–117, 1988.
7. Lopez, A, et al: Suitability of solid-phase chemistry for quantification of leukocytes in cerebrospinal, seminal and peritoneal fluid. Clin Chem 33(8):1475–1476, 1987.
8. Makler, A: The improved ten-micrometer chamber for rapid sperm count and motility. Fertil Steril 33(3):337–338, 1980.
9. Marshburn, PB, and Kutteh, WH: The role of antisperm antibodies in infertility. Fertil Steril 61:799–811, 1994.
10. Overstreet, JW, and Katz, DF: Semen analysis. Urol Clin North Am 14(3):441–449, 1987.
11. Sampson, JH, and Alexander, NJ: Semen analysis: A laboratory approach. Lab Med 13(4):218–223, 1982.
12. Sarhar, S, and Henry, JB: Andrology laboratory and fertility assessment. In Henry, JB (ed): Clinical Diagnosis and Management by Laboratory Methods. WB Saunders, Philadelphia, 1996.
13. World Health Organization: WHO Laboratory Manual for the Examination of Human Semen and Sperm-Cervical Interaction. Cambridge University Press, London, 1999.
14. Yablonsky, T: Male fertility testing. Lab Med 27(6):378–383, 1996.

STUDY QUESTIONS

1. State the primary sites of sperm production and maturation.
2. List the four reproductive structures that produce components of the semen, and state the components produced.
3. How will failure to collect the first portion of the semen specimen affect the analysis?
4. If an initial semen analysis report contains an abnormal result, what should be the next instruction given to the patient?
5. Why is the time a semen specimen is collected recorded on the requisition form?
6. Should a semen specimen for fertility analysis received in a routine condom be accepted? Why or why not?
7. What safety precautions should be observed when performing semen analysis? Why?
8. State a possible cause of a semen specimen appearing red, yellow, or white and turbid.
9. Which parameter of the routine semen analysis would be most critically affected in a low-volume specimen that was improperly collected? Why?
10. Will sperm motility be affected by a specimen that produces droplets when dispensed from a pipette? Why or why not?
11. What is the significance of a semen specimen with a pH of 6.5?
12. Calculate the sperm concentration and count using the following information:
    a. Specimen diluted 1:20
    b. Number of sperm in the 5 RBC squares = 78 and 84
    c. Specimen volume = 3 mL
13. Using the preceding information, calculate the sperm concentration and count when the sperm are counted in two WBC squares.
14. Which of the preceding results is normal, and which is abnormal?
15. In addition to diluting the specimen, what two other functions can diluting fluid perform?
16. What two parameters are evaluated when grading sperm motility?
17. Describe a sperm motility evaluation graded as 2.0.
18. Define and state the purpose of CASA.
19. Describe and state the function of the sperm acrosomal cap.
20. How do sperm head and tail morphologic abnormalities affect fertilization?
21. How do Kruger's strict criteria differ from routine morphology criteria?
22. Ten neutrophils are counted in conjunction with 100 sperm during morphology analysis of a specimen with a 30 million per milliliter concentration. Is this normal or abnormal? Why?
23. What is the significance of an eosin-nigrosin stain report of 75 percent nonviable sperm and a sperm concentration of 60 million per milliliter?
24. List three possible causes of the development of male antisperm antibodies.
25. Explain how the addition of AHG and immunoglobulin-coated RBCs to a semen specimen will detect the presence of antisperm antibodies.
26. State two advantages of the immunobead antisperm antibody test.
27. What chemical test is performed to determine if semen is present in a specimen? Why?
28. How does the performance of a postvasectomy semen analysis differ from a fertility analysis?
29. Name a sperm function test that might be performed following an abnormal eosin-nigrosin stain.
30. What procedures are available to ensure appropriate quality control of the semen analysis?

CASE STUDIES AND CLINICAL SITUATIONS

1. A repeat semen analysis for fertility testing is reported as follows:

VOLUME: 3.5 mL	SPERM CONCENTRATION: 6 million/mL
VISCOSITY: Normal	SPERM MOTILITY: 30%—grade 1.0
PH: 7.5	MORPHOLOGY: <30% normal forms—30 spermatids/100 sperm

   The results correspond with the first analysis.
   a. List three abnormal parameters.
   b. What is the sperm count? Is this normal?
   c. What chemical test could provide additional information? Why?
   d. How would a laboratorian safely prepare the reagent for this test?
2. A semen analysis on a postvasovasectomy patient has a normal sperm concentration; however, motility is decreased, and clumping is observed on the wet preparation.
   a. Explain the possible connection between these observations and the patient's recent surgery.
   b. What tests could be performed to further evaluate the patient's infertility?

c. State three ways in which a positive result on these tests could be affecting male fertility.
d. Name two sperm function tests that could be affected by a positive result and explain why.

3. A yellow-colored semen specimen is received in the laboratory. The analysis is normal except for decreased sperm motility. Explain the possible connection between the two abnormal findings.

4. Abnormal results of a semen analysis are volume = 1.0 mL and sperm concentration = 1 million per milliliter. State a nonpathologic cause of these abnormal results.

5. A semen specimen with normal initial appearance fails to liquefy after 60 minutes.
   a. Would a specimen pH of 8.2 be consistent with this observation? Why or why not?
   b. State three chemical tests that would be of value in this analysis.
   c. How does this abnormality affect fertility?

CHAPTER 12

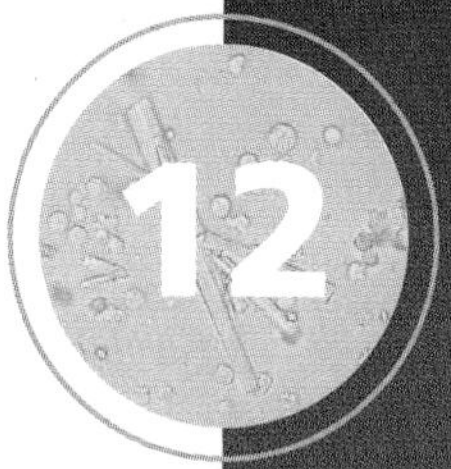

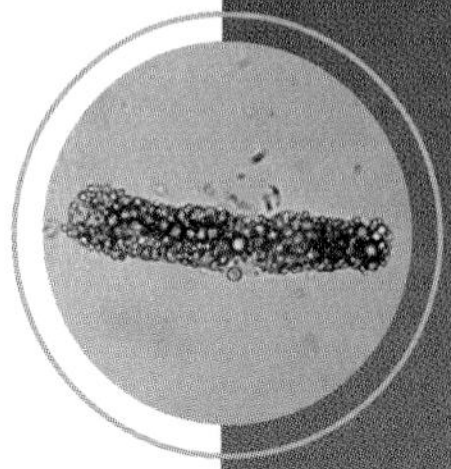

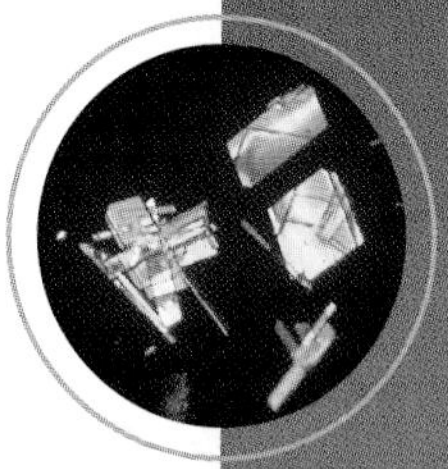

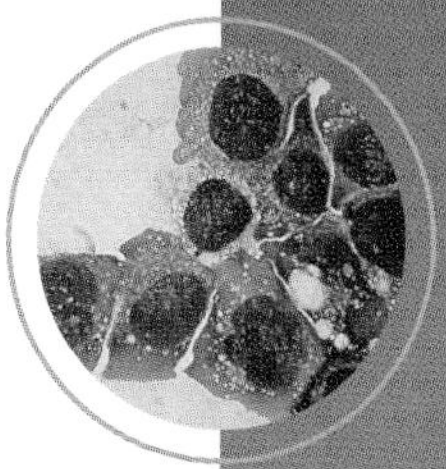

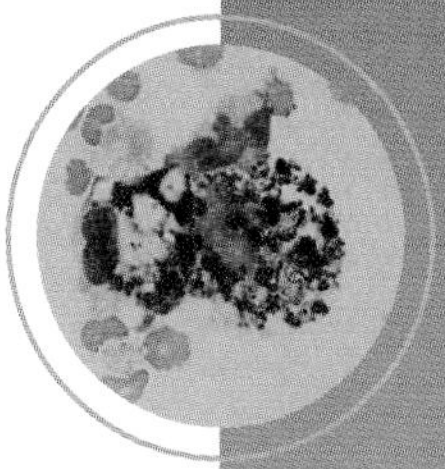

Synovial Fluid

LEARNING OBJECTIVES

Upon completion of this chapter, the reader will be able to:

1. Describe the formation and function of synovial fluid.
2. Relate laboratory test results to the four common classifications of joint disorders.
3. Determine the appropriate collection tubes for requested laboratory tests on synovial fluid.
4. Describe the appearance of synovial fluid in normal and abnormal states.
5. Discuss the normal and abnormal cellular composition of synovial fluid.
6. List and describe six crystals found in synovial fluid.
7. Explain the differentiation of monosodium urate and calcium pyrophosphate crystals using polarized and compensated polarized light.
8. State the clinical significance of glucose and lactate tests on synovial fluid.
9. List four genera of bacteria most frequently found in synovial fluid.
10. Describe the relationship of serologic testing of serum to joint disorders.

KEY TERMS

arthritis
arthrocentesis
hyaluronic acid
synovial fluid

Physiology

Synovial fluid, often referred to as "joint fluid," is a viscous liquid found in the cavities of the movable joints (**diarthroses**) or synovial joints. As shown in Figure 12–1, the bones in the synovial joints are lined with articular cartilage and separated by a cavity containing the synovial fluid. The smooth articular cartilage and synovial fluid reduce friction between the bones during joint movement. In addition to providing lubrication in the joints, synovial fluid provides nutrients to the articular cartilage and lessens the shock of joint compression occurring during activities such as walking and jogging.

Synovial fluid is formed as an ultrafiltrate of plasma across the synovial membrane. The filtration is nonselective except for the exclusion of high molecular weight proteins. Therefore, the majority of the chemical constituents have concentrations similar to plasma values. Cells lining the synovial membrane (**synoviocytes**) secrete a mucopolysaccharide containing ***hyaluronic acid*** and a small amount of protein into the fluid. This substance causes the noticeable viscosity of synovial fluid. Normal values for synovial fluid analysis are shown in Table 12–1.

Damage to the articular membranes produces pain and stiffness in the joints, collectively referred to as ***arthritis***. A variety of conditions including infection, inflammation, metabolic disorders, trauma, physical stress, and advanced age are associated with arthritis. Laboratory results of synovial fluid analysis can be used to determine the pathologic origin of arthritis. Disorders are frequently classified into four groups, as shown in Table 12–2. Some overlap of test results among the groups may occur (Table 12–3), and the patient's clinical history must also be considered when assigning a category. The most frequently performed tests are the WBC count, differential, Gram stain, culture, and polarized microscopy examination for crystals.[9]

TABLE 12–1 **Normal Synovial Fluid Values[10]**

Volume	<3.5 mL
Color	Pale yellow
Clarity	Clear
Viscosity	Able to form a string 4–6 cm long
Erythrocyte count	<2000 cells/μL
Leukocyte count	<200 cells/μL
Neutrophils	<20% of the differential
Lymphocytes	<15% of the differential
Monocytes and macrophages	65% of the differential
Crystals	None present
Glucose	<10 mg/dL lower than the blood glucose
Lactate	<250 mg/dL
Total protein	<3 g/dL
Uric acid	Equal to blood value

Specimen Collection and Handling

Synovial fluid is collected by needle aspiration called ***arthrocentesis***. The amount of fluid present will vary with the size of the joint and the degree of fluid buildup in the joint. For example, the normal amount of fluid in the large knee cavity is less than 3.5 mL, but can increase to greater than 25 mL with inflammation. In some instances, only a few drops of fluid are obtained, but these can still be used for microscopic analysis or culturing. The volume of fluid collected should be recorded.

Normal synovial fluid does not clot; however, fluid from a diseased joint may contain fibrinogen and will clot. Therefore, fluid is usually collected in a syringe that has been moistened with heparin. When sufficient fluid is collected, it should be distributed into three tubes—a sterile

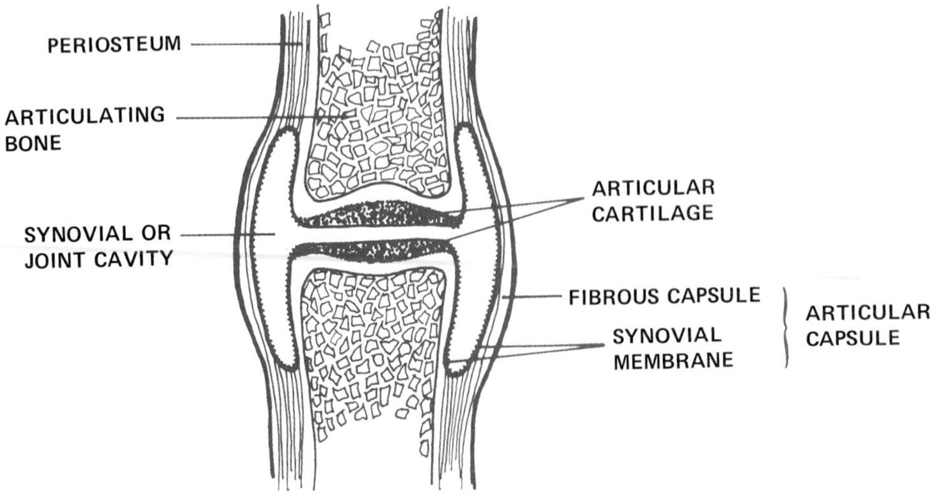

FIGURE 12–1 Diagram of a synovial joint.

TABLE 12–2 Classification and Pathologic Significance of Joint Disorders

Group Classification	Pathologic Significance
I. Noninflammatory	Degenerative joint disorders
II. Inflammatory	Immunologic problems, including rheumatoid arthritis and lupus erythematosus
	Crystal-induced gout and pseudogout
III. Septic	Microbial infection
IV. Hemorrhagic	Traumatic injury
	Coagulation deficiencies

heparinized tube for the microbiology laboratory, a liquid ethylenediaminetetraacetic acid (**EDTA**) tube for the hematology laboratory, and a nonanticoagulated tube for other tests. Powdered anticoagulants should not be used because they may produce artifacts that will interfere with crystal analysis. The nonanticoagulated tube must be centrifuged and separated to prevent cellular elements from interfering with chemical and serologic analyses. Ideally, all testing should be done as soon as possible to prevent cellular lysis and possible changes in crystals.

TABLE 12–3 Laboratory Findings in Joint Disorders[7,10]

Group Classification	Laboratory Findings
I. Noninflammatory	Clear, yellow fluid Good viscosity WBCs <2000 µL Neutrophils <30% Normal glucose (similar to blood glucose)
II. Inflammatory (immunologic origin)	Cloudy, yellow fluid Poor viscosity WBCs 2000–5000 µL Neutrophils >50% Decreased glucose level Possible autoantibodies present
(crystal-induced origin)	Cloudy or milky fluid Poor viscosity WBCs up to 50,000 µL Neutrophils <90% Decreased glucose level Elevated uric acid level Crystals present
III. Septic	Cloudy, yellow-green fluid Poor viscosity WBCs 10,000–200,000 µL Neutrophils >90% Decreased glucose level Positive culture and Gram stain
IV. Hemorrhagic	Cloudy, red fluid Poor viscosity WBCs <5000 µL Neutrophils <50% Normal glucose level RBCs present

Appearance and Viscosity

A report of the gross appearance is an essential part of the synovial fluid analysis.[4] Normal synovial fluid appears clear and pale yellow. The color often becomes a deeper yellow in the presence of inflammation and may have a greenish tinge with bacterial infection. As with cerebrospinal fluid, in synovial fluid the presence of blood from a hemorrhagic arthritis must be distinguished from blood from a traumatic aspiration. This is accomplished primarily by observing the uneven distribution of blood in the specimens obtained from a traumatic aspiration.

Turbidity is frequently associated with the presence of WBCs; however, synovial cell debris and fibrin also produce turbidity. The fluid may appear milky when crystals are present.

Viscosity of the synovial fluid comes from the polymerization of the hyaluronic acid and is essential for the proper lubrication of the joints. Arthritis affects both the production of hyaluronate and its ability to polymerize, thus decreasing the viscosity of the fluid. Several methods are available to measure the viscosity of the fluid, the simplest being to observe the ability of the fluid to form a string from the tip of a syringe, and can be done at the bedside. A string that measures 4 to 6 cm is considered normal.

Measurement of the degree of hyaluronate polymerization can be performed using a Ropes, or mucin clot, test. When added to a solution of 2 to 5 percent acetic acid, normal synovial fluid will form a solid clot surrounded by clear fluid. As the ability of the hyaluronate to polymerize decreases, the clot becomes less firm, and the surrounding fluid increases in turbidity. The mucin clot test is reported in terms of good (solid clot), fair (soft clot), poor (friable clot), and very poor (no clot). The mucin clot test is not routinely performed, because all forms of arthritis decrease viscosity and little diagnostic information is obtained. Formation of a mucin clot following the addition of acetic acid can be used to identify a questionable fluid as synovial fluid.

Cell Counts

The total leukocyte count is the most frequently performed cell count on synovial fluid. However, red blood cell counts may be requested unless evidence of a traumatic tap exists. To prevent cellular disintegration, counts should be performed as soon as possible or the specimen should be refrigerated. Very viscous fluid may need to be pretreated by adding a pinch of hyaluronidase to 0.5 mL of fluid or one drop of 0.05 percent hyaluronidase in phosphate buffer per milliliter of fluid and incubating at 37°C for 5 minutes.[5]

Manual counts on thoroughly mixed specimens are done using the Neubauer counting chamber in the same manner as cerebrospinal fluid counts. Clear fluids can usually be counted undiluted, but dilutions are necessary when fluids are turbid or bloody. Dilutions can be made using the procedure presented in Chapter 10; however, traditional WBC diluting fluid cannot be used because it contains acetic acid, which will cause the formation of mucin clots. Normal saline can be used as a diluent. If it is necessary to lyse the RBCs, hypotonic saline (0.3 percent) or saline that contains saponin is a suitable diluent. Methylene blue added to the normal saline will stain the WBC nuclei, permitting separation of the RBCs and WBCs during counts performed on mixed specimens. Automated cell counters can be used for synovial fluid counts; however, highly viscous fluid may block the apertures, and the presence of debris and tissue cells may falsely elevate counts. As described previously, incubation of the fluid with hyaluronidase will decrease the specimen viscosity. Analysis of scattergrams can aid in the detection of tissue cells and debris. Properly controlled automated counts provide higher precision than manual counts.[8]

WBC counts less than 200 cells/μL are considered normal and may reach 100,000 cells/μL or higher in severe infections.[6] There is, however, considerable overlap of elevated leukocyte counts between septic and inflammatory forms of arthritis.

Differential Count

Differential counts should be performed on cytocentrifuged preparations or on thinly smeared slides. Fluid should be incubated with hyaluronidase prior to slide preparation. Mononuclear cells, including monocytes, macrophages, and synovial tissue cells, are the primary cells seen in normal synovial fluid. Neutrophils should account for less than 20 percent of the differential count and lymphocytes less than 15 percent. Increased neutrophils indicate a septic condition, whereas an elevated cell count with a predominance of lymphocytes suggests a nonseptic inflammation. In both normal and abnormal specimens, cells may appear more vacuolated than they do on a blood smear.[5] Besides increased numbers of these usually normal cells, other cell abnormalities include the presence of eosinophils, LE cells, **Reiter cells** (vacuolated macrophages with ingested neutrophils), and RA cells or **ragocytes** (neutrophils with small, dark, cytoplasmic granules that consist of precipitated rheumatoid factor).[1] Lipid droplets may be present following crush injuries, and hemosiderin granules are seen in cases of **pigmented villonodular synovitis**. The most frequently encountered cells and inclusions seen in synovial fluid are summarized in Table 12–4.

Crystal Identification

Microscopic examination of synovial fluid for the presence of crystals is an important diagnostic test in the evaluation of arthritis. Crystal formation in a joint frequently results in an acute, painful inflammation. Causes of crystal formation include metabolic disorders and decreased renal excretion that produce elevated blood levels of crystallizing chemicals, degeneration of cartilage and bone, and injection of medications, such as corticosteroids into a joint.

TABLE 12–4 **Cells and Inclusions Seen in Synovial Fluid**

Cell/Inclusion	Description	Significance
Neutrophil	Polymorphonuclear leukocyte	Bacterial sepsis Crystal-induced inflammation
Lymphocyte	Mononuclear leukocyte	Nonseptic inflammation
Macrophage (monocyte)	Large mononuclear leukocyte, may be vacuolated	Normal Viral infections
Synovial lining cell	Similar to macrophage, but may be multinucleated, resembling a mesothelial cell	Normal
LE cell	Neutrophil containing characteristic ingested: "round body"	Lupus erythematosus
Reiter cell	Vacuolated macrophage with ingested neutrophils	Reiter's syndrome Nonspecific inflamation
RA cell (ragocyte)	Neutrophil with dark cytoplasmic granules containing immune complexes	Rheumatoid arthritis Immunologic inflammation
Cartilage cells	Large, multinucleated cells	Osteoarthritis
Rice bodies	Macroscopically resemble polished rice Microscopically show collagen and fibrin	Tuberculosis, septic and rheumatoid arthritis
Fat droplets	Refractile intracellular and extracellular globules Stain with Sudan dyes	Traumatic injury
Hemosiderin	Inclusions within clusters of synovial cells	Pigmented villonodular synovitis

The primary crystals seen in synovial fluid are monosodium urate (uric acid) (**MSU**) found in cases of gout and calcium pyrophosphate (**CPPD**) seen with pseudogout. Increased serum uric acid resulting from impaired metabolism of nucleic acid associated with myeloproliferative disorders and decreased renal excretion of uric acid are the most frequent causes of gout. Pseudogout is most often associated with degenerative arthritis, resulting in cartilage calcification and endocrine disorders producing elevated serum calcium levels.

Additional crystals that may be present include hydroxyapatite (basic calcium phosphate) associated with calcified cartilage degeneration, cholesterol crystals, corticosteroids following injections, and calcium oxalate crystals in renal dialysis patients. The patient history must always be considered. Microscopic characteristics of the commonly encountered crystals are presented in Table 12–5. Artifacts present may include talc and starch from gloves, precipitated anticoagulants, dust, and scratches on slides and coverslips. Slides and coverslips should be examined and cleaned prior to use.

Ideally crystal examination should be performed soon after fluid collection to ensure that crystals are not affected by changes in temperature and pH. Both MSU and CPPD crystals are reported as being located extracellularly and intracellularly (within neutrophils); therefore, fluid must be examined prior to WBC disintegration.

Fluid is examined unstained under polarized and compensated polarized light for detection and identification of MSU and CPPD crystals. Crystals may be observed in Wright's stained preparations (Figure 12–2); however, this should not replace the wet preparation examination. Slides are first scanned under low power with direct polarized light, then focused using high power, and finally examined under compensated polarized light. MSU crystals are seen routinely as needle-shaped crystals, appearing extracellularly and within the cytoplasm of neutrophils (Figures 12–3 through 12–5). CPPD crystals usually appear rhombic-shaped (Figures 12–6 and 12–7) and are found as intracellular inclusions.

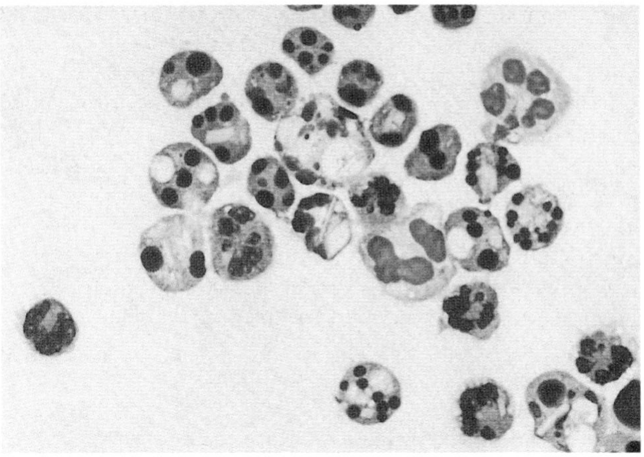

FIGURE 12–2 Wright's stained neutrophils containing CPPD crystals (×1000).

Once the presence of the crystals has been determined using direct polarization, positive identification is made using compensated polarized light. A control slide for the

TABLE 12–5 **Characteristics of Synovial Fluid Crystals**

Crystal	Shape		Compensated Polarized Light	Location
Monosodium urate	Needles	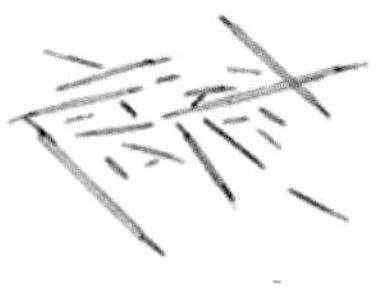	Negative birefringence	Intracellular and extracellular
Calcium pyrophosphate	Rod Needles Rhombics	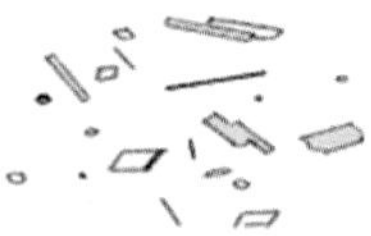	Positive birefringence	Intracellular and extracellular
Cholesterol	Notched rhombic plates	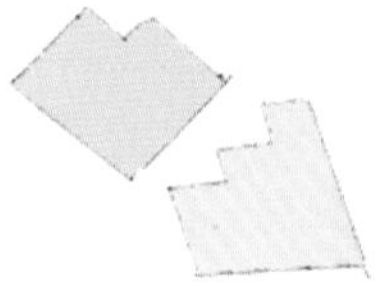	Negative birefringence	Extracellular
Corticosteroid	Flat, variable-shaped plates	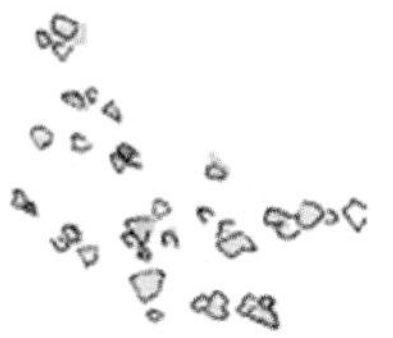	Positive and negative birefringence	Primarily intracellular

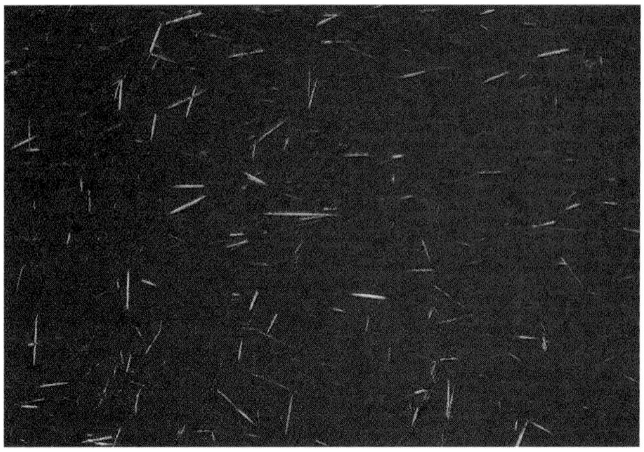

FIGURE 12–3 Extracellular MSU crystals under compensated polarized light: Notice the change in color with crystal alignment (×100).

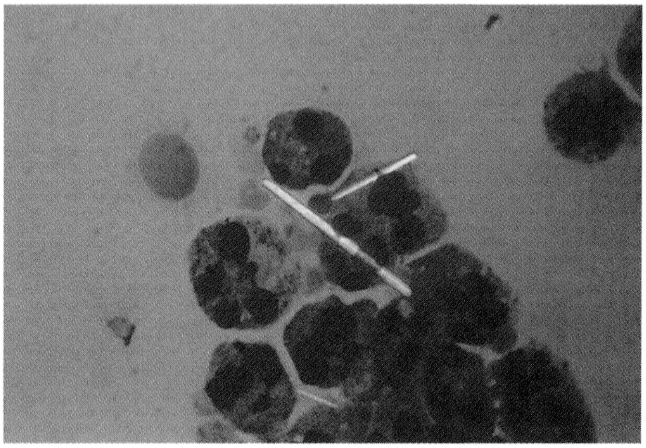

FIGURE 12–4 Highly birefringent MSU crystals under polarized light (×500).

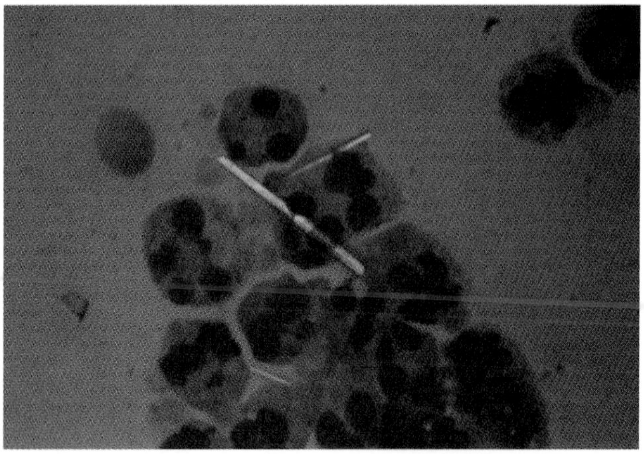

FIGURE 12–5 MSU crystals under compensated polarized light, the yellow crystal is aligned with the slow vibration (×500).

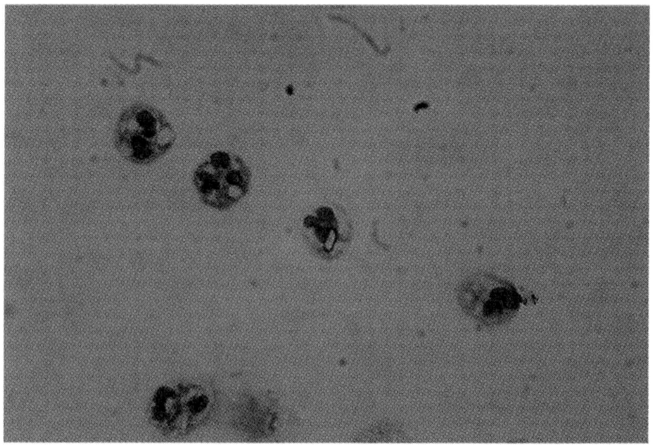

FIGURE 12–6 Weakly birefringent CPPD crystals under polarized light (×1000).

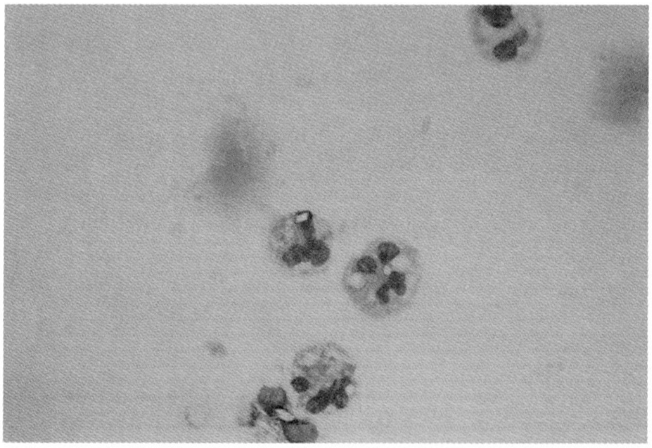

FIGURE 12–7 CPPD crystals under compensated polarized light, the blue crystal is aligned with the slow vibration (×1000).

polarization properties of MSU can be prepared using betamethasone acetate corticosteroid.

Both MSU and CPPD crystals have the ability to polarize light as discussed in Chapter 6; however, MSU is more hightly birefringent and will appear brighter against the dark background.

When compensated polarized light is used, a red compensator crystal is placed in the microscope between the crystal and the analyzer (Figure 12–8). The compensator separates the light ray into slow-moving and fast-moving vibrations and produces a red background.

Owing to differences in the linear structure of the molecules in MSU and CPPD crystals, the color produced by each crystal when it is aligned with the slow vibration can be used to identify the crystal. The molecules in MSU crystals run parallel to the long axis of the crystal and, when aligned with the slow vibration, the velocity of the slow light passing through the crystal is not impeded as

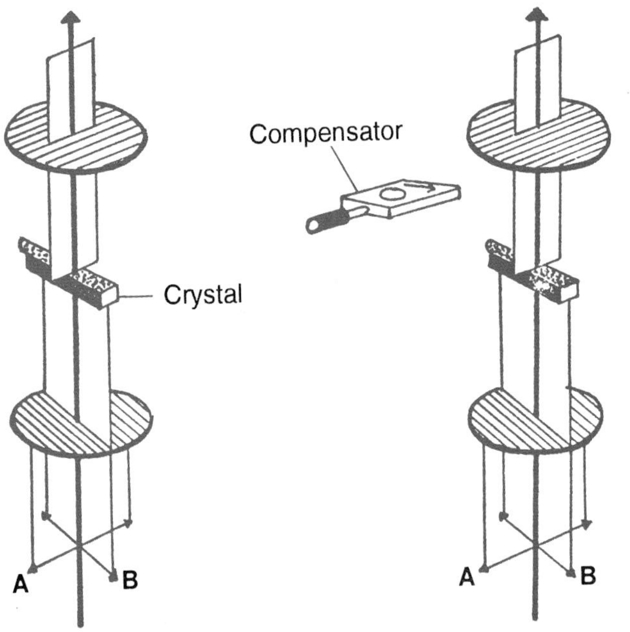

FIGURE 12–8 *(Left)* Direct polarized light. *(Right)* Compensated polarized light. (Adapted from Phelps, Steele, and McCarty: Compensated polarized light microscopy: Identification of crystals in synovial fluid from gout and pseudogout. JAMA 203(7):167, 1969.)

much as the fast light, which runs against the grain and produces a yellow color. This is considered negative birefringence (subtraction of velocity from the fast ray). In contrast, the molecules in CPPD crystals run perpendicular to the long axis of the crystal and when aligned with the slow axis of the compensator, the velocity of the fast light passing through the crystal is much quicker, producing a blue color and positive birefringence.[2] Care must be taken to ensure crystals being analyzed are aligned in accordance with the compensator axis. Notice how the colors of the MSU crystals in Figure 12–9 vary with the alignment.

Crystal shapes and patterns of birefringence that vary from the standard MSU and CPPD patterns may indicate the presence of one of the less commonly encountered crystals and further investigation is required.

Chemistry Tests

Because synovial fluid is chemically an ultrafiltrate of plasma, chemistry test values are approximately the same as serum values. Therefore, few chemistry tests are considered clinically important. The most frequently requested test is the glucose determination, because markedly decreased values are indicative of inflammatory (group II) or septic (group III) disorders. Because normal synovial fluid glucose values are based on the blood glucose level, simultaneous blood and synovial fluid samples should be obtained, preferably after the patient has fasted for 8 hours to allow equilibration between the two fluids. Under these conditions, normal synovial fluid glucose should not be more than 10 mg/dL lower than the blood value. To prevent falsely decreased values caused by glycolysis, specimens should be analyzed within 1 hour or preserved with sodium fluoride.

Measurement of synovial fluid lactate levels has been shown to provide rapid differentiation between inflammatory and septic arthritis and does not require equilibration and comparison with blood lactate levels. Synovial fluid lactate levels greater than 250 mg/dL are found consistently with septic arthritis, but may also be seen in rheumatoid arthritis.[3,10]

Other chemistry tests that may be requested are the total protein and uric acid determinations. Because the large protein molecules are not filtered through the synovial membranes, normal synovial fluid contains less than 3 g/dL of protein (approximately one-third of the serum value). Increased levels are found in inflammatory and hemorrhagic disorders; however, measurement of synovial fluid protein does not contribute greatly to the classification of these disorders. When requested, the analysis is performed using the same methods used for serum protein determinations. The elevation of serum uric acid in cases of gout is well known; therefore, demonstration of an elevated synovial fluid uric acid level may be used to confirm the diagnosis when the presence of crystals cannot be demonstrated in the fluid.

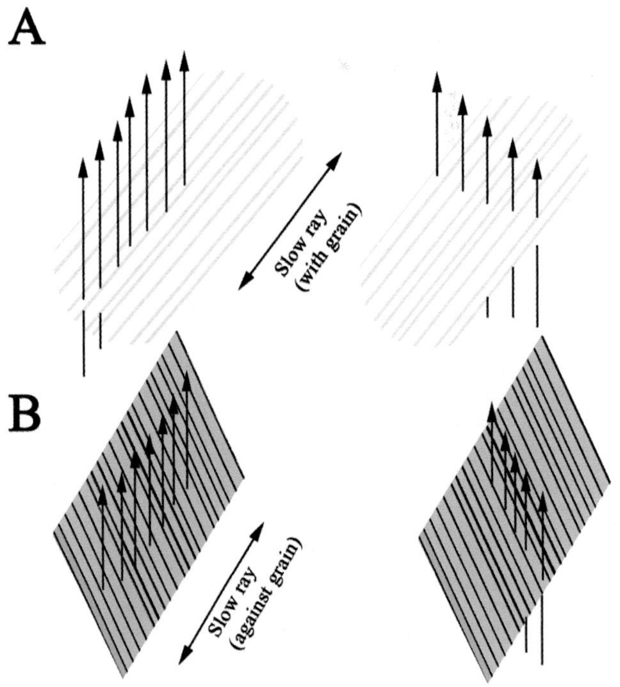

FIGURE 12–9 Diagram of negative and positive birefringence in MSU and CPPD crystals. *(A)* MSU crystal with grain running parallel to the long axis. The slow ray passes with the grain producing negative (yellow) birefringence. *(B)* CPPD crystal with grain running perpendicular to the long axis. The slow ray passes against the grain and is retarded producing positive (blue) birefringence.

Microbiologic Tests

An infection may occur as a secondary complication of inflammation; therefore, Gram stains and cultures are two of the most important tests performed on synovial fluid. Gram stains should be performed on all specimens. Bacterial infections are most frequently seen; however, fungal, tubercular, and viral infections also can occur. When they are suspected, special culturing procedures should be used. Routine bacterial cultures should always include an enrichment medium, such as chocolate agar, because in addition to *Staphylococcus* and *Streptococcus*, the most common organisms that infect synovial fluid are the fastidious *Hemophilus* species and *Neisseria gonorrhoeae*.

Serologic Tests

Because of the association of the immune system to the inflammation process, serologic testing plays an important role in the diagnosis of joint disorders. However, the majority of the tests are performed on serum, with actual analysis of the synovial fluid serving as a confirmatory measure in cases that are difficult to diagnose. The autoimmune diseases rheumatoid arthritis and lupus erythematosus cause very serious inflammation of the joints and are diagnosed in the serology laboratory by demonstrating the presence of their particular autoantibodies in the patient's serum. These same antibodies can also be demonstrated in the synovial fluid, if necessary. Arthritis is a frequent complication of Lyme disease. Therefore, demonstration of antibodies to the causative agent *Borrelia burgdorferi* in the patient's serum can confirm the cause of the arthritis.

REFERENCES

1. Broderick, PA, et al: Exfoliative cytology: Interpretation of synovial fluid in disease. J Bone Joint Surg Am 58(3):396–399, 1976.
2. Cornbleet, PJ: Synovial fluid crystal analysis. Lab Med 28(12):774–779, 1997.
3. Gratacos, J, et al: d-lactic acid in synovial fluid: A rapid diagnostic test for bacterial synovitis. J Rheumatol 22(8):1504–1508, 1995.
4. Hasselbacher, P: Variation in synovial fluid analysis by hospital laboratories. Arthritis Rheum 30(6):637–642, 1987.
5. Kjeldsberg, CR, and Knight, JA: Body Fluids: Laboratory Examination of Amniotic, Cerebrospinal, Seminal, Serous and Synovial Fluids: A Textbook Atlas. ASCP, Chicago, 1993.
6. Naib, ZM: Cytology of synovial fluids. Acta Cytol 17(4):299–309, 1973.
7. Rippey, J: Synovial fluid analysis. Lab Med 10(3):140–145, 1979.
8. Salinas, M, et al: Comparison of manual and automated cell counts in EDTA preserved synovial fluids. Am Rheum Dis 56(10):622–626, 1997.
9. Shmerling, RH: Synovial fluid analysis. A critical reappraisal. Rheum Dis Clin North Am 20(2):503–512, 1994.
10. Smith, GP, and Kjeldsberg, CR: Cerebrospinal, synovial, and serous body fluids. In Henry, JB (ed): Clinical Diagnosis and Management by Laboratory Methods. WB Saunders, Philadelphia, 1996.

STUDY QUESTIONS

1. State three functions of synovial fluid.
2. List the four classifications of joint disease and a pathologic cause of each.
3. List the five most frequently performed laboratory tests on synovial fluid.
4. What procedure is performed to collect synovial fluid?
5. Why is synovial fluid collected in liquid rather than powdered anticoagulant?
6. What is the clinical significance of the following synovial fluid colors: dark yellow, milky, blood streaked, green?
7. Why is hyaluronic acid an important constituent of synovial fluid? How is its presence determined?
8. How is synovial fluid diluted when performing a WBC count? Why?
9. What is the significance of the following in a synovial fluid differential: increased neutrophils, increased lymphocytes, ragocytes?
10. Name the two primary crystals seen in synovial fluid, and state the pathologic significance of each.
11. Under what conditions might calcium oxalate crystals be seen in synovial fluid? Corticosteroid crystals?
12. What is the recommended slide preparation for the detection and identification of synovial fluid crystals?
13. Under polarized light, do MSU or CPPD crystals appear brighter? Which appears blue when aligned with the slow axis of the red compensator?
14. Are fast light rays more impeded when passing through MSU or CPPD crystals? Why?
15. If an MSU crystal is aligned perpendicular to the slow axis, what color will it be?
16. Why are synovial fluid glucose levels compared with serum glucose levels and synovial fluid protein levels not compared?
17. What is the significance of an elevated synovial fluid lactate level?
18. Why is chocolate agar routinely included in synovial fluid cultures?
19. Name two causes of arthritis in which autoantibodies may be found in the patient's serum.
20. What is the significance of a patient's serum containing antibodies to *Borrelia burgdorferi*?

CASE STUDIES AND CLINICAL SITUATIONS

1. A 50-year-old man presents in the emergency room with severe pain and swelling in the right knee.

Arthrocentesis is performed and 20 mL of milky synovial fluid is collected. The physician orders a STAT Gram stain and crystal examination of the fluid and a serum uric acid. He requests that the fluid be saved for possible additional tests.

a. Describe the tubes into which the fluid would be routinely placed.
b. If the patient's serum uric acid level is elevated, what type of crystals and disorder are probable?
c. Describe the appearance of these crystals under direct and compensated polarized light.
d. Why was the Gram stain ordered?

2. A medical technology student dilutes a synovial fluid prior to performing a WBC count. The fluid forms a clot.

a. Why did the clot form?
b. How can the student perform a correct dilution of the fluid?
c. What two concerns might the student have when performing the count using an automated cell counter? How can they be prevented?

3. Fluid obtained from the knee of an obese 65-year-old woman being evaluated for a possible knee replacement has the following results:

APPEARANCE: Pale yellow and hazy
WBC COUNT: 500 cells/μL
GRAM STAIN: Negative
GLUCOSE: 110 mg/dL (SERUM GLUCOSE: 115 mg/dL)

a. What classification of joint disorder do these results suggest?
b. Under electron microscopy, what crystals might be detected?
c. How does the glucose result aid in the disorder classification?
d. Are the test results consistent with a probable candidate for a knee replacement? Why or why not?

CHAPTER 13

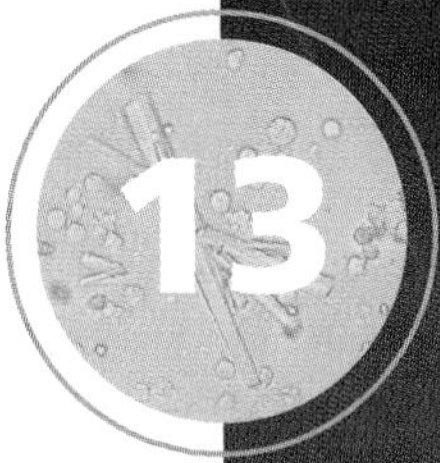

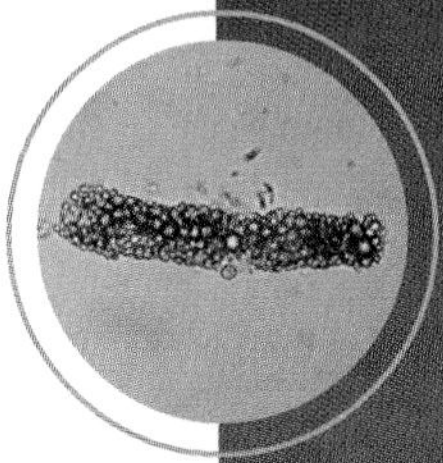

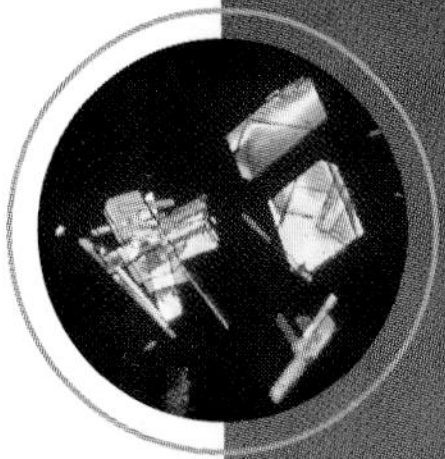

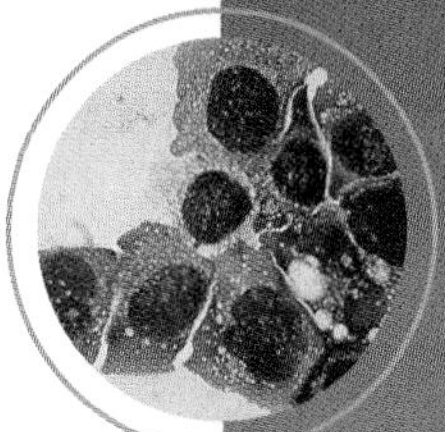

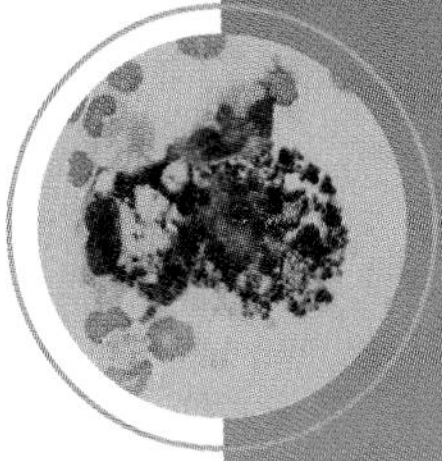

Serous Fluid

LEARNING OBJECTIVES

Upon completion of this chapter, the reader will be able to:

1. Describe the normal formation of serous fluid.
2. Describe four primary causes of serous effusions.
3. Differentiate between a transudate and an exudate, including etiology, appearance, and laboratory tests.
4. Differentiate between a hemothorax and a hemorrhagic exudate.
5. Differentiate between a chylous and a pseudochylous exudate.
6. State the significance of increased neutrophils, lymphocytes, eosinophils, and plasma cells in pleural fluid.
7. Describe the morphologic characteristics of mesothelial cells and malignant cells.
8. List three common chemistry tests performed on pleural fluid, and state their significance.
9. State the common etiologies of pericardial effusions.
10. Discuss the diagnostic significance of peritoneal lavage.
11. Calculate a serum-ascites gradient, and state its significance.
12. Differentiate between ascitic effusions of hepatic and peritoneal origin.
13. State the clinical significance of the carcinoembryonic antigen and CA 125 tests.
14. List four chemical tests performed on ascitic fluid, and state their significance.

KEY TERMS

ascites
effusion
exudate
paracentesis
pericardiocentesis
pericarditis
parietal membrane
peritonitis
serous fluid
thoracentesis
transudate
visceral membrane

The closed cavities of the body—namely, the pleural, pericardial, and peritoneal cavities—are each lined by two membranes referred to as the serous membranes. One membrane lines the cavity wall (***parietal membrane***), and the other covers the organs within the cavity (***visceral membrane***). The fluid between the membranes, which provides lubrication as the surfaces move against each other, is called ***serous fluid***. Normally, only a small amount of serous fluid is present, because production and reabsorption take place at a constant rate.

Formation

Serous fluids are formed as ultrafiltrates of plasma, with no additional material contributed by the membrane cells. Production and reabsorption are subject to hydrostatic and colloidal (oncotic) pressures from the capillaries serving the cavities and the capillary permeability. Under normal conditions, colloidal pressure from serum proteins is the same in the capillaries on both sides of the membrane. Therefore, the greater hydrostatic pressure in the systemic capillaries on the parietal side favors fluid production through the parietal membrane and reabsorption into the lymphatic system through the visceral membrane. In Figure 13–1, the normal formation and absorption of pleural fluid are demonstrated.

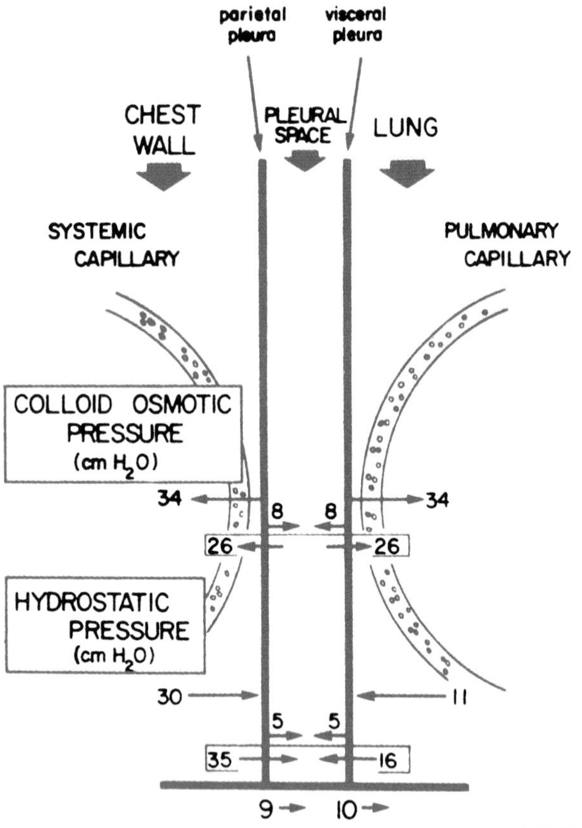

FIGURE 13–1 The normal formation and absorption of pleural fluid. (From Fraser, RG, and Pare, JAP: Diagnosis of Diseases of the Chest, vol. 1. WB Saunders, Philadelphia, 1977, p. 2069, with permission.)

Disruption of the mechanisms of serous fluid formation and reabsorption causes an increase in fluid between the membranes. This is termed an ***effusion***. Primary causes of effusions include increased hydrostatic pressure (congestive heart failure), decreased oncotic pressure (hypoproteinemia), increased capillary permeability (inflammation and infection), and lymphatic obstruction (tumors).

Specimen Collection and Handling

Fluids for laboratory examination are collected by needle aspiration from the respective cavities. These aspiration procedures are referred to as ***thoracentesis*** (pleural), ***pericardiocentesis*** (pericardial), and **paracentesis** (peritoneal). Abundant fluid (greater than 100 mL) is usually collected; therefore, suitable specimens are available for each section of the laboratory.

An ethylenediaminetetraacetic acid (EDTA) tube is used for cell counts and the differential. The remaining fluid can be heparinized (green-top evacuated tubes) for chemical, serologic, microbial, and cytologic analysis. Specimens for pH must be maintained anaerobically in ice. For better recovery of microorganisms and abnormal cells, at least 100 mL of the fluid is concentrated by centrifugation and used for these analyses.

Chemical tests performed on serous fluids are frequently compared with plasma chemical concentrations because the fluids are essentially plasma ultrafiltrates. Therefore, blood specimens should be obtained at the time of collection.

Transudates and Exudates

A general classification of the cause of an effusion can be accomplished by separating the fluid into the category of ***transudate*** or ***exudate***. Effusions that form because of a systemic disorder that disrupts the balance in the regulation of fluid filtration and reabsorption—such as the changes in hydrostatic pressure created by congestive heart failure or the hypoproteinemia associated with the nephrotic syndrome—are called transudates. Exudates are produced by conditions that directly involve the membranes of the particular cavity, including infections and malignancies. Classification of a serous fluid as a transudate or exudate can provide a valuable initial diagnostic step and aid in the course of further laboratory testing, because testing of transudate fluids is usually not necessary.[4] Traditionally, a variety of laboratory tests have been used to differentiate between transudates and exudates, including appearance, total protein, lactic dehydrogenase, cell counts, and spontaneous clotting. However, the most reliable differentiation is obtained by determining the fluid-to-blood ratios for protein and lactic dehydrogenase.[3] Differential values for these parameters are shown in Table 13–1. Additional tests are available for specific fluids and will be discussed in the following sections.

TABLE 13–1 **Laboratory Differentiation of Transudates and Exudates**[9]

	Transudate	Exudate
Appearance	Clear	Cloudy
Fluid:serum protein ratio	<0.5	>0.5
Fluid:serum LD ratio	<0.6	>0.6
White blood cell count	<1000/µL	>1000/µL
Spontaneous clotting	No	Possible
Pleural fluid cholesterol	<60 mg/dL	>60 mg/dL
Pleural fluid:serum cholesterol ratio	<0.3	>0.3
Pleural fluid:bilirubin ratio	<0.6	>0.6
Serum-ascites albumin gradient	>1.1	<1.1

General Laboratory Procedures

Serous fluid examination—including classification as a transudate or exudate, appearance, cell count and differential, and chemistry, microbiology, and cytology procedures—is performed in the same manner on all serous fluids. However, the significance of the test results and the need for specialized tests vary among fluids. Therefore, the interpretation of routine and special procedures will be discussed individually for each of the three serous fluids.

Tests that are usually performed on all serous fluids include evaluation of the appearance and differentiation between a transudate and an exudate. Effusions of exudative origin are then examined for the presence of microbiologic and cytologic abnormalities. Additional tests are ordered based on specific clinical symptoms.

Red blood cell (RBC) and white blood cell (WBC) counts are not frequently performed on serous fluids because they provide little diagnostic information.[5] In general, WBC counts greater than 1000/µL and RBC counts greater than 100,000/µL are indicative of an exudate. Serous fluid cell counts can be performed manually by using a Neubauer counting chamber and the methods discussed in Chapter 10 or by electronic cell counters. The Model 500 Yellow IRIS workstation contains a cell-counting component for serous and other body fluids (see Appendix A). Inclusion of tissue cells and debris in the count must be considered when electronic counters are used, and care must be taken to prevent the blocking of tubing with debris.

Differential cell counts are routinely performed on serous fluids, preferably on Wright's stained, cytocentrifuged specimens or on slides prepared from the sediment of centrifuged specimens. Smears must be examined not only for WBCs, but also for normal and malignant tissue cells. Any suspicious cells seen on the differential are referred to the cytology laboratory or the pathologist.

Pleural Fluid

Pleural fluid is obtained from the pleural cavity, located between the parietal pleural membrane lining the chest wall and the visceral pleural membrane covering the lungs. Pleural effusions may be of either transudative or exudative origin. In addition to the tests routinely performed to differentiate between transudates and exudates, two additional procedures are helpful when analyzing pleural fluid. These are the pleural fluid cholesterol and fluid–to–serum cholesterol ratio and the pleural fluid–to–serum total bilirubin ratio. A pleural fluid cholesterol greater than 60 mg/dL or a pleural fluid–to–serum cholesterol ratio greater than 0.3 provides reliable information that the fluid is an exudate.[11] A fluid–to–serum total bilirubin ratio of 0.6 or more also indicates the presence of an exudate.

APPEARANCE

Considerable diagnostic information concerning the etiology of a pleural effusion can be learned from the appearance of the specimen (Table 13–2). Normal and transudate pleural fluids are clear and pale yellow. Turbidity is usually related to the presence of WBCs and indicates bacterial infection, tuberculosis, or an immunologic disorder, such as rheumatoid arthritis. The presence of blood in the pleural fluid can signify a **hemothorax** (traumatic injury), membrane damage such as occurs in malignancy, or a traumatic aspiration. As seen with other fluids, blood from a traumatic tap appears streaked and uneven.

To differentiate between a hemothorax and hemorrhagic exudate, a hematocrit can be run on the fluid. If the blood is from a hemothorax, the fluid hematocrit will be similar to the whole blood hematocrit, because the effusion is actually occurring from the inpouring of blood from the injury. A chronic membrane disease effusion will contain both blood and increased pleural fluid, resulting in a much lower hematocrit.

The appearance of a milky pleural fluid may be due to the presence of **chylous material** from thoracic duct leakage or to **pseudochylous material** produced in chronic inflammatory conditions. Chylous material contains a high concentration of triglycerides, whereas pseudochylous material has a higher concentration of cholesterol. Therefore, Sudan III staining will be strongly positive with chylous material. In contrast, pseudochylous effusions will contain cholesterol crystals.[10] Differentiation between chylous and pseudochylous effusions is summarized in Table 13–3.

TABLE 13–2 **Correlation of Pleural Fluid Appearance and Disease**

Appearance	Disease
Clear, pale yellow	Normal
Turbid, white	Microbial infection (tuberculosis)
Bloody	Hemothorax
	Hemorrhagic effusion
Milky	Chylous material from thoracic duct leakage
	Pseudochylous material from chronic inflammation

TABLE 13–3 **Differentiation Between Chylous and Pseudochylous Pleural Effusions**[9]

	Chylous Effusion	Pseudochylous Effusion
Cause	Thoracic duct leakage	Chronic inflammation
Appearance	Milky/white	Milky/green tinge
Leukocytes	Predominantly lymphocytes	Mixed cells
Cholesterol crystals	Absent	Present
Triglycerides	>110 mg/dL	<50 mg/dL
Sudan III staining	Strongly positive	Negative/weakly positive

HEMATOLOGY TESTS

As mentioned previously, the differential cell count is the most diagnostically significant hematology test performed on serous fluids. Primary cells associated with pleural fluid include neutrophils, lymphocytes, eosinophils, mesothelial cells, plasma cells, and malignant cells (Table 13–4). These same cells are also found in pericardial and peritoneal fluids.

Similar to other body fluids, an increase in pleural fluid neutrophils is indicative of a bacterial infection, such as pneumonia. Neutrophils are also increased in effusions resulting from pancreatitis and pulmonary infarction.

Lymphocytes are normally noticeably present in both transudates and exudates in a variety of forms, including small, large, and reactive. More prominent nucleoli and cleaved nucleii may be present. Elevated lymphocyte counts are seen in effusions resulting from tuberculosis, viral infections, malignancy, and autoimmune disorders such as lupus erythematosus. LE cells also may be seen (Figure 13–2).

TABLE 13–4 **Significance of Cells Seen in Pleural Fluid**

Cell	Significance
Neutrophils	Pneumonia Pancreatitis Pulmonary infarction
Lymphocytes	Tuberculosis Viral infection Autoimmune disorders Malignancy
Mesothelial cells	Normal and reactive forms have no clinical significance Decreased mesothelial cells are associated with tuberculosis
Plasma cells	Tuberculosis
Malignant cells	Primary adenocarcinoma and small-cell carcinoma Metastatic carcinoma

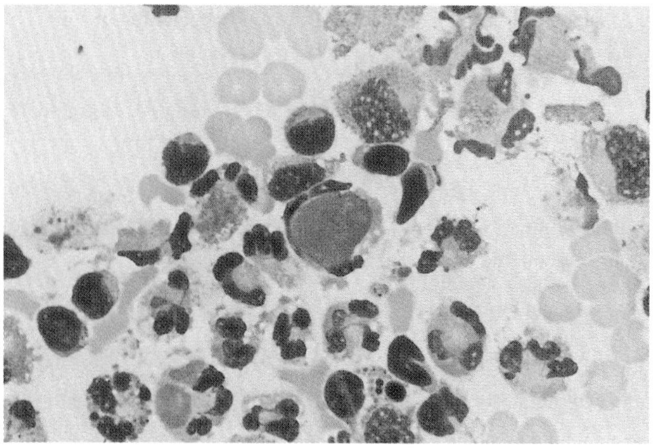

FIGURE 13–2 LE cell in pleural fluid. Notice the ingested "round body" (×1000).

Increased eosinophil levels (greater than 10 percent) may be associated with trauma resulting in the presence of air or blood in the pleural cavity. They are also seen in allergic reactions and parasitic infections.

The membranes lining the serous cavities contain a single layer of mesothelial cells; therefore, it is not unusual to find these cells in the serous fluids. Mesothelial cells are pleomorphic; they resemble lymphocytes, plasma cells, and malignant cells, frequently making identification difficult. They often appear as single, small or large round cells with abundant blue cytoplasm and round nucleii with uniform dark purple cytoplasm and may be referred to as "normal" mesothelial cells (Figures 13–3 and 13–4). In contrast, "reactive" mesothelial cells may appear in clusters, have varying amounts of cytoplasm, eccentric nucleii, and prominent nucleoli, and be multinucleated, therefore, more closely resembling malignant cells (Figures 13–5 and 13–6). An increase in mesothelial cells is not a diagnostically significant finding; however, they may be increased in pneumonia and malignancy. Of more significance is the noticeable lack of mesothelial cells associated with tuberculosis, which results from exudate covering the pleural

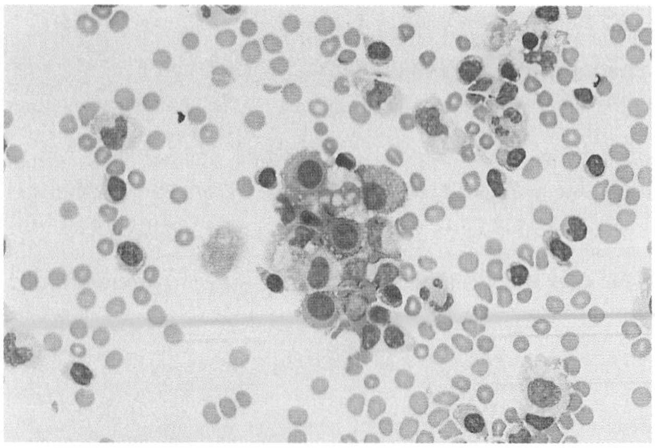

FIGURE 13–3 Normal pleural fluid mesothelial cells, lymphocytes, and monocytes (×250).

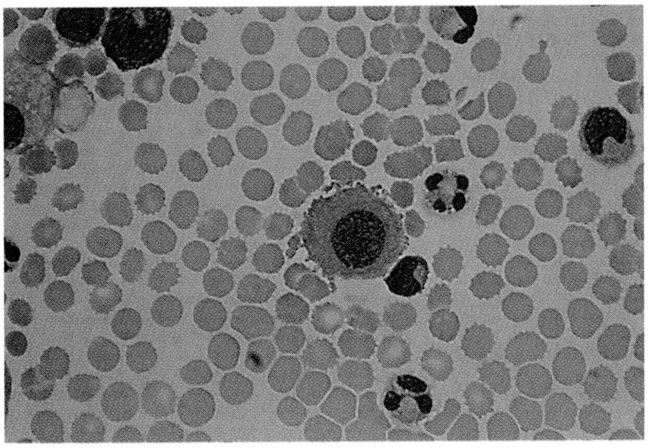

FIGURE 13–4 Normal mesothelial cell (×500).

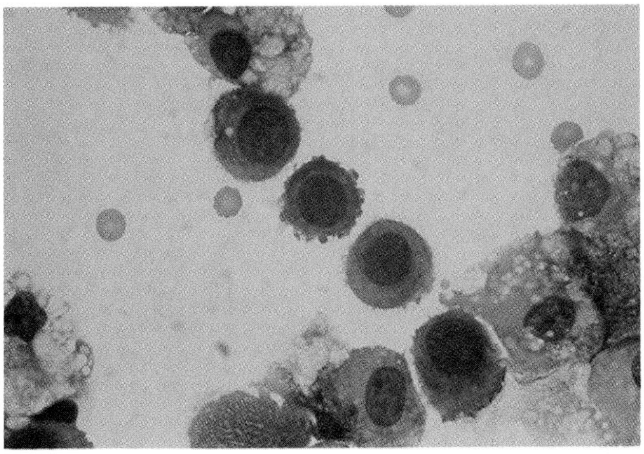

FIGURE 13–5 Reactive mesothelial cells showing eccentric nuclei and vacuolated cytoplasm (×500).

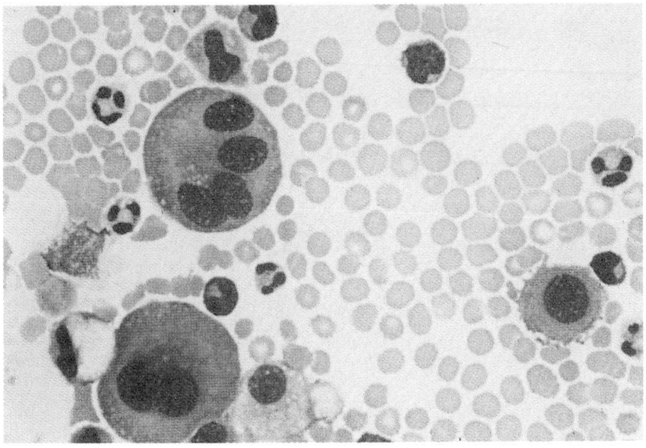

FIGURE 13–6 One normal and two reactive mesothelial cells with a multinucleated form (×500).

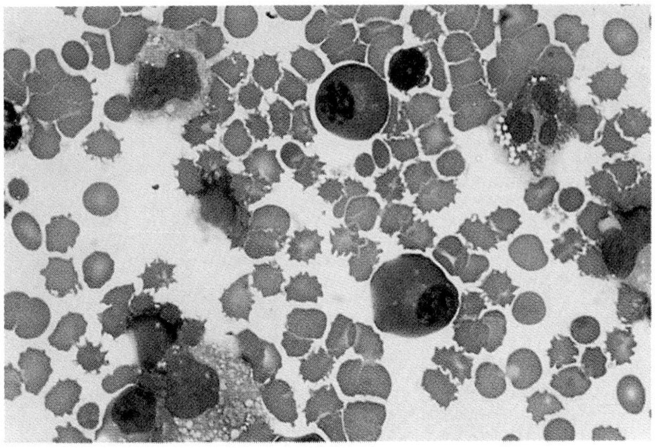

FIGURE 13–7 Pleural fluid plasma cells seen in a case of tuberculosis (×1000).

membranes. Also associated with tuberculosis is an increase in the presence of pleural fluid plasma cells (Figure 13–7).

A primary concern in the examination of all serous effusions is detecting the presence of malignant cells. Differentiation among mesothelial cells and other tissue cells and malignant cells is often difficult. Distinguishing characteristics of malignant cells may include nuclear and cytoplasmic irregularities, hyperchromatic nucleoli, cellular clumps with cytoplasmic molding (community borders), and abnormal nuclear-to-cytoplasmic ratios (Figures 13–8 through 13–10). Malignant effusions most frequently contain large, irregular adenocarcinoma cells, small or oatcell carcinoma cells resembling large lymphocytes, and clumps of metastatic breast carcinoma cells (Figures 13–11 through 13–13). Special staining techniques and flow cytometry may be used for positive identification of tumor cells.

CHEMISTRY TESTS

In addition to the chemical tests performed to differentiate between a pleural transudate and exudate, the most common chemical tests performed on pleural fluid are glucose, pH, and amylase. Triglyceride levels also may be measured to confirm the presence of a chylous effusion (Table 13–5).

Decreased glucose levels are seen with rheumatoid inflammation and purulent infections. As an ultrafiltrate of plasma, pleural fluid glucose levels parallel plasma levels with values less than 60 mg/dL considered decreased. Fluid values should be compared with plasma values. Pleural fluid lactate levels are elevated in bacterial infections and can be considered in addition to the glucose level.

Pleural fluid pH lower than 7.3 may indicate the need for chest-tube drainage, in addition to administration of antibiotics in cases of pneumonia. The finding of a pH as low as 6.0 indicates an esophageal rupture that is allowing the influx of gastric fluid.[2]

As with serum, elevated amylase levels are associated with pancreatitis, and amylase is often elevated first in the

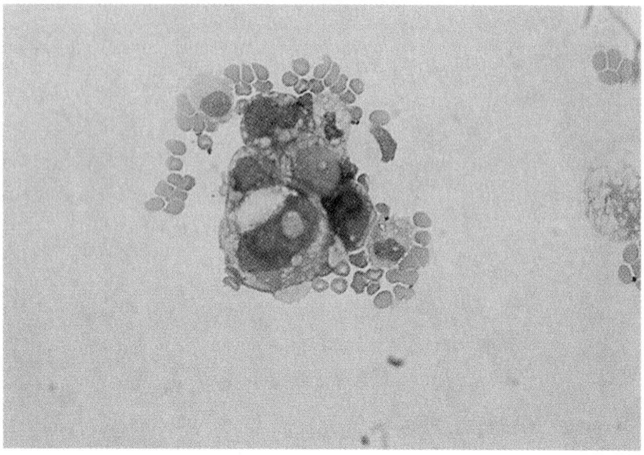

FIGURE 13–8 Pleural fluid adenocarcinoma showing cytoplasmic molding (×250).

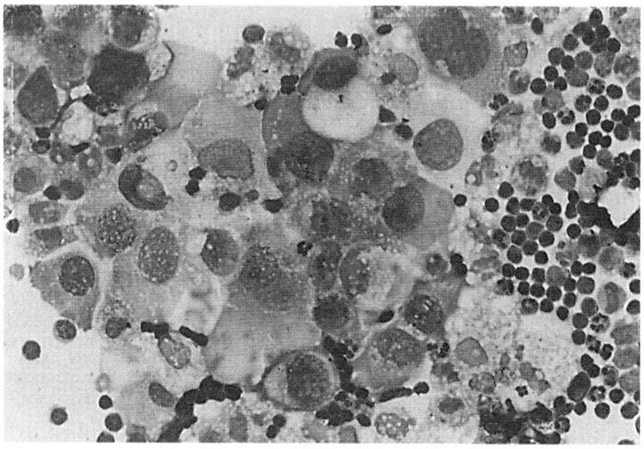

FIGURE 13–9 Pleural fluid adenocarcinoma showing fine nuclear chromatin, nuclear and cytoplasmic molding, and vacuolated cytoplasm (×1000).

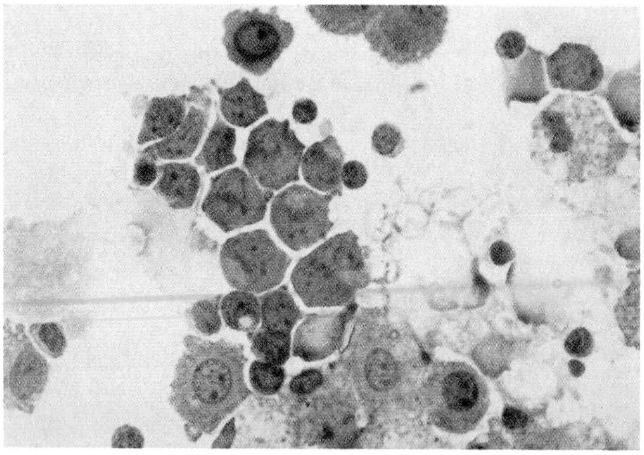

FIGURE 13–10 Enhancement of nuclear irregularities using a toluidine blue stain (×250).

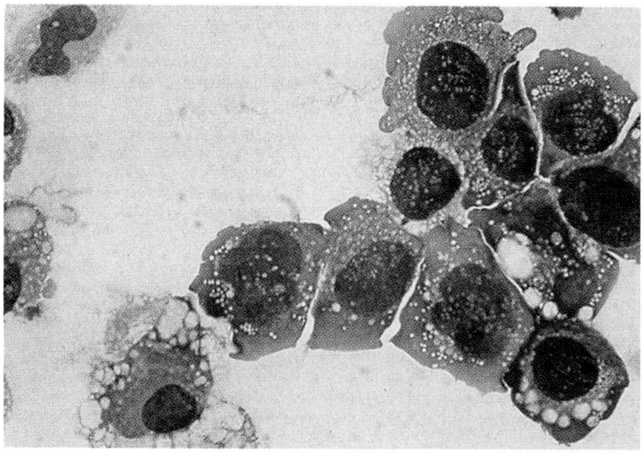

FIGURE 13–11 Poorly differentiated pleural fluid adenocarcinoma showing nuclear irregularities and cytoplasmic vacuoles (×500).

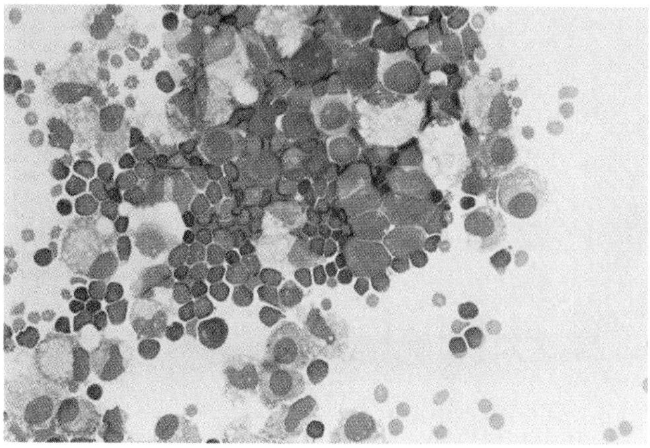

FIGURE 13–12 Pleural fluid small-cell carcinoma showing nuclear molding (×250).

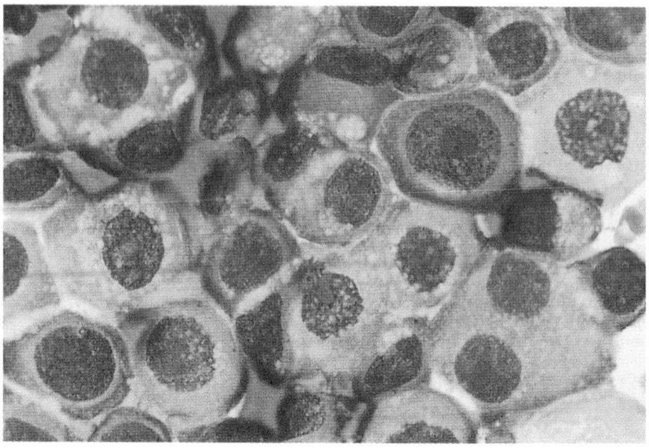

FIGURE 13–13 Metastatic breast carcinoma cells in pleural fluid. Notice the hyperchromatic nucleoli (×1000).

TABLE 13–5 **Significance of Chemical Testing of Pleural Fluid**

Test	Significance
Glucose	Decreased in rheumatoid inflammation Decreased in purulent infection
Lactate	Elevated in bacterial infection
Triglyceride	Elevated in chylous effusions
pH	Decreased in pneumonia not responding to antibiotics Markedly decreased with esophageal rupture
Amylase	Elevated in pancreatitis, esophageal rupture, and malignancy

pleural fluid. Pleural fluid amylase, including salivary amylase, also may be elevated in esophageal rupture and malignancy.

MICROBIOLOGIC AND SEROLOGIC TESTS

Microorganisms primarily associated with pleural effusions include *Staphylococcus aureus*, Enterobacteriaceae, anaerobes, and *Mycobacterium tuberculosis*. Gram stains, cultures (both aerobic and anaerobic), acid-fast stains, and *Mycobacteria* cultures are performed on pleural fluid when clinically indicated. Serologic testing of pleural fluid is used to differentiate effusions of immunologic origin from noninflammatory processes. Tests for antinuclear antibody (**ANA**) and rheumatoid factor (**RF**) are the most frequently performed.

Detection of the tumor marker carcinoembryonic antigen (**CEA**) provides valuable diagnostic information in effusions of malignant origin.

Pericardial Fluid

Normally, only a small amount (10 to 50 mL) of fluid is found between the pericardial serous membranes. Pericardial effusions are primarily the result of changes in the permeability of the membranes due to infection (***pericarditis***), malignancy, trauma, or metabolic disorders, such as uremia (Table 13–6). The presence of an effusion is suspected when cardiac compression is noted during the physician's examination.

APPEARANCE

Normal and transudate pericardial fluid appears clear and pale-yellow. Effusions resulting from infection and malignancy are turbid, and malignant effusions frequently are blood streaked. Grossly bloody effusions are associated with accidental cardiac puncture and misuse of anticoagulant medications. Milky fluids representing chylous and pseudochylous effusions may also be present.

TABLE 13–6 **Significance of Pericardial Fluid Testing**

Test	Significance
Appearance	
Clear, pale yellow	Normal
Blood-streaked	Infection, malignancy
Grossly bloody	Cardiac puncture, anticoagulant medications
Milky	Chylous and pseudochylous material
Differential	
Increased neutrophils	Bacterial endocarditis
Malignant cells	Metastatic carcinoma
Carcinoembryonic antigen	Metastatic carcinoma
Gram stain and culture	Bacterial endocarditis
Acid-fast stain	Tubercular effusion
Adenosine deaminase	Tubercular effusion

LABORATORY TESTS

Tests performed on pericardial fluid are primarily directed at determining if the fluid is a transudate or an exudate and include the fluid–to–serum protein and lactic dehydrogenase (LD) ratios. Like pleural fluid, WBC counts are of little clinical value, although a count of greater than 1000 WBCs/µL with a high percentage of neutrophils can be indicative of **bacterial endocarditis**.

Cytologic examination of pericardial exudates for the presence of malignant cells is an important part of the fluid analysis. Cells most frequently encountered are the result of metastatic lung or breast carcinoma and resemble those found in pleural fluid (Figure 13–14). Pericardial fluid CEA levels correlate well with cytologic studies.[6]

Bacterial cultures and Gram stains are performed on concentrated fluids when endocarditis is suspected. Effusions of tubercular origin are increasing as the result of acquired immunodeficiency syndrome (AIDS). Therefore, acid-fast stains and chemical tests for adenosine deaminase are often requested on pericardial effusions.

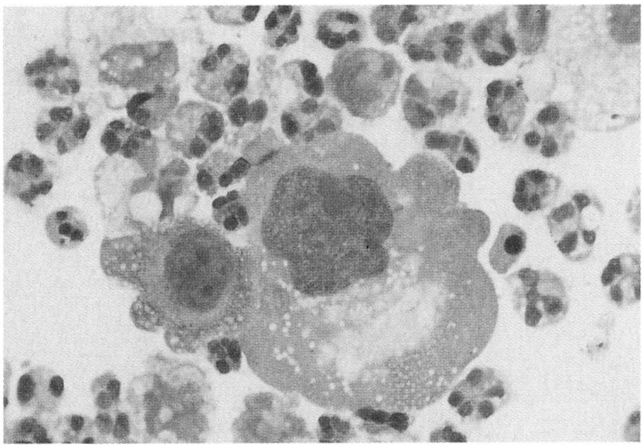

FIGURE 13–14 Malignant pericardial effusion showing cytoplasmic molding and hyperchromatic nucleoli (×1000).

Peritoneal Fluid

Accumulation of fluid in the peritoneal cavity is called ***ascites***, and the fluid is commonly referred to as ascitic fluid rather than peritoneal fluid. In addition to the causes of transudative effusions discussed previously, hepatic disorders, such as cirrhosis, are frequent causes of ascitic transudates. Bacterial infections (***peritonitis***) often as a result of intestinal perforation or a ruptured appendix and malignancy are the most frequent causes of exudative fluids (Table 13–7).

Normal saline is sometimes introduced into the peritoneal cavity to act as a lavage for the detection of abdominal injuries that have not yet resulted in the accumulation of fluid. **Peritoneal lavage** is a particularly sensitive test for the detection of intra-abdominal bleeding in blunt trauma cases, and results of the RBC count are used to aid in determining the need for surgery.[1] RBC counts greater than 100,000/μL are indicative of blunt trauma injuries.

TRANSUDATES VERSUS EXUDATES

Differentiation between ascitic fluid transudates and exudates is more difficult than for pleural and pericardial effusions. The serum-ascites albumin gradient is recommended over the fluid to serum total protein and LD ratios for the detection of transudates of hepatic origin.[8] Fluid and serum albumin levels are measured concurrently, and the fluid albumin level is then subtracted from the serum albumin level. A difference (gradient) of 1.1 or greater suggests a transudate effusion of hepatic origin, and lower gradients are associated with exudative effusions.

EXAMPLE:
Serum albumin = 3.8 mg/dL
Fluid albumin = 1.2 mg/dL
Gradient = 2.6 indicating hepatic effusion

TABLE 13–7 Significance of Peritoneal Fluid Testing

Test	Significance
Appearance	
Clear, pale yellow	Normal
Turbid	Microbial infection
Green	Gallbladder, pancreatic disorders
Blood-streaked	Trauma, infection, or malignancy
Milky	Lymphatic trauma and blockage
Peritoneal lavage	>100,000 RBCs/μL indicates blunt trauma injury
WBC count	
<500 cells/μL	Normal
>500 cells/μL	Bacterial peritonitis, cirrhosis
Differential	Bacterial peritonitis Malignancy
Carcinoembryonic antigen	Malignancy of gastrointestinal origin
CA 125	Malignancy of ovarian origin
Glucose	Decreased in tubercular peritonitis, malignancy
Amylase	Increased in pancreatitis, gastrointestinal perforation
Alkaline phosphatase	Increased in gastrointestinal perforation
Blood urea nitrogen/creatinine	Ruptured or punctured bladder
Gram stain and culture	Bacterial peritonitis
Acid-fast stain	Tubercular peritonitis
Adenosine deaminase	Tubercular peritonitis

APPEARANCE

Like pleural and pericardial fluids, normal peritoneal fluid is clear and pale yellow. Exudates are turbid with bacterial or fungal infections and may appear green when bile is present. The presence of bile can be confirmed using standard chemical tests for bilirubin. Blood-streaked fluid is seen following trauma and with intestinal disorders and malignancy. Chylous or pseudochylous material may be present with trauma or blockage of lymphatic vessels.

LABORATORY TESTS

Normal WBC counts are less than 500 cells/μL, and the count increases with bacterial peritonitis and cirrhosis. To distinguish between those two conditions, an absolute neutrophil count should be performed. An absolute neutrophil count greater than 250 to 500 cells/μL or greater than 50 percent of the total WBC count is indicative of infection.[9]

Examination of ascitic exudates for the presence of malignant cells is important for the detection of tumors of primary and metastatic origin. Malignancies are most frequently of gastrointestinal or ovarian origin. Cells present in ascitic fluid include leukocytes, abundant mesothelial cells, macrophages including lipophages (Figure 13–15), and malignant cells (Figures 13–16 and 13–17). Malignant

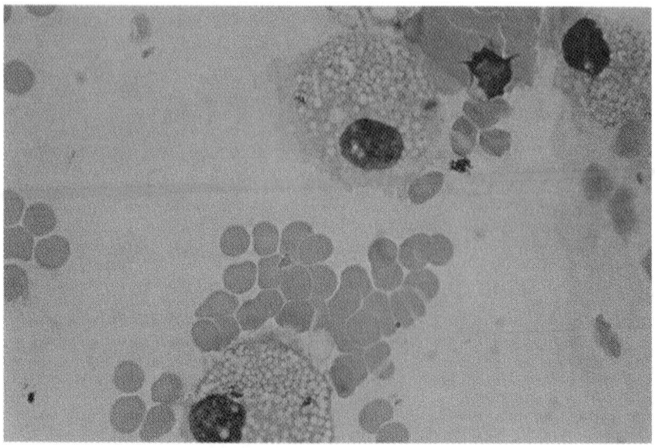

FIGURE 13–15 Lipophages (macrophages containing fat droplets) in peritoneal fluid (×500).

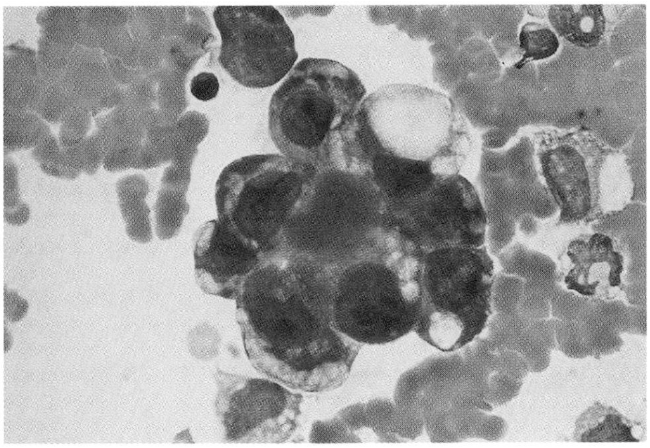

FIGURE 13–16 Ovarian carcinoma showing community borders, nuclear irregularity, and hyperchromatic nucleoli (×500).

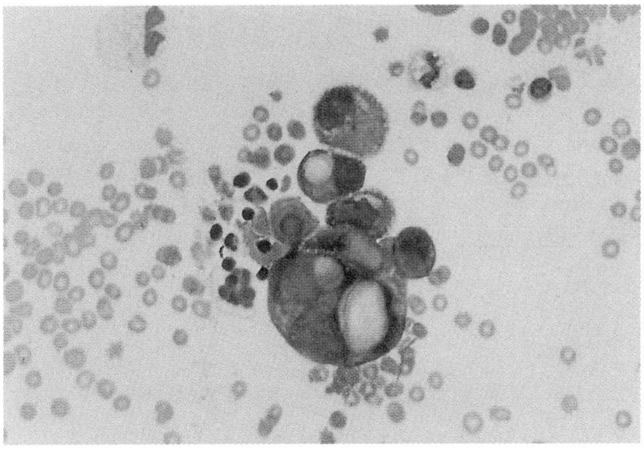

FIGURE 13–19 Colon carcinoma cells containing mucin vacuoles and nuclear irregularities (×500).

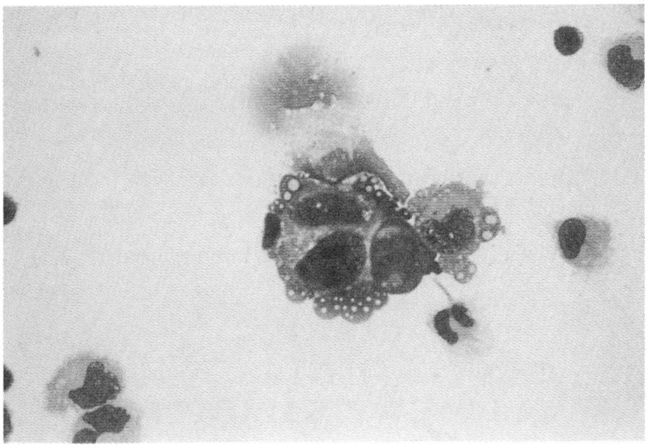

FIGURE 13–17 Adenocarcinoma of the prostate showing cytoplasmic vacuoles, community borders, and hyperchromatic nucleoli (×500).

cells often contain mucin-filled vacuoles (Figures 13–18 and 13–19). Psammoma bodies containing concentric striations of collagen-like material can be seen in benign conditions and are also associated with ovarian and thyroid malignancies (Figure 13–20). Measurement of the tumor markers CEA and CA 125 is a valuable procedure for identifying the primary source of tumors producing ascitic exudates. The presence of CA 125 antigen with a negative CEA suggests the source is from the ovaries, fallopian tubes, or endometrium.[7]

Chemical examination of ascitic fluid consists primarily of glucose, amylase, and alkaline phosphatase determinations. Glucose is decreased below serum levels in tubercular peritonitis and malignancy. Amylase is determined on ascitic fluid to ascertain cases of pancreatitis, and it may be elevated in patients with gastrointestinal perforations. An elevated alkaline phosphatase level is also highly diagnostic of intestinal perforation.

Measurements of blood urea nitrogen and creatinine in the fluid are requested when a ruptured bladder or acciden-

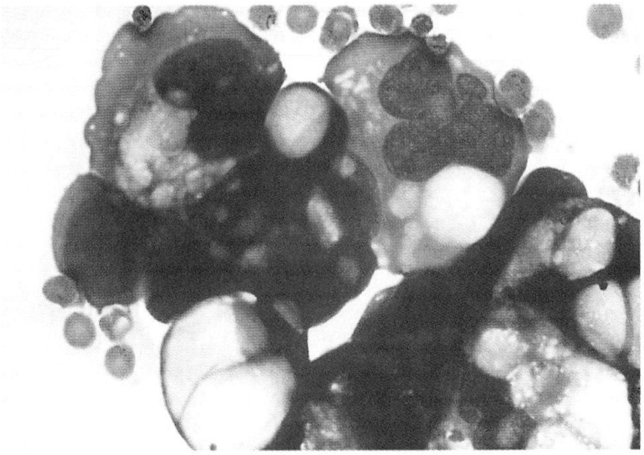

FIGURE 13–18 Ovarian carcinoma cells with large mucin-containing vacuoles (×500).

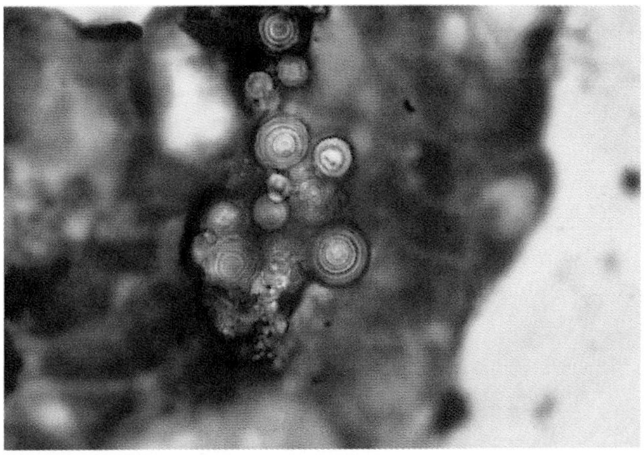

FIGURE 13–20 Psammoma bodies exhibiting concentric striations (×500).

tal puncture of the bladder during the paracentesis is of concern.

Gram stains and bacterial cultures for both aerobes and anaerobes are performed when bacterial peritonitis is suspected. Inoculation of fluid into blood culture bottles at the bedside increases the recovery of anaerobic organisms. Acid-fast stains, adenosine deaminase, and cultures for tuberculosis may also be requested.

REFERENCES

1. Feied, CF: Diagnostic peritoneal lavage. Postgrad Med 85(4):40–49, 1989.
2. Houston, MC: Pleural fluid pH: Diagnostic, therapeutic and prognostic value. Am J Surg 154(3):333–337, 1987.
3. Jain, AP, Gupta, OP, and Khan, N: Comparative diagnostic efficiency of criteria used for differentiating transudate and exudate pleural effusions. J Assoc Physicians India 30(11):823–825, 1982.
4. Jay, SJ: Pleural effusions: Definitive evaluation of the exudate. Postgrad Med 80(5):180–188, 1986.
5. Kjeldsberg, CR, and Knight, JA: Body Fluids: Laboratory Examination of Amniotic, Cerebrospinal, Seminal, Serous and Synovial Fluids. A Textbook Atlas. ASCP, Chicago, 1993.
6. Pinto,MM: Carcinoembryonic antigen in pericardial effusion. Lab Med 18(10): 671–672, 1987.
7. Pinto, MM, et al: Immunoradiometric assay of CA 125 in effusions. Cancer 59(2):218–222, 1987.
8. Runyan, BA, et al. The serum-ascites albumin gradient is superior to the exudate transudate concept in the differential diagnosis of ascites. Ann Intern Med 117:215–218, 1992.
9. Smith, GP, and Kjeldsberg, CR: Cerebrospinal, synovial and serous body fluids. In Henry, JB (ed): Clinical Diagnosis and Management by Laboratory Methods. WB Saunders, Philadelphia, 1996.
10. Stogner, SW, and Campbell, GD: Pleural effusions: What you can learn from the results of a "tap." Postgrad Med 91(5):439–454, 1992.
11. Valdez, L, et al: Cholesterol: A useful parameter for distinguishing between pleural exudates and transudates. Chest 99(5):1097–1102, 1991.

STUDY QUESTIONS

1. What is the purpose of serous fluid?
2. Explain why each of the following conditions will cause a serous effusion: congestive heart failure, hypoproteinemia, inflammation, and lymphatic tumor.
3. What type of serous fluid is obtained by thoracentesis? Paracentesis?
4. Why is differentiation of a serous fluid as a transudate or an exudate of diagnostic significance?
5. State a pathologic condition that causes production of a transudate. An exudate.
6. Describe the characteristic appearance, fluid–to–serum protein and LD ratios, and cell count of a transudate. Which result(s) are most reliable?
7. How can performing a hematocrit aid in determining the cause of a bloody pleural fluid?
8. How can the laboratory determine if a milky pleural fluid is caused by thoracic duct leakage?
9. State a pathologic cause of increased pleural fluid neutrophils. Lymphocytes. Eosinophils. Plasma cells.
10. Why are mesothelial cells routinely seen in pleural fluid differentials?
11. Is it more clinically significant to observe increased or decreased mesothelial cells? Why?
12. State four characteristics of malignant cells.
13. Should pleural fluid glucose levels be compared with plasma levels? Why or why not?
14. Why is the pH of pleural fluid decreased following esophageal rupture?
15. Describe two clinically significant cellular observations in pericardial fluid.
16. Define ascites.
17. Under what circumstance might a peritoneal lavage be performed?
18. The ascitic fluid albumin is 2.8 mg/dL and the patient's serum albumin is 3.5 mg/dL. Is this fluid a transudate or an exudate? Why?
19. What is the significance of an ascitic fluid that is positive for CA 125 antigen?
20. How should cultures of ascitic fluid be incubated?

CASE STUDIES AND CLINICAL SITUATIONS

1. Fluid from a patient with congestive heart failure is collected by thoracentesis and sent to the laboratory for testing. It appears clear and pale yellow and has a WBC count of 450/μL, fluid to serum protein ratio of 0.35, and fluid to serum LD ratio of 0.46.
   a. What type of fluid was collected?
   b. Based on the laboratory results, would this fluid be considered a transudate or an exudate? Why?
   c. List two other tests that could be performed to aid in classifying this fluid.
2. A cloudy pleural fluid has a glucose level of 30 mg/dL (serum glucose level is 100 mg/dL) and a pH of 6.8.
   a. What condition do these results indicate?
   b. What additional treatment might the patient receive based on these results?
3. A cloudy pericardial fluid from a patient with AIDS is received in the laboratory. Gram stain and routine cultures are negative. What additional tests should be performed on this fluid?
4. Paracentesis is performed on a patient with ascites. The fluid appears turbid and has an elevated WBC count. Additional tests ordered include an absolute

granulocyte count, amylase, creatinine, CEA, and CA 125.

a. What is the purpose for the absolute granulocyte count? If it is less than 250 cells/μL, what condition is indicated?
b. If the amylase level is elevated, what is its significance? State an additional test that might be ordered.
c. Explain the significance of an elevated creatinine level.

5. Describe a situation in which paracentesis might be performed on a patient who does not have ascites. If the RBC count is 300,000/μL, what does this indicate?

6. Microscopic examination of an ascitic fluid shows many cells with nuclear and cytoplasmic irregularities containing Psammoma bodies. The CEA test result is normal. What additional test would be helpful?

CHAPTER 14

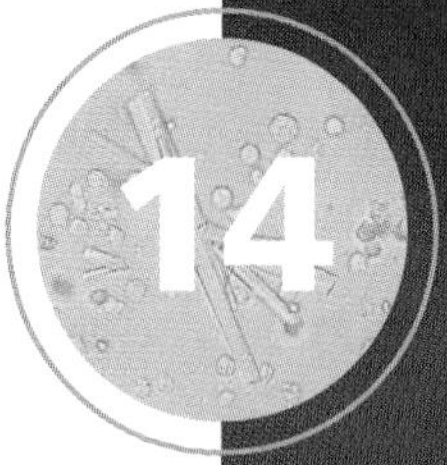

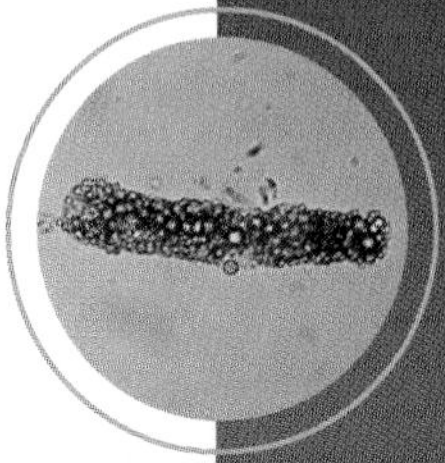

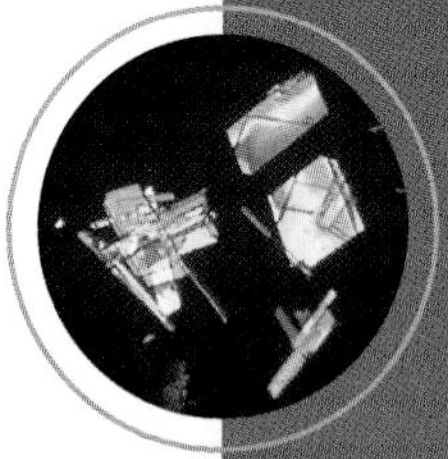

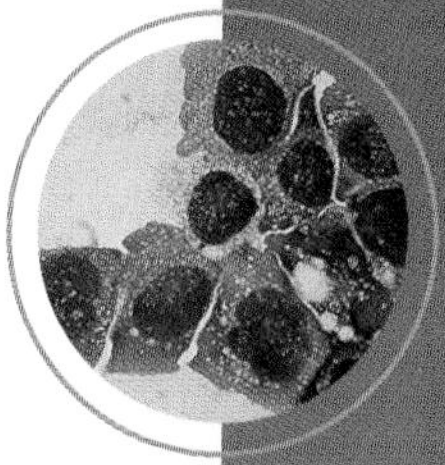

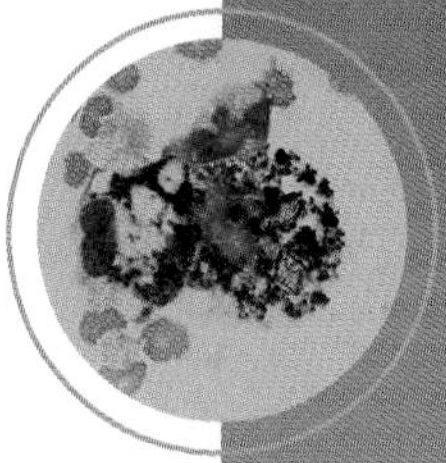

Amniotic Fluid

LEARNING OBJECTIVES

Upon completion of this chapter, the reader will be able to:

1 State the functions of amniotic fluid.
2 Describe the formation and composition of amniotic fluid.
3 Describe the specimen handling and processing procedures for testing of amniotic fluid for bilirubin, fetal lung maturity (FLM), and cytogenetic analysis.
4 Discuss the principle of the spectrophotometric analysis for evaluation of hemolytic disease of the newborn.
5 Interpret a Liley graph.
6 Describe the analysis of amniotic fluid for the detection of neural tube disorders.
7 Explain the physiologic significance of the lecithin-sphingomyelin (L/S) ratio.
8 State the relationship of phosphatidyl glycerol to FLM.
9 Discuss the principle of and sources of error for the L/S ratio, Amniostat-FLM, Foam Stability Index, and microviscosity tests for FLM.
10 Describe the relationship of lamellar bodies to FLM and the laboratory tests performed.

KEY TERMS

amniocentesis
cytogenetic analysis
fetal lung maturity
hemolytic disease of the newborn
lamellar body
lecithin-sphingomyelin ratio
surfactants

Although the testing of amniotic fluid is frequently associated with ***cytogenetic analysis***, the clinical laboratory also performs several significant tests on amniotic fluid. Because amniotic fluid is a product of fetal metabolism, the constituents that are present in the fluid provide information about the metabolic processes taking place and the progress of fetal maturation. When conditions that adversely affect the fetus arise, the danger to the fetus must be measured against the ability of the fetus to survive an early delivery. The tests covered in this chapter are used to determine the extent of fetal distress and fetal maturity (Table 14–1).

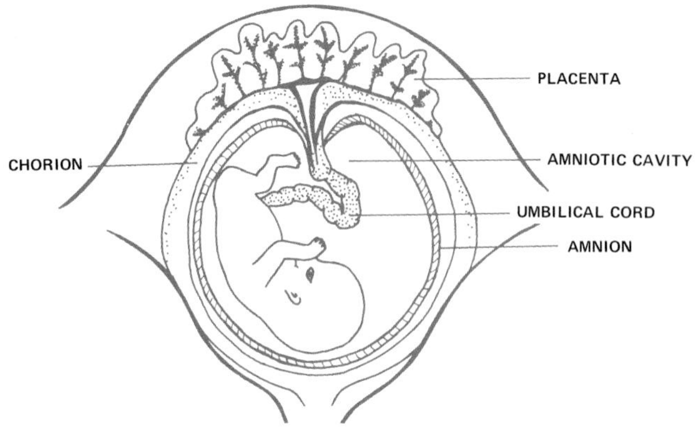

FIGURE 14–1 Fetus in amniotic sac.

Physiology

Amniotic fluid is present in the **amnion**, a membranous sac that surrounds the fetus (Figure 14–1). The primary function of the fluid is to provide a protective cushion for the fetus and allow movement. Exchanges of water and chemicals also take place between the fluid, the fetus, and the maternal circulation.

The amount of amniotic fluid increases throughout pregnancy, reaching a peak of approximately 1 L during the third trimester, and then gradually decreases prior to delivery. During the first trimester, the approximately 35 mL of amniotic fluid is derived primarily from the maternal circulation. The fluid has a composition similar to that of the maternal plasma and contains a small amount of sloughed fetal cells. These cells provide the basis for cytogenetic analysis.

After the first trimester, fetal urine is the major contributor to the amniotic fluid volume. At the time that fetal urine production occurs, fetal swallowing of the amniotic fluid begins and regulates the increase in fluid from the fetal urine. Failure of the fetus to begin swallowing results in excessive accumulation of amniotic fluid (**hydramnios**) and is an indication of fetal distress, often associated with neural tube disorders. Increased fetal swallowing, urinary tract deformities, and membrane leakage are possible causes of decreased amniotic fluid (**oligohydramnios**).

As would be expected, the chemical composition of the amniotic fluid changes when fetal urine production begins. The concentrations of creatinine, urea, and uric acid increase, whereas glucose and protein concentrations decrease. Concentrations of electrolytes, enzymes, hormones, and metabolic end products also vary but are of little clinical significance. Measurement of amniotic fluid creatinine has been used to determine fetal age. Prior to 36 weeks' gestation, the amniotic fluid creatinine level ranges between 1.5 and 2.0 mg/dL. It then rises above 2.0 mg/dL, thereby providing a means of determining fetal age as greater than 36 weeks.[15]

Differentiation between amniotic fluid and maternal urine may be necessary to determine possible premature membrane rupture or accidental puncture of the maternal bladder during specimen collection. Chemical analysis of creatinine, urea, glucose, and protein will aid in the differentiation. Levels of creatinine and urea are much lower in amniotic fluid than in urine. Creatinine does not exceed 3.5 mg/dL and urea 30 mg/dL in amniotic fluid, whereas values as high as 10 mg/dL for creatinine and 300 mg/dL for urea may be found in urine.[16] Measurement of glucose and protein is a less reliable indicator, because glucose and protein are not uncommon urine constituents during pregnancy. However, under normal circumstances, the presence of glucose, protein, or both is associated more closely with amniotic fluid.

TABLE 14–1 **Tests for Fetal Well-Being and Maturity**

Test	Normal Values at Term[16]	Significance
Bilirubin scan	$\Delta A_{450} > .025$	Hemolytic disease of the newborn
Alpha-fetoprotein	<2.0 MoM	Neural tube disorders
Lecithin-sphingomyelin ratio	≥2.0	Fetal lung maturity
Amniostat-fetal lung maturity	Positive	Fetal lung maturity/phosphatidyl glycerol
Foam Stability Index	≥47	Fetal lung maturity
Microviscosity	≥70 mg/g	Fetal lung maturity
Optical density 650 nm	≥0.150	Fetal lung maturity
Lamellar body count	≥32,000/μL	Fetal lung maturity

Specimen Collection

Amniotic fluid is obtained by needle aspiration into the amniotic sac, a procedure called ***amniocentesis***. The procedure most frequently performed is a transabdominal amniocentesis. Vaginal amniocentesis may also be performed; however, this method carries a greater risk of infection. In general, amniocentesis is a safe procedure, particularly when performed after the 14th week of gestation. Fluid for chromosome analysis is usually collected at approximately 16 weeks' gestation, whereas tests for fetal distress and maturity are performed later in the third trimester.

A maximum of 30 mL of amniotic fluid is collected in sterile syringes. The first 2 or 3 mL collected can be contaminated by maternal blood, tissue fluid, and cells and are discarded. Fluid for bilirubin analysis in cases of ***hemolytic disease of the newborn*** **(HDN)** must be protected from light at all times. This can be accomplished by placing the specimens in amber-colored tubes.

Specimen Handling and Processing

Handling and processing of amniotic fluid vary with the tests requested. However, in all circumstances, special handling procedures should be performed immediately and the specimen delivered promptly to the laboratory. Fluid for ***fetal lung maturity*** **(FLM)** tests should be placed in ice for delivery to the laboratory and refrigerated prior to testing. Specimens for cytogenetic studies are maintained at room temperature or body temperature (37°C incubation) prior to analysis to prolong the life of the cells needed for analysis.

All fluid for chemical testing should be separated from cellular elements and debris as soon as possible to prevent distortion of chemical constituents by cellular metabolism or disintegration. This can be performed using centrifugation or filtration. Low-speed centrifugation (500 to 1000 g) for no longer than 5 minutes is required for FLM testing, because at higher speeds some of the phospholipids measured in the tests may be lost in the sediment. Filtration is often recommended for FLM methods to prevent loss of the phospholipids.

Color and Appearance

Normal amniotic fluid is colorless and may exhibit slight to moderate turbidity from cellular debris, particularly in later stages of fetal development. Blood-streaked fluid may be present as the result of a traumatic tap, abdominal trauma, or intra-amniotic hemorrhage. The source of the blood (maternal or fetal) can be determined using the Kleihauer-Betke test for fetal hemoglobin and is important for further case management.

The presence of bilirubin gives the fluid a yellow color and is indicative of red blood cell destruction resulting from HDN. **Meconium**, which is usually defined as a newborn's first bowel movement, may be present in the amniotic fluid as the result of fetal intestinal secretions. It produces a dark green color. Fetal aspiration of meconium during fetal swallowing is a concern when increased amounts are present in the fluid. A very dark red-brown fluid is associated with fetal death.

Summary of Amniotic Fluid Color

Color	Significance
Colorless	Normal
Blood-streaked	Traumatic tap, abdominal trauma, intra-amniotic hemorrhage
Yellow	Hemolytic disease of the newborn (bilirubin)
Dark green	Meconium
Dark red-brown	Fetal death

Tests for Fetal Distress

HEMOLYTIC DISEASE OF THE NEWBORN

The oldest routinely performed laboratory test on amniotic fluid evaluates the severity of the fetal anemia produced by HDN. The incidence of this disease has been decreasing rapidly since the development of methods to prevent anti-Rh antibody production in postpartum mothers. However, antibodies against other red cell antigens are also capable of producing HDN, and immunization of Rh-negative mothers may not be effective or even performed in all cases. When antibodies present in the maternal circulation cross the placenta, the destruction of fetal red blood cells results in the appearance of the red blood cell degradation product, bilirubin, in the amniotic fluid. By measuring the amount of bilirubin in the fluid, the degree of hemolysis taking place may be determined and the danger this anemia presents to the fetus may be assessed.

The measurement of amniotic fluid bilirubin is performed by spectrophotometric analysis. As illustrated in Figure 14–2, the optical density **(OD)** of the fluid is mea-

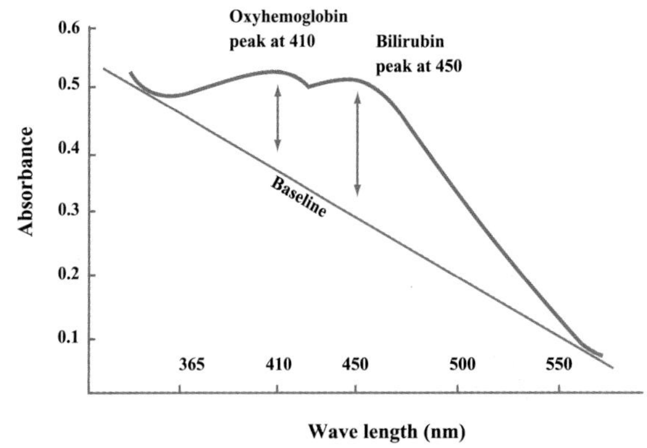

FIGURE 14–2 Spectrophotometric bilirubin scan showing bilirubin and oxyhemoglobin peaks.

sured in intervals between 365 nm and 550 nm and the readings plotted on semilogarithmic graph paper. In normal fluid, the OD will be highest at 365 nm and decrease linearly to 550 nm. When bilirubin is present, a rise in OD will be seen at 450 nm because this is the wavelength of maximum bilirubin absorption. The difference between the OD of the theoretic baseline and the OD at 450 nm represents the amniotic fluid bilirubin concentration. This difference in OD, referred to as the absorbance difference at 450 nm (ΔA_{450}), is then plotted on a Liley graph to determine the severity of the hemolytic disease (Figure 14–3).[9]

Notice that the Liley graph plots the ΔA_{450} against gestational age and is divided into three zones that represent the degree of hemolytic severity. Values falling in zone I indicate no more than a mildly affected fetus; those in zone II require careful monitoring, whereas a value in zone III suggests a severely affected fetus. Intervention through induction of labor or intrauterine exchange transfusion must be considered when a ΔA_{450} is plotted in zone III.

As mentioned previously, specimens must be protected from light at all times. Markedly decreased values will be obtained with as little as 30 minutes of exposure to light. Care must be taken to ensure that contamination of the fluid by cells, hemoglobin, meconium, or other debris does not interfere with the spectrophotometric analysis. Specimens should be immediately centrifuged to remove particulate interference. Maximum absorbance of oxyhemoglobin occurs at 410 nm and can interfere with the bilirubin absorption peak (see Fig. 14–2). This interference can be removed by extraction with chloroform if necessary.[13] A control may be prepared by diluting commercial chemistry control sera 1 to 10 with normal saline and treating it in the same manner as the patient specimen. Bilirubin and protein levels approximate those in amniotic fluid and can be varied by using low or high control sera.[10]

NEURAL TUBE DEFECTS

Increased levels of alpha-fetoprotein (**AFP**) in both the maternal circulation and the amniotic fluid can be indicative of fetal neural tube defects, such as anencephaly and spina bifida. AFP is the major protein produced by the fetal liver during early gestation (prior to 18 weeks). It is found in the maternal serum due to the combined fetal-maternal circulations and in the amniotic fluid from diffusion and excretion of fetal urine. Increased levels are found in the maternal serum and amniotic fluid when the skin fails to close over the neural tissue, as occurs in anencephaly and spina bifida.

Measurement of amniotic fluid AFP levels is indicated when maternal serum levels are elevated or a family history of previous neural tube defects exists. The possibility of a multiple pregnancy also must be investigated when serum levels are elevated. Normal values are based on the week of gestational age, as the fetus produces maximal AFP between 12 and 15 weeks' gestation, after which levels in amniotic fluid then begin to decline. Both serum and amniotic fluid AFP levels are reported in terms of multiples of the median (**MoM**). The median is the laboratory's reference level for a given week of gestation. A value two times

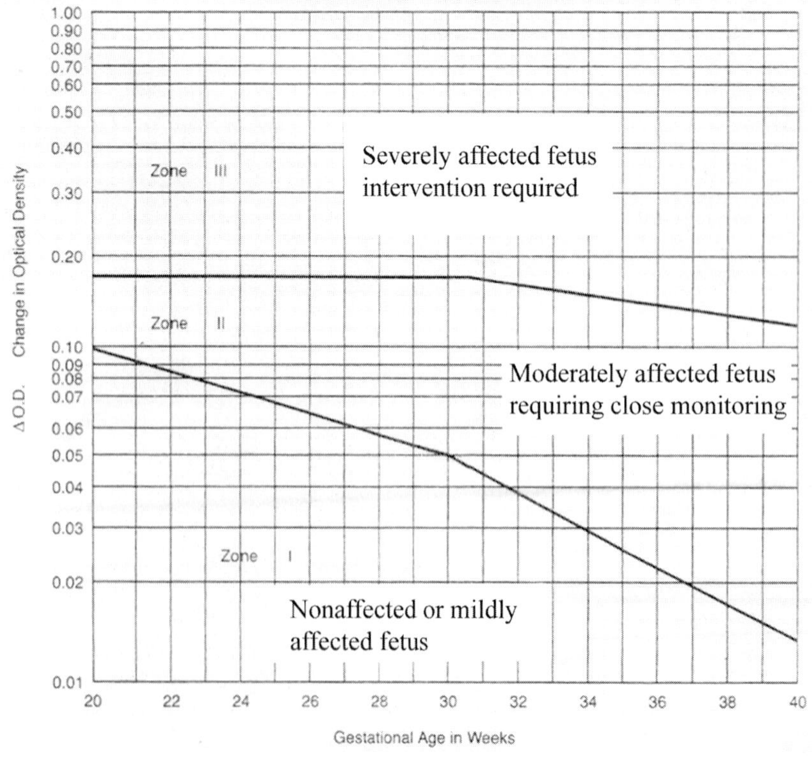

FIGURE 14–3 Example of a Liley graph. (Adapted from Harmening, DM: Modern Blood Banking and Transfusion Practices, ed 4. FA Davis, Philadelphia, 1999, p. 427)

the median value is considered abnormal (greater than two MoM) for both maternal serum and amniotic fluid. Testing for AFP has been automated by the Access Immunoassay System (Beckman Coulter, Inc., Fullerton, CA.).

Elevated amniotic fluid AFP levels are followed by measurement of amniotic acetylcholinesterase (**AChE**). The test is more specific for neural tube disorders than AFP, provided it is not performed on a bloody specimen, because blood contains AChE.[16]

Tests for Fetal Maturity

Fetal distress, whether caused by HDN or other conditions, forces the obstetrician to consider a preterm delivery. At this point, fetal maturity must be assessed.

FETAL LUNG MATURITY

Respiratory distress is the most frequent complication of early delivery. Therefore, laboratory tests must be performed to determine the maturity of the fetal lungs. Several laboratory tests are available to measure FLM.

LECITHIN-SPHINGOMYELIN RATIO

The reference method to which tests of FLM are compared is the ***lecithin-sphingomyelin* (L/S) *ratio***. Lecithin is the primary component of the ***surfactants*** (phospholipids, neutral lipids, and proteins) that make up the alveolar lining and account for alveolar stability.

Lecithin is produced at a relatively low and constant rate until the 35th week of gestation, at which time a noticeable increase in its production occurs, resulting in the stabilization of the fetal lung alveoli. Sphingomyelin is a lipid that is produced at a constant rate after about 26 weeks' gestation; therefore, it can serve as a control on which to base the rise in lecithin. Both lecithin and sphingomyelin appear in the amniotic fluid in amounts proportional to their concentrations in the fetus.[7] Prior to 35 weeks' gestation, the L/S ratio is usually less than 1.6 because large amounts of lecithin are not being produced at this time. It will rise to 2.0 or higher when lecithin production increases. Therefore, when the L/S ratio reaches 2.0, a preterm delivery is usually considered to be a relatively safe procedure. Falsely elevated results are encountered in fluid contaminated with blood or meconium because both these substances contain lecithin and sphingomyelin.

Quantitative measurement of lecithin and sphingomyelin is performed using thin-layer chromatography. The procedure is labor intensive and subject to high coefficients of variation. Many laboratories have replaced the L/S ratio with the more cost-effective phosphatidyl glycerol immunoassays, fluorescence polarization, and ***lamellar body*** density procedures.[4]

AMNIOSTAT-FLM

The presence of another lung surface lipid, phosphatidyl glycerol, is also essential for adequate lung maturity. The production of phosphatidyl glycerol normally parallels that of lecithin, but its production is delayed in diabetic mothers. In this circumstance, respiratory distress will occur in the presence of an L/S ratio of 2.0. Therefore, a thin-layer chromatography lung profile must include lecithin, sphingomyelin, and phosphatidyl glycerol to provide an accurate measurement.[8]

Development of an immunologic agglutination test for phosphatidyl glycerol has provided a more rapid method for assessment of fetal maturity that does not require a laboratory to be equipped to perform thin-layer chromatography. The Aminostat-FLM (Irving Scientific, Santa Ana, CA) uses antisera specific for phosphatidyl glycerol and is not affected by specimen contamination with blood and meconium.[5] Studies have shown good correlation with thin-layer chromatography but with a slightly higher incidence of false-negative results that may need to be followed up with further testing.[3,11]

FOAM STABILITY

Until the development of biochemical techniques to measure the individual lung-surface lipid concentrations, a mechanical screening test, called the "foam" or "shake" test, was used to determine their presence. Because it can be performed at the bedside or in the laboratory, the test is still in use. Amniotic fluid is mixed with 95 percent ethanol, shaken for 15 seconds, and then allowed to sit undisturbed for 15 minutes. At the end of this time, the surface of the fluid is observed for the presence of a continuous line of bubbles around the outside edge. The presence of bubbles indicates that a sufficient amount of phospholipid is available to reduce the surface tension of the fluid even in the presence of alcohol, an antifoaming agent.

A modification of the foam test uses 0.5 mL of amniotic fluid added to increasing amounts of 95 percent ethanol, providing a gradient of ethanol/fluid ratios ranging from 0.42 mL to 0.55 mL in 0.01-mL increments, which can be used to provide a semiquantitative measure of the amount of surfactant present. A value of 47 or higher indicates FLM. The Foam Stability Index has shown good correlation with the L/S ratio and tests for phosphatidyl glycerol. The test cannot be used with contaminated amniotic fluid because blood and meconium will also reduce surface tension.

PROCEDURE

Foam Shake Test Procedure

1. Mix equal parts of amniotic fluid with 95% ethanol.
2. Vigorously shake for 15 seconds.
3. Allow to sit undisturbed for 15 minutes.
4. Observe for the presence of a continuous line of bubbles around the outside edge.

PROCEDURE

Procedure for Foam Stability Index

1. Add 0.5 mL of amniotic fluid to tubes containing increasing amounts of 95% ethanol ranging from 0.42–0.55 mL in 0.01-mL increments.
2. Vigorously shake for 15 seconds.
3. Allow to sit undisturbed for 15 minutes.
4. Observe for the presence of a continuous line of bubbles around the outside edge.
5. Values >47 indicate fetal lung maturity.

MICROVISCOSITY

The presence of phospholipids decreases the microviscosity of the amniotic fluid. This change in microviscosity can be measured using the principle of fluorescence polarization employed by the Abbott TDx analyzer (Abbott Laboratories, Abbott Park, IL). The instrument measures the polarization of a fluorescent dye that combines with both surfactants and albumin. Dye bound to surfactant exhibits low polarization, whereas dye bound to albumin has high polarization. Albumin is used as an internal standard in the same manner as sphingomyelin because it remains at a constant level throughout gestation. The recorded changes in polarization produce a surfactant/albumin ratio expressed in milligrams surfactant to grams albumin that is compared with a standard curve that includes phosphatidyl glycerol and ranges from 0 to 160 mg/g (Figure 14–4). A ratio of 70 or greater provides a conservative prediction of FLM and lower values may be considered.[2, 14] Fluid should be filtered rather than centrifuged prior to examination to prevent sedimentation of the lipids, and use of contaminated fluid is not recommended.

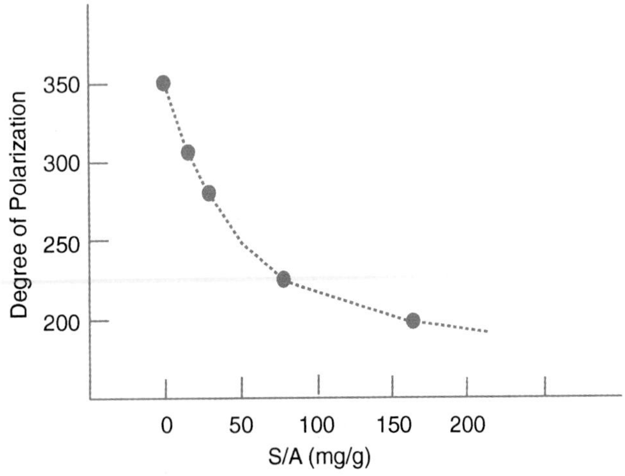

FIGURE 14–4 Sample TDx FLM calibration curve. (Adapted from Ashwood, et al.[1])

LAMELLAR BODIES AND OPTICAL DENSITY

The surfactants responsible for FLM are produced and secreted by the type II pneumocytes of the fetal lung in the form of structures termed lamellar bodies. The lamellar bodies enter the alveolar spaces to provide surfactant and also enter the amniotic fluid. Therefore, the number of lamellar bodies present in the amniotic fluid correlates with the amount of phospholipid present in the fetal lungs.

The presence of lamellar bodies increases the OD of the amniotic fluid. Specimens are centrifuged at 2000 g for 10 minutes and examined using a wavelength of 650 nm, which rules out interference from hemoglobin but not other contaminants, such as meconium. An OD of 0.150 has been shown to correlate well with an L/S ratio of greater than or equal to 2.0 and the presence of phosphatidyl glycerol.[12]

Lamellar bodies can be counted using resistance-pulse counting, such as that employed by Coulter cell-counting instruments (Beckman Coulter, Inc., Fullerton, CA.). Ranging in size from 1.7 to 7.3 fL, lamellar bodies can be counted using the platelet channel.[1] This technique is easily performed; however, samples must be free of particle contamination such as meconium and blood. A count of 32,000 or more particles per microliter represents adequate FLM.[6]

REFERENCES

1. Ashwood, ER, et al: Measuring the number of lamellar body particles in amniotic fluid. Obstet Gynecol 75:289–292, 1990.
2. Ashwood, ER, Palmer, SE, and Lenke, RR: Rapid FLM testing: Commercial versus NBD-phosphatidylcholine assay. Obstet Gynecol 80(6):1048–1053, 1992.
3. Chapman, JF: Current methods for evaluating FLM. Lab Med 17(10):597–602, 1986.
4. Dubin, SB: Assessment of FLM: Practice parameter. Am J Clin Pathol 110:723–732, 1998.
5. Eisenbrey, AB, et al: Phosphatidyl glycerol in amniotic fluid: Comparison of an "ultrasensitive" immunologic assay with TLC and enzymatic assay. Am J Clin Pathol 91(3):293–297, 1989.
6. Fakhoury, G, et al: Lamellar body concentrations and the prediction of fetal pulmonary maturity. Am J Obstet Gynecol 170:72, 1994.
7. Gluck, L, et al: Diagnosis of the respiratory distress syndrome by amniocentesis. Am J Obstet Gynecol 109(3):440–445, 1971.
8. Kulovich, MV, Hallman, MB, and Gluck, L: The lung profile: Normal pregnancy. Am J Obstet Gynecol 135:57–60, 1979.
9. Liley, AW: Liquor amnii analysis in the management of the pregnancy complicated by Rhesus sensitization. Am J Obstet Gynecol 82:1359, 1961.
10. McDonald, OL, and Watts, MT: Use of commercially prepared control sera as quality control materials for spectrophotometric bilirubin determinations in amniotic fluid. Am J Clin Pathol 84(4):513–517, 1985.
11. Saad, SA, et al: The reliability and clinical use of a rapid phosphatidylglycerol assay in normal and diabetic pregnancies. Am J Obstet Gynecol 157(6):1516–1520, 1987.
12. Sbarra, AJ, et al: Correlation of amniotic fluid optical density at 650 nm and lecithin/sphingomyelin ratios. Obstet Gynecol 48:613, 1976.
13. Spinnato, JA, et al: Amniotic bilirubin and fetal hemolytic disease. Am J Obstet Gynecol 165(4):1030–1035, 1991.
14. Steinfeld, JD, et al: The utility of the TDx test in the assessment of FLM. Obstet Gynecol 79(3):460–464, 1992.
15. Weiss, RR, et al: Amniotic fluid uric acid and creatinine as measures of fetal maturity. Obstet Gynecol 44(2):208–214, 1974.
16. Wenk, RE, and Rosenbaum, JM: Examination of amniotic fluid. In Henry, JB (ed): Clinical Diagnosis and Management by Laboratory Methods. WB Saunders, Philadelphia, 1996.

STUDY QUESTIONS

1. State two functions of amniotic fluid.
2. What is the primary cause of the normal increase in amniotic fluid as a pregnancy progresses?
3. State reasons for increased and decreased amounts of amniotic fluid.
4. Why might a creatinine level be requested on an amniotic fluid?
5. What is the purpose of placing a specimen of amniotic fluid in an amber-colored tube prior to sending it to the laboratory?
6. How are specimens for FLM testing delivered to and stored in the laboratory?
7. Why are specimens for cytogenetic analysis incubated prior to analysis?
8. What is the first processing procedure that the laboratory performs on amniotic fluid?
9. State the significance of the following colors in amniotic fluid: dark green, colorless, yellow, and red-brown.
10. What is the significance of a rise in the OD of amniotic fluid at 450 nm? 410 nm?
11. What is the purpose of plotting the amniotic fluid ΔA_{450} on a Liley graph?
12. Why do neural tube disorders such as spina bifida and anencephaly produce increased amniotic fluid AFP?
13. Define MoM.
14. Explain the relationship between evaluation of amniotic fluid for HDN and FLM.
15. What is the role of lecithin in FLM?
16. Prior to 35 weeks' gestation, what is the normal L/S ratio? Why?
17. State two advantages of the Aminostat-FLM over the L/S ratio.
18. Does the failure to produce bubbles in the Foam Stability Index indicate increased or decreased lecithin? Why?
19. Relate the principle of the microviscosity test to the principle of the L/S ratio.
20. Does an L/S ratio of 2.0 correlate with a surfactant/albumin ratio of 40 mg/g? Why or why not?
21. What is the relationship of lamellar bodies and fluid OD at 650 nm to FLM?
22. Which test for FLM is least affected by contamination with hemoglobin and meconium? Why?

CASE STUDIES AND CLINICAL SITUATIONS

1. Amniocentesis is performed on a woman believed to be in approximately the 31st week of gestation. This is the second pregnancy for this Rh-negative, woman with diabetes. Spectrophotometric analysis of the fluid shows a ΔA_{450} of 0.3.
   a. Based on the Liley graph, should the physician consider inducing labor?
   b. What else must the physician consider prior to inducing labor?

   The physician decides to induce labor based on a positive Aminostat-FLM.
   c. What information did this test provide for the physician?
   d. Why did the physician prefer an Aminostat-FLM over an L/S ratio in this situation?
2. Amniocentesis is performed following a maternal serum AFP level of 2.2 MoM at 15 weeks' gestation.
   a. What fetal condition is suspected?
   b. If the amniotic fluid AFP is 2.5 MoM, what additional test could be performed?
   c. In what situation would this additional test not be performed?
3. If the degree of fluorescence polarization in an amniotic fluid is decreased, does this represent increased or decreased lecithin?
4. Amniotic fluid for FLM testing is centrifuged for 10 minutes at 5000 g. How will this affect the test results?
5. How might a dark green amniotic fluid affect the results of the following tests?
   a. Foam Stability Index
   b. L/S ratio
   c. Aminostat-FLM
   d. OD_{650}
6. How might a blood-streaked amniotic fluid affect the results of the following tests?
   a. L/S ratio
   b. AChE
   c. Bilirubin analysis
   d. Aminostat-FLM

CHAPTER 15

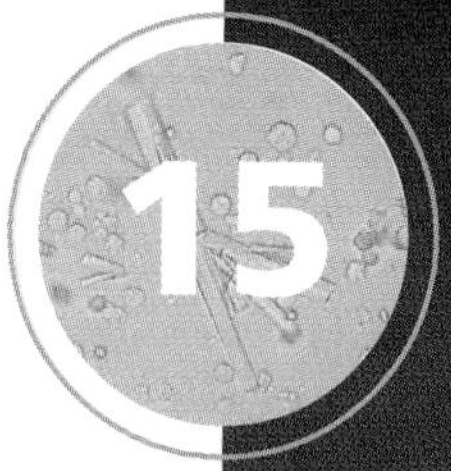

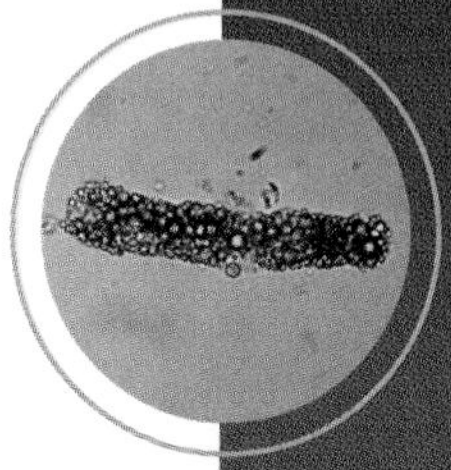

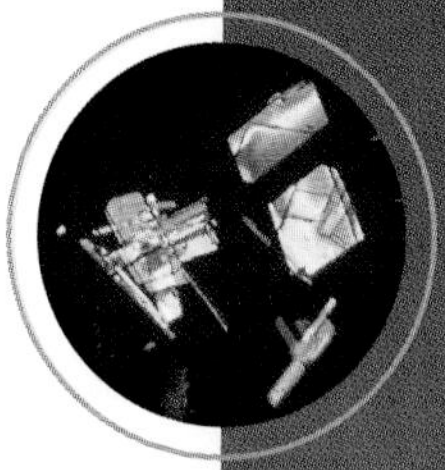

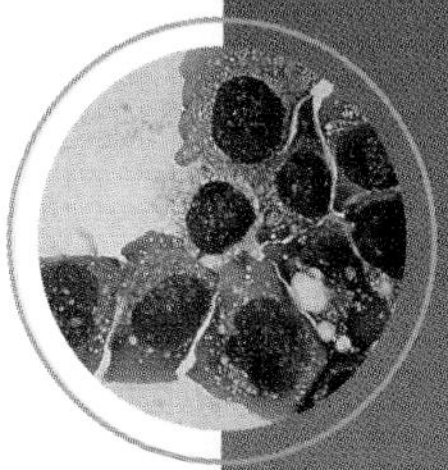

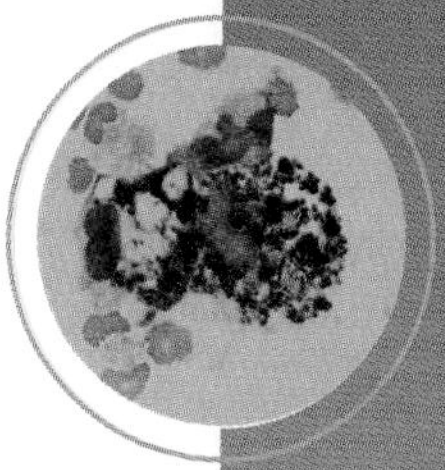

Fecal Analysis

LEARNING OBJECTIVES

Upon completion of this chapter, the reader will be able to:

1. Describe the normal composition of feces.
2. Differentiate between secretory and osmotic diarrhea.
3. Instruct patients in the collection of random and quantitative stool specimens.
4. State a pathogenic and a nonpathogenic cause for stools colored red, black, and pale yellow.
5. State the significance of bulky, ribbon-like, and mucus-containing stools.
6. State the significance of increased neutrophils in a stool specimen.
7. Describe a positive microscopic examination for muscle fibers.
8. Name the fecal fats stained by Sudan III, and give the conditions under which they will stain.
9. Describe and interpret the microscopic results that will be seen when a specimen from a patient with steatorrhea is stained with Sudan III.
10. Explain the principle of the guaiac test for occult blood and the reasons that guaiac is the reagent of choice.
11. Instruct a patient in the collection of specimens for occult blood, including providing an explanation of dietary restrictions.
12. Briefly describe a chemical screening test performed on feces for each of the following: fetal hemoglobin, pancreatic insufficiency, and carbohydrate intolerance.

KEY TERMS

malabsorption
maldigestion
occult blood
osmotic diarrhea
pancreatic insufficiency
secretory diarrhea
steatorrhea

In the minds of most laboratory personnel, analysis of fecal specimens fits into the category of a "necessary evil." However, as an end product of body metabolism, feces do provide valuable diagnostic information. Routine fecal examination includes macroscopic, microscopic, and chemical analyses for the early detection of gastrointestinal bleeding, liver and biliary duct disorders, ***maldigestion/ malabsorption*** syndromes, and inflammation. Of equal diagnostic value is the detection and identification of pathogenic bacteria and parasites; however, these procedures are best covered in a microbiology textbook and will not be discussed here.

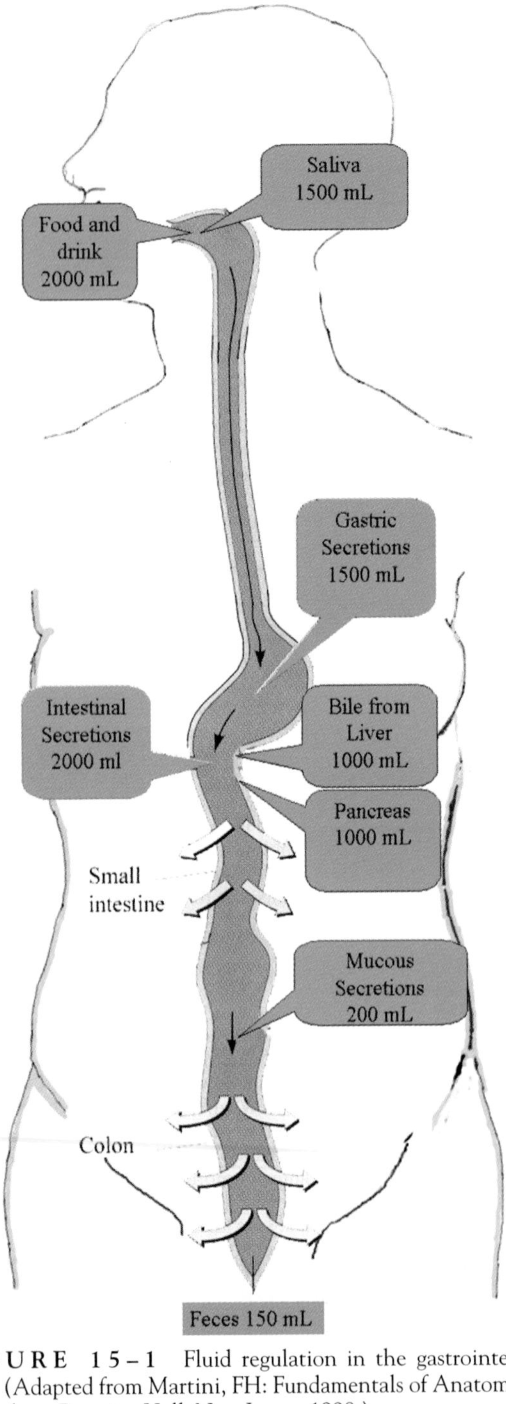

FIGURE 15–1 Fluid regulation in the gastrointestinal tract. (Adapted from Martini, FH: Fundamentals of Anatomy and Physiology. Prentice Hall, New Jersey, 1998.)

Physiology

The normal fecal specimen contains bacteria, cellulose and other undigested foodstuffs, gastrointestinal secretions, bile pigments, cells from the intestinal walls, electrolytes, and water. Many species of bacteria make up the normal flora of the intestines. Bacterial metabolism produces the strong odor associated with feces and intestinal gas or **flatus**.

Although digestion of ingested proteins, carbohydrates, and fats takes place throughout the **alimentary tract**, the small intestine is the primary site for the final breakdown and reabsorption of these compounds. Digestive enzymes secreted into the small intestine by the pancreas include trypsin, chymotrypsin, amino peptidase, and lipase. Bile salts provided by the liver aid in the digestion of fats. A deficiency in any of these substances causes the inability to digest and, therefore, reabsorb certain foods. Excess undigested or unreabsorbed material will then appear in the feces, and patients exhibit symptoms of maldigestion and malabsorption. As shown in Figure 15–1, approximately 9000 mL of ingested fluid, saliva, gastric, liver, pancreatic, and intestinal secretions enter the digestive tract each day. Under normal conditions, only between 500 to 1500 mL of this fluid reaches the large intestine, and only about 150 mL is excreted in the feces. Water and electrolytes are readily absorbed in both the small and large intestines, resulting in a fecal electrolyte content that is similar to that of plasma.

The large intestine is capable of absorbing approximately 3000 mL of water. When the amount of water reaching the large intestine exceeds this amount, it is excreted with the solid fecal material, producing **diarrhea**. **Constipation**, on the other hand, provides time for additional water to be reabsorbed from the fecal material, producing small, hard **stools**.

Bacterial, viral, and protozoan infections produce increased secretion of water and electrolytes, which override the reabsorptive ability of the large intestine (***secretory diarrhea***). Incomplete breakdown or reabsorption of foodstuffs presents increased fecal material to the large intestine resulting in the retention of water and electrolytes in the large intestine (***osmotic diarrhea***). Laboratory testing of feces is frequently performed to aid in determining the cause of diarrhea (Table 15–1).

Specimen Collection

Collection of a fecal specimen, frequently called a stool specimen, is not an easy task for patients. Detailed instructions and appropriate containers should be provided.

Patients should be instructed to collect the specimen in a clean container, such as a bedpan or disposable container, and transfer the specimen to the laboratory container. Patients should understand that the specimen must not be contaminated with urine or toilet water that may contain chemical disinfectants. Some kits provided for the collec-

TABLE 15–1 Common Fecal Tests for Diarrhea

Secretory	Osmotic
Stool cultures	Microscopic fecal fats
Ova and parasite examinations	Muscle fiber detection
Rotavirus immunoassay	Qualitative fecal fats
Fecal leukocytes	Trypsin screening
	Microscopic fecal fats
	Muscle fiber detection
	Quantitative fecal fats
	Clinitest
	D-xylose tolerance test
	Lactose tolerance test

tion of specimens for ***occult blood*** contain paper that can be floated in the toilet bowl to collect the specimen. This method should only be used when collecting specimens to be tested using the kit in which they are included. Containers containing preservatives for ova and parasites must not be used to collect specimens for other tests.

Random specimens suitable for qualitative testing for blood and microscopic examination for leukocytes, muscle fibers, and fecal fats are usually collected in plastic or glass containers with screw-capped tops similar to those used for urine specimens. Material collected on a physician's glove and samples applied to filter paper in occult blood testing kits are also received.

For quantitative testing, such as for fecal fats, timed specimens are required. Because of the variability of bowel habits and the transit time required for food to pass through the digestive tract, the most representative sample is a 3-day collection. These specimens are frequently collected in paint cans to accommodate the specimen quantity and facilitate emulsification prior to testing. Care must be taken when opening any fecal specimen to slowly release gas that has accumulated within the container. Also, patients must be cautioned not to contaminate the outside of the container.

Macroscopic Screening

The first indication of gastrointestinal disturbances can often be provided by changes in the brown color and formed consistency of the normal stool. Of course, the appearance of abnormal fecal color may also be caused by the ingestion of highly pigmented foods and medications, so a differentiation must be made between this and a possible pathologic cause.

COLOR

The brown color of the feces results from intestinal oxidation of urobilinogen to urobilin. As discussed in Chapter 5, urobilinogen formed in the degradation of hemoglobin passes through the bile duct to the small intestine. Therefore, stools appearing pale in color may signify a blockage of the bile duct. Pale stools are also associated with diagnostic procedures using barium sulfate.

A primary concern is the presence of blood in a stool specimen. Depending on the area of the intestinal tract from which bleeding is occurring, the color can range from bright to dark red to black. Blood originating from the esophagus, stomach, or duodenum takes approximately 3 days to appear in the stool; during this time, degradation of hemoglobin produces the characteristic black, tarry stool. Likewise, blood from the lower gastrointestinal tract requires less time to appear and will retain its original red color. Both black and red stools should be chemically tested for the presence of blood, because ingestion of iron, charcoal, or bismuth will often produce a black stool, and medications and foods, including beets, will produce a red stool.

Green stools may be observed in patients taking oral antibiotics owing to oxidation of fecal bilirubin to biliverdin. Ingestion of increased amounts of green vegetables or food coloring also will produce green stools.

APPEARANCE

Besides variations in color, additional abnormalities that may be observed during the macroscopic examination include the watery consistency present in diarrhea and the small, hard stools seen with constipation. Slender, ribbon-like stools suggest an obstruction of the normal passage of material through the intestine.

Pale stools associated with biliary obstruction will appear bulky and frothy and frequently have a foul odor. Absence of bile salts that assist pancreatic lipase in the breakdown and subsequent reabsorption of triglycerides produces an increase in stool fat termed ***steatorrhea***. Likewise, pan-

TABLE 15–2 Macroscopic Stool Characteristics[1,5]

Color/Appearance	Possible Cause
Black	Upper gastrointestinal bleeding Iron therapy Charcoal Bismuth (antacids)
Red	Lower gastrointestinal bleeding Beets and food coloring Rifampin
Pale yellow, white, gray	Bile-duct obstruction Barium sulfate
Green	Biliverdin/oral antibiotics Green vegetables
Bulky/frothy	Bile-duct obstruction Pancreatic disorders
Ribbon-like	Intestinal constriction
Mucus/blood-streaked mucus	Colitis Dysentery Malignancy Constipation

creatic disorders, including cystic fibrosis, chronic pancreatitis, and carcinoma that decrease the production of pancreatic enzymes, are also associated with steatorrhea.

The presence of mucus-coated stools is indicative of intestinal inflammation or irritation. Mucus-coated stools may be caused by pathologic colitis or excessive straining during elimination. Blood-streaked mucus suggests damage to the intestinal walls, possibly caused by bacterial or amebic **dysentery** or malignancy. The presence of mucus should be reported (Table 15–2).

PROCEDURE

Methylene Blue Stain Procedure for Fecal Leukocytes

1 Place mucus or a drop of liquid stool on a slide.
2 Add two drops Löffler methylene blue.
3 Mix with a wooden applicator stick.
4 Allow to stand 2–3 minutes.
5 Examine for neutrophils under high power.

Microscopic Examination of Feces

Microscopic screening of fecal smears is performed to detect the presence of leukocytes associated with microbial diarrhea and undigested muscle fibers and fats associated with steatorrhea.

FECAL LEUKOCYTES

Leukocytes, primarily neutrophils, are seen in the feces in conditions that affect the intestinal mucosa, such as ulcerative colitis and bacterial dysentery. Microscopic screening is performed as a preliminary test to determine whether diarrhea is being caused by invasive bacterial pathogens including *Salmonella, Shigella, Campylobacter, Yersinia,* and enteroinvasive *Escherichia coli.* Bacteria that cause diarrhea by toxin production, such as *Staphylococcus aureus* and *Vibrio* sp., viruses, and parasites usually do not cause the appearance of fecal leukocytes. Therefore, the presence or absence of fecal neutrophils can provide the physician with diagnostic information prior to the receiving of a culture report.

Specimens can be examined as wet preparations stained with methylene blue or as dried smears stained with Wright's or Gram stain. Methylene blue staining is the faster procedure but may be more difficult to interpret. Dried preparations stained with either Wright's or Gram stains provide permanent slides for evaluation. An additional advantage of the Gram stain is the observation of gram-positive and gram-negative bacteria, which could aid in the initial treatment.[8] All slide preparations must be performed on fresh specimens. When examining preparations under high power, as few as three neutrophils per high power field can be indicative of an invasive condition.[1] Using oil immersion, the finding of any neutrophils has approximately 70 percent sensitivity for the presence of invasive bacteria.[10]

A lactoferrin latex agglutination test is available for the detection of fecal leukocytes and remains sensitive in refrigerated and frozen specimens. The presence of lactoferrin, a component of granulocyte secondary granules, is indicative of an invasive bacterial pathogen.[9]

MUSCLE FIBERS

Microscopic examination of the feces for the presence of undigested striated muscle fibers can be helpful in the diagnosis and monitoring of patients with ***pancreatic insufficiency***, such as in cases of cystic fibrosis. It is frequently ordered in conjunction with microscopic examinations for fecal fats. Increased amounts of striated fibers may also be seen in biliary obstruction and **gastrocolic fistulas**.

Slides for muscle fiber detection are prepared by emulsifying a small amount of stool in 10 percent alcoholic eosin, which enhances the muscle fiber striations. The entire slide is examined for exactly 5 minutes, and the number of red-stained fibers with well-preserved striations is counted. Care must be taken to correctly classify the fibers observed. Undigested fibers have visible striations running both vertically and horizontally. Partially digested fibers exhibit striations in only one direction, and digested fibers have no visible striations. Only undigested fibers are counted, and the presence of more than 10 is reported as increased.

To produce a representative sample, patients should be instructed to include red meat in their diet prior to collecting the specimen. Specimens should be examined within 24 hours of collection.

QUALITATIVE FECAL FATS

Specimens from suspected cases of steatorrhea can be screened microscopically for the presence of excess fecal fat. The procedure can also be used to monitor patients undergoing treatment for malabsorption disorders.[15] In general, correlation between the qualitative and quantitative fecal fat procedures is good; however, additional unstained phospholipids and cholesterol esters are measured by the quantitative procedure.[6,12] Lipids included in the microscopic examination of feces are neutral fats (triglycerides), fatty acid salts (soaps), fatty acids, and cholesterol. Their presence can be observed microscopically by staining with

PROCEDURE

Muscle Fiber Procedure

1 Emulsify a small amount of stool in two drops of 10% eosin in alcohol.
2 Coverslip and let stand 3 minutes.
3 Examine under high power for 5 minutes.
4 Count the number of undigested fibers.

PROCEDURE

Neutral Fat Stain Procedure

1. Homogenize one part stool with two parts water.
2. Mix emulsified stool with one drop 95% ethyl alcohol on slide.
3. Add two drops saturated Sudan III in 95% ethanol.
4. Mix and coverslip.
5. Examine under high power.
6. Count orange droplets per high-power field.

the dyes Sudan III, Sudan IV, or oil red O, of which Sudan III is the most routinely used. The staining procedure consists of two parts, the neutral fat stain and the split fat stain.

Neutral fats are readily stained by Sudan III and appear as large orange-red droplets, often located near the edge of the coverslip.[14] Observation of more than 60 droplets/hpf can be indicative of steatorrhea; however, the split fat stain representing total fat content can provide a better indication.[4] The breakdown of neutral fats by bacterial lipase and the spontaneous hydrolysis of neutral fats may lower the neutral fat count. This also prevents using comparison of the two slide tests to determine whether maldigestion or malabsorption is causing steatorrhea.

Soaps and fatty acids do not stain directly with Sudan III. Therefore, a second slide must be examined after the specimen has been mixed with acetic acid and heated. Examination of this slide will reveal stained droplets that represent not only the free fatty acids but also the fatty acids produced by hydrolysis of the soaps and the neutral fats. When examining this split fat slide, both the number and size of the fat droplets must be considered. Normal specimens may contain as many as 100 small droplets, less than 4 μm in size, per hpf. The same number of droplets measuring 1 to 8 μm is considered slightly increased, and 100 droplets measuring 6 to 75 μm is increased.[3]

Cholesterol is stained by Sudan III after heating and as the specimen cools forms crystals that can be identified microscopically.

PROCEDURE

Split Fat Stain Procedure

1. Mix emulsified stool with one drop of 36% acetic acid.
2. Add two drops saturated Sudan III.
3. Mix and coverslip.
4. Heat gently almost to boiling.
5. Examine under high power.
6. Count and measure the orange droplets per high-power field.

Chemical Testing of Feces

OCCULT BLOOD

By far the most frequently performed fecal analysis is the chemical screening test for the detection of occult blood. As discussed previously, bleeding in the upper gastrointestinal tract may produce a black, tarry stool, and bleeding in the lower gastrointestinal tract may result in an overtly bloody stool. However, because any bleeding in excess of 2.5 mL/150 g of stool is considered pathologically significant, and no visible signs of bleeding may be present with this amount of blood, fecal occult blood testing (**FOBT**) is necessary. Originally used primarily to test suspected cases of gastrointestinal disease, FOBT has currently become widely used as a mass screening procedure for the early detection of colorectal cancer. Testing for occult blood has a high positive predictive value for detection of colorectal cancer in the early stages and is recommended by the American Cancer Society, particularly for persons older than age 50.

The most frequently encountered screening tests for occult blood are based on detection of the pseudoperoxidase activity of hemoglobin. This is the same principle as the reagent strip test for urinary blood, but uses a different indicator chromogen. The reaction uses the pseudoperoxidase activity of hemoglobin reacting with hydrogen peroxide to oxidize a colorless compound to a colored compound:

$$\text{Hemoglobin} \xrightarrow[\text{Peroxidase}]{\text{Pseudo}} H_2O_2 \xrightarrow{(0)} \text{Guaiac} \rightarrow \underset{\text{(Blue color)}}{\text{Oxidized guaiac}} + H_2O$$

Several different indicator chromagens have been used to detect occult blood. All react in the same chemical manner but vary in their sensitivity. Listed in order of decreasing sensitivity, these compounds include benzidine, ortho-tolidine, and gum guaiac. Contrary to most chemical testing, the least sensitive reagent, guaiac, is preferred for routine testing. Considering that a normal stool can contain up to 2.5 mL of blood, a less sensitive chemical reactant is understandably more desirable. In addition, pseudoperoxidase activity is present from hemoglobin and myoglobin in ingested meat and fish, certain vegetables and fruits, and some intestinal bacteria. Therefore, to prevent false-positive reactions, the sensitivity of the test must be decreased. This can be accomplished by varying the amount and purity of the guaiac reagent used in the test.

Many commercial testing kits are available for occult blood testing with guaiac reagent. The kits contain guaiac-impregnated filter paper, to which the fecal specimen and hydrogen peroxide are added. Two or three filter paper areas are provided for application of material taken from different areas of the stool, and positive and negative controls are also included. Obtaining samples from the center of the stool will avoid false-positives from external contamination. Addition of hydrogen peroxide to the back of the filter paper that contains stool produces a blue color with guaiac reagent when pseudoperoxidase activity is present.

Packaging of the guaiac-impregnated filter paper in individually sealed containers has facilitated the screening pro-

Summary of Occult Blood Testing Interference

False-Positive

Aspirin and anti-inflammatory medications
Red meat
Horseradish
Raw broccoli, cauliflower, radishes, turnips
Melons
Menstrual and hemorrhoid contamination

False-Negative

Vitamin C >250 mg/d
Iron supplements containing vitamin C

gram for colorectal cancer by allowing persons at home to place the specimen on the filter paper and bring or mail it to the laboratory for testing. To prevent false-positive reactions, specimens mailed to the laboratory should not be rehydrated prior to adding the hydrogen peroxide, unless specifically instructed by the kit manufacturer (Hemocult II Sansa, Smith Kline Diagnostics, Sunnyvale, CA). Specimens applied to the paper in the laboratory should be allowed to dry prior to testing. The specimens should be tested within 6 days of collection. Two samples from three different stools should be tested before a negative result is confirmed. Patients should be instructed to avoid eating red meats, horseradish, melons, raw broccoli, cauliflower, radishes, and turnips for 3 days prior to specimen collection. This will prevent the presence of dietary pseudoperoxidases in the stool. Aspirin and nonsteroidal anti-inflammatory agents, other than acetaminophen, should not be taken for 7 days prior to specimen collection to prevent possible gastrointestinal irritation. Vitamin C and iron supplements containing vitamin C should be avoided for 3 days prior to collections, because ascorbic acid is a strong reducing agent that will interfere with the peroxidase reaction.[7]

Additional more sensitive and specific methods for the detection of occult blood have been developed. Hemoquant (Smith Kline Diagnostics, Sunnyvale, CA) provides a fluorometric test for hemoglobin and porphyrin. As hemoglobin progresses through the intestinal tract, bacterial actions degrade it to porphyrin that the guaiac test cannot detect. This can result in some false-negative results from upper gastrointestinal bleeding when using the guaiac test. The immunologic tests, HemeSelect and FlexSure OBT (Smith Kline Diagnostics, Sunnyvale, CA) are specific for human hemoglobin and do not require dietary restrictions. They are more sensitive to lower gastrointestinal bleeding and can be used for patients who are taking aspirin and other anti-inflammatory medications. Collection kits are similar to those used for guaiac testing and can be provided to patients for home collection.

QUANTITATIVE FECAL FAT TESTING

Quantitative fecal fat analysis is used as a confirmatory test for steatorrhea. As discussed previously, quantitative fecal analysis requires the collection of at least a 3-day specimen.

PROCEDURE

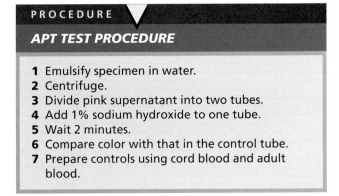

APT TEST PROCEDURE

1 Emulsify specimen in water.
2 Centrifuge.
3 Divide pink supernatant into two tubes.
4 Add 1% sodium hydroxide to one tube.
5 Wait 2 minutes.
6 Compare color with that in the control tube.
7 Prepare controls using cord blood and adult blood.

The patient must also maintain a regulated intake of fat (100 g/d) prior to and during the collection period. Paint cans make excellent collection containers because the specimen must be homogenized prior to analysis, and this can be accomplished by placing the container on a conventional paint-can shaker. The method routinely used for fecal fat measurement is the Van de Kamer titration, although gravimetric methods are available.[14] Fecal lipids are converted to fatty acids and titrated to a neutral end point with sodium hydroxide. The fat content is reported as grams of fat or the coefficient of fat retention per 24 hours. Normal values based on a 100 g/d intake are 1 to 6 g/d or a coefficient of fat retention of at least 95 percent. The coefficient of fat retention is calculated as follows:

$$\frac{(\text{dietary fat} - \text{fecal fat})}{(\text{dietary fat})} \times 100$$

APT TEST (FETAL HEMOGLOBIN)

Grossly bloody stools and vomitus are sometimes seen in neonates as the result of swallowing maternal blood during delivery. Should it be necessary to distinguish between the presence of fetal blood or maternal blood in an infant's stool or vomitus, the Apt test may be requested.

The material to be tested is emulsified in water to release hemoglobin, and after centrifugation, 1 percent sodium hydroxide is added to the pink hemoglobin-containing supernatant. In the presence of alkali-resistant fetal hemoglobin, the solution will remain pink, whereas denaturation of the maternal hemoglobin will produce a yellow-brown supernatant after standing for 2 minutes. The Apt test distinguishes not only between fetal hemoglobin and hemoglobin A but also between maternal hemoglobins AS, CS, and SS and fetal hemoglobin. The presence of maternal thalassemia major would produce erroneous results owing to the high concentration of hemoglobin F. Stool specimens should be tested when fresh. They may appear bloody but should not be black and tarry, because this would indicate already denatured hemoglobin.[2]

FECAL ENZYMES

Enzymes supplied to the gastrointestinal tract by the pancreas are essential for the digestion of dietary proteins,

TABLE 15–3 **Summary of Fecal Screening Tests**

Test	Methodology/Principle	Interpretation
Examination for neutrophils	Microscopic count of neutrophils in smear stained with methylene blue, Gram stain, or Wright's stain	Three per high-power field indicates condition affecting intestinal wall
Qualitative fecal fats	Microscopic examination of direct smear stained with Sudan III	60 large orange-red droplets indicates malabsorption
	Microscopic examination of smear heated with acetic acid and Sudan III	100 orange-red droplets measuring 6–75 µm indicates malabsorption
Occult blood	Pseudoperoxidase activity of hemoglobin liberates oxygen from hydrogen peroxide to oxidize guaiac reagent	Blue color indicates gastrointestinal bleeding
Apt test	Addition of sodium hydroxide to hemoglobin-containing emulsion determines presence of maternal or fetal blood	Pink color indicates presence of fetal blood
Trypsin	Emulsified specimen placed on x-ray paper determines ability to digest gelatin	Inability to digest gelatin indicates lack of trypsin
Clinitest	Addition of Clinitest tablet to emulsified stool detects presence of reducing substances	Reaction of 0.5 g/dL reducing substances suggests carbohydrate intolerance

carbohydrates, and fats. A decrease in production of these enzymes (pancreatic insufficiency) is associated with disorders such as chronic pancreatitis and cystic fibrosis. Steatorrhea and the presence of undigested foodstuffs are present in the feces.

Analysis of the feces focuses primarily on the proteolytic enzymes, trypsin, chymotrypsin, and elastase I. Historically, absence of trypsin has been screened for by exposing x-ray paper to stool emulsified in water. When trypsin is present in the stool, it will digest the gelatin on the paper, leaving a clear area. Inability to digest the gelatin indicates a deficiency in trypsin production. The gelatin test is an insensitive procedure that detects only severe cases of pancreatic insufficiency. In addition, false-negative results may occur as the result of intestinal degradation of trypsin and the possible presence of trypsin inhibitors in the feces. The proteolytic activity of bacteria enzymes may produce false-positive results in old specimens.

Fecal chymotrypsin is more resistant to intestinal degradation and is a more sensitive indicator of less severe cases of pancreatic insufficiency. It also will remain stable in fecal specimens for up to 10 days at room temperature. Chymotrypsin is capable of gelatin hydrolysis but is most frequently measured by spectrophotometric methods.

Elastase I is an isoenzyme of the enzyme elastase and is the enzyme form that the pancreas produces. It is present in high concentrations in pancreatic secretions and is strongly resistant to degradation. Elastase I can be measured by immunoassay and provides a very sensitive indicator of pancreatic insufficiency.[11,13]

CARBOHYDRATES

The presence of increased carbohydrates in the stool will produce an osmotic diarrhea. Carbohydrates in the feces may be present as a result of intestinal inability to reabsorb carbohydrates, as is seen in celiac disease, or caused by lack of digestive enzymes such as lactase resulting in lactose intolerance. Carbohydrate malabsorption or intolerance (maldigestion) is primarily analyzed by serum and urine tests; however, an increased concentration of carbohydrate can be detected by performing a copper reduction test on the fecal specimen. Fecal carbohydrate testing is most valuable in assessing cases of infant diarrhea and may be accompanied by a pH determination. Normal stool pH is between 7 and 8; however, increased use of carbohydrates by intestinal bacteria will lower the pH to below 5.5 in cases of carbohydrate disorders.

The copper reduction test is performed using a Clinitest tablet (Bayer Diagnostics, Elkhart, IN) and one part stool emulsified in two parts water. A result of 0.5 g/dL is considered indicative of carbohydrate intolerance. As discussed in Chapter 5, this is a general test for the presence of reducing substances, and a positive result would be followed by more specific serum carbohydrate tolerance tests, the most common being the D-xylose test for malabsorption and the lactose tolerance test for maldigestion.

A summary of fecal screening tests is presented in Table 15–3.

REFERENCES

1. Bradley, GM: Fecal analysis: Much more than an unpleasant necessity. Diagn Med 3(2):64–75, 1980.
2. Croak, M: Haemoglobin in stools from neonates: Measurement by a modified Apt test. Med Lab Sci 48(4):346–350, 1991.
3. Drummey, GD, Benson, JA, and Jones, CM: Microscopic examination of the stool for steatorrhea. N Engl J Med 264:85–87, 1961.
4. Freeman, JA, and Beeler, MF: Laboratory Medicine: Urinalysis and Medical Microscopy. Lea & Febiger, Philadelphia, 1983.
5. Kao, YS, Liu, FJ, and Alexander, DR: Laboratory diagnosis of gastrointestinal tract and exocrine pancreatic disorders. In Henry, JB (ed): Clinical Diagnosis and Management by Laboratory Methods. WB Saunders, Philadelphia, 1996.
6. Khouri, MR, Huang, G, and Shiau, YF: Sudan stain of fecal fat: New insight into an old test. Gastroenterology 96(2 Pt 1):421–427, 1990.

7. Knight, KK, Fielding, JE, and Battista, RN: Occult blood screening for colorectal cancer. JAMA 261:587–590, 1989.
8. Koepke, JA: Tips from the clinical experts. MLO Sept. p. 15, 1995.
9. McCray, WH, and Krevsky, B: Diagnosing diarrhea in adults: A practical approach. Hosp Med 34(4):27–36, 1998.
10. Novak, R, et al: How useful are fecal neutrophil determinations? Lab Med 26(11):433, 1995.
11. Phillips, IJ, et al: Faecal elastase I: A marker of exocrine pancreatic insufficiency in cystic fibrosis. Ann Clin Chem 36:739–742, 1999.
12. Simko, V: Fecal fat microscopy. Am J Gastroenterol 75(3):204–208, 1981.
13. Thorne, D, and O'Brien, C: Diagnosing chronic pancreatitis. Advance 12(14):8–12, 2000.
14. Van de Kamer, JH, et al: A rapid method for determination of fat in feces. J Biol Chem 177:347–355, 1949.
15. Walters, MP, et al: Clinical monitoring of steatorrhea in cystic fibrosis. Arch Dis Child 65:99–102, 1990.

STUDY QUESTIONS

1. In what part of the digestive tract do pancreatic enzymes and bile salts contribute to digestion?
2. What is the primary digestive process taking place in the large intestine?
3. State whether the following tests are performed to detect secretory or osmotic diarrhea: fecal fats, Clinitest, fecal neutrophils, and muscle fiber examination.
4. State three methods of collection by which the laboratory might receive specimens for occult blood testing.
5. Why is a 3-day specimen recommended for quantitative fecal testing?
6. How can a laboratory accident be avoided when a quantitative fecal collection is received?
7. How does blockage of the bile duct affect the color and appearance of a stool? Why do these changes occur?
8. How does the significance of a bloody stool differ from that of a black, tarry stool?
9. A patient being treated for a sinus infection produces a green-colored stool. Is this significant? Why or why not?
10. State a pathologic and nonpathologic cause of mucus-containing stools.
11. Why does constipation cause production of small, hard stools?
12. What is the significance of fecal neutrophils?
13. Would the presence of fecal neutrophils be expected with diarrhea caused by a rotavirus? *Salmonella*?
14. How can a fecal specimen that has been refrigerated overnight be tested for the presence of neutrophils?
15. Describe the appearance of a microscopic slide that is positive for muscle fibers. What other microscopic test might be requested?
16. How does performance of microscopic examination for triglycerides differ from that performed to detect fatty acids?
17. Describe a slide that is positive for neutral fats and one that is positive for fatty acids.
18. Why is guaiac the reagent of choice for fecal occult blood testing? What is the principle of this test?
19. What is the recommended number of samples that should be tested to confirm a negative occult blood result? From what part of the stool should the samples be taken? Why?
20. What are the advantages of the Hemoquant and the FlexSure FOBT tests over the guaiac test? Which is more sensitive to upper gastrointestinal bleeding? Why?
21. Define steatorrhea. Would a coefficient of fat retention of 85 percent be considered indicative of steatorrhea? Why or why not?
22. What is the significance of an Apt test that remains pink after addition of sodium hydroxide?
23. Is failure of a stool sample to digest the gelatin on x-ray film associated with pancreatic insufficiency? How could you confirm that this is not a false-negative result?
24. What would cause the pH of a specimen collected in a case of infant diarrhea to be low?
25. State two reasons why increased carbohydrates may be present in a stool.

CASE STUDIES AND CLINICAL SITUATIONS

1. Microscopic screening of a stool from a patient exhibiting prolonged diarrhea shows increased fecal neutrophils and normal qualitative fecal fats and meat fibers.
   a. What type of diarrhea do these results suggest?
   b. Name an additional test that could provide more diagnostic information.
   c. Name one probable result for this test and one improbable result.
   d. If the test for fecal neutrophils was negative and the fecal fat concentration increased, what type of diarrhea is suggested?
2. Laboratory studies are being performed on a 5-year-old boy to determine whether there is a metabolic reason for his continued failure to gain weight. In addition to having blood drawn, the patient has a sweat chloride collected, provides a random stool sample, and is asked to collect a 72-hour stool sample.
   a. How can the presence of steatorrhea be screened for by testing the random stool sample?
   b. How does this test distinguish among neutral fats, soaps, and fatty acids?

c. What confirmatory test should be performed?
d. Describe the appearance of the stool specimens if steatorrhea is present.
e. If a diagnosis of cystic fibrosis is suspected, state two screening tests that could be performed on a stool specimen to aid in the diagnosis.
f. State a possible reason for a false-negative reaction in each of these tests.
g. What confirmatory test could be performed?

3. A physician's office laboratory is experiencing inconsistencies in the results of patient-collected specimens for FOBT. Patients are instructed to submit samples from two areas of three different stools. Positive and negative controls are producing satisfactory results. Patient #1 is a 30-year-old woman taking over-the-counter medications for gastric reflux who has reported passing frequent black stools. The results of all three specimens are negative for occult blood. Patient #2 is a 70-year-old woman suffering from arthritis. She is taking the test as part of a routine physical. The results of all three specimens are positive for occult blood. Patient #3 is a 50-year-old man advised by the doctor to lose 30 lb. He has been doing well on a high-protein, low-carbohydrate diet. Two of his three specimens are positive for occult blood.
a. What is the possible nonpathologic cause of the unexpected results for patient #1? Patient #2? Patient #3?
b. How could the physician's office staff avoid these discrepancies?
c. What testing methodology could be used for patients #2 and #3?

4. A watery black stool from a neonate is received in the laboratory with requests for an Apt test, fecal pH, and a Clinitest.
a. Can all three tests be performed on this specimen? Why?
b. If the Clinitest is positive, what pH reading can be expected? Why?
c. The infant's hemoglobin remains constant at 18 g/dL. What was the significance of the black stool?
d. Would this infant be expected to have ketonuria? Why or why not?

APPENDIX A

Urinalysis Automation

Studies have shown that the biggest variable in urinalysis testing is the conscientiousness of the laboratory personnel in their interpretations of the color reactions. This subjectivity associated with visual discrimination among colors has been alleviated by the development of automated reagent strip readers that use a spectrophotometric measurement of light reflection termed reflectance photometry. Reflectance photometry uses the principle that light reflection from the test pads decreases in proportion to the intensity of color produced by the concentration of the test substance. A monochromatic light source is directed toward the reagent pads by placing a filter between the light source and the reflective surface of the pad or by using a light-emitting diode (**LED**) to provide the specific wavelength needed for each test pad color reaction. The light is reflected to a photodetector and an analog/digital converter. The instruments compare the amount of light reflection with that of known concentrations and display or print concentration units or transmit data to a laboratory information system (**LIS**). The ultimate goal of automation is to improve reproducibility and color discrimination while increasing productivity and standardization for reporting urinalysis results.

Several automated instruments are currently available to standardize sample processing, analyze test strips, and report results with consistent quality free of visual discrimination. Additional features include on-line computer capability; bar coding; manual entry of color, clarity, and microscopic results to be included on the printed report; flagging of abnormal results, storing of patient and control results; and minimal calibration, cleaning, and maintenance.

Automated instruments in urinalysis include individual strip readers, semiautomated analyzers, fully automated chemistry analyzers, and the complete urinalysis workstations. Semiautomated instruments are still dependent on an operator for specimen mixing, test strip dipping, and inputting physical and microscopic results. The fully automated chemistry analyzers add urine to the reagent strip, and the workstations have a "walk-away" capability for a complete urinalysis.

The major automated chemistry urine analyzers are the Clinitek 50 and 100 strip readers, semiautomated Clinitek 200/200+, Clinitek 500, and the fully automated Clinitek Atlas (Bayer Diagnostics, Elkhart, IN/Dublin, Ireland) as well as the semiautomated Chemstrip 101, Chemstrip Criterion II, Chemstrip Urine Analyzer, and the fully automated Chemstrip Super Automated Urine Analyzer (Roche-Boehringer Mannheim Diagnostics, Indianapolis, IN), and the semiautomated Rapimat II/T (Behring Diagnostics Inc. Somerville, NJ). A variety of International Remote Imaging Systems workstations are available (Chatsworth, CA). All instruments use reflectance photometry to determine each analyte concentration. The automated urinalysis instruments currently available are listed in Table A–1.

The Bayer Clinitek 50 and 100 strip readers are well suited for small volume laboratories and physician's offices (Figure A–1) and meet the Clinical Laboratory Improvement Amendments (CLIA)-waived standards. Reagent strips are manually dipped and placed on the strip reader, and results are displayed or printed. Patient identification and specimen color and clarity may be manually entered, abnormal results may be flagged, up to 100 test results may be stored in memory, and computer interfacing is available. An additional feature of these strip readers is their ability to provide automated reading of Bayer microalbumin/creatinine and human chorionic gonadotrophin strips.

The Clinitek 200+ is designed for medium-volume to large-volume urine laboratories with a high specimen output of one strip every 10 seconds. Multistix reagent tests strips are used, and the instrument has the ability to report semiquantitative (mg/dL) results or plus (+) and Système International units. All positive results are flagged to indicate a patient sample that requires additional confirmation testing or microscopic evaluation. The operator manually enters urine color and clarity observations and the patient identification number from a keyboard or an optional barcode reader. Bidirectional interface is available to upload and download patient identification information with the host computer. The reflectometer is calibrated daily and

TABLE A–1 **Urinalysis Automation**

Equipment	Manufacturer
Semiautomated Chemistry Instruments	
Clinitek 200/200+	Bayer Diagnostics
Clinitek 500	Bayer Diagnostics
Chemstrip 101	Roche-Boehringer Mannheim Diagnostics
Chemstrip Criterion II	Roche-Boehringer Mannheim Diagnostics
Chemstrip Urine Analyzer	Roche-Boehringer Mannheim Diagnostics
Rapimat II/T	Behring Diagnostics Inc.
Fully Automated Chemistry Instruments	
Clinitek Atlas	Bayer Diagnostics
Chemstrip Super Automated Urine Analyzer	Roche-Boehringer Mannheim Diagnostics
Automated Microscopy	
UF-100 Urine Cell Analyzer	International Remote Imaging Systems
Workstations	
Yellow IRIS	International Remote Imaging Systems
Model 300 Urinalysis Workstation	International Remote Imaging Systems
Model 500 Urinalysis Workstation	International Remote Imaging Systems
Model 939UDx Urine Pathology System	International Remote Imaging Systems

maintenance is required each day for all areas in contact with urine test strips.

The Clinitek 500 is the most recent Bayer benchtop analyzer (Figure A–2). It features an advanced read head design that determines urine color automatically and nonhemolyzed trace blood detection. Specific gravity is measured in 0.005 increments and pH is measured in 0.5 increments. The Clinitek 500 contains a bar-code reader that provides rapid entry of sample identification, color, and clarity values. This instrument includes automatic reagent strip detection, automatic calibration, confirmatory and microscopic sieve functions to flag results for quick review, and a user-friendly interface with a touch-screen display to provide a high-volume throughput of 500 strips per hour. Parameters for each analyte are set at installation to meet laboratory-specific protocol. Memory stores 500 patient results and 200 control results. Results are easily edited and reported by internal storing, transferring to the computer, or by printing. Calibration is automatic and maintenance is minimal.

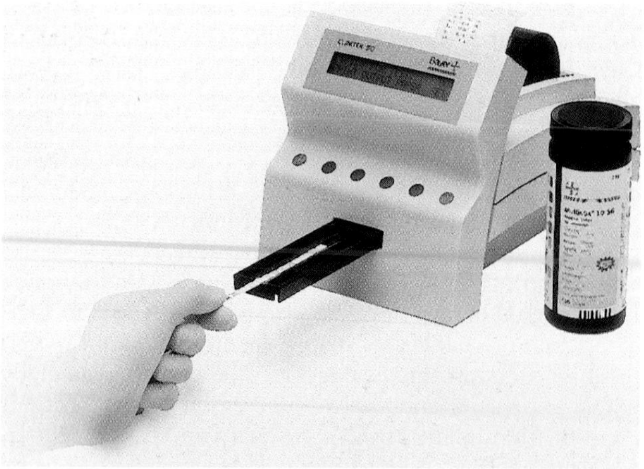

FIGURE A–1 Clinitek 50 Urine Chemistry Analyzer. (Courtesy of Bayer Diagnostics, Elkhart, IN.)

The fully automated Clinitek Atlas, which is designed for a high-volume urinalysis laboratory, performs 12 tests automatically including urine chemistries using reflectance colorimetry, specific gravity using a fiberoptic refractive index method, color, and clarity (Figure A–3). This instrument offers a "walk-away" capability for urine chemistry testing producing a throughput of 225 samples per hour. Regular urine sample tubes are used and can be placed in a circular 50-position tray or in up to 20 (10-position) linear racks that are compatible with the IRIS/Symex UF-100 Urine Cell Analyzer. Two milliliters of urine are required. STATS may be performed at any time. A reagent pack containing a roll of 490 dry chemistry reagents on a continuous roll minimizes reagent handling. An exact volume of urine sample is pipetted onto the reagent test pad. Reagent pads advance automatically to the reflectance photometer to measure the color change of each reagent pad. Reagent pads then advance automatically to the disposal area. The Atlas uses bar-code sample identification and allows abnormal ranges to be selected for identification and flagging of samples requiring microscopic examination or confirmatory testing. One thousand patient results and 200 control results and calibrations are stored for visual display, printout, or transmission to a laboratory computer system. Standardized controls are run as set by laboratory protocol and a 24-hour within-lot calibration is performed.

Roche-Boehringer Mannheim Diagnostics Chemstrip 101 compact urine analyzer provides simple test strip evaluation. It is designed for small laboratories or physician office laboratories and has a 50-test per hour throughput. Test strips are dipped and placed in a tray, and the start button initiates testing. Incubation timing, analyte mea-

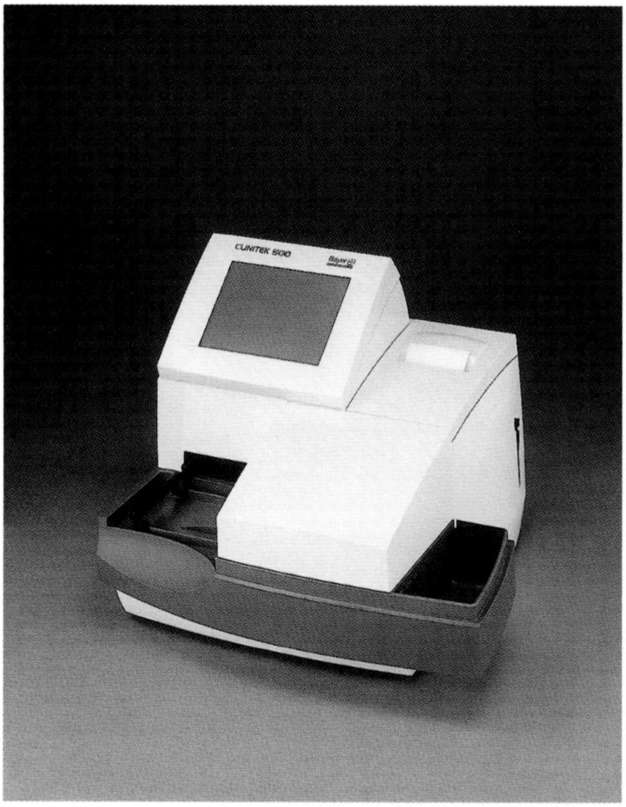

FIGURE A–2 Clinitek 500 Urine Chemistry Analyzer. (Courtesy of Bayer Diagnostics, Dublin, Ireland.)

surement by reflectance photometry, result calculation, and printout are automatic. Software options are available. One hundred patient samples are held in memory, and minimal calibration or maintenance is required. All Roche-Boehringer Mannheim instruments have urine compensation color pads.

The Chemstrip Criterion II, a semiautomated urine test strip analyzer with upgraded software capability, is convenient for mid-sized laboratories. This instrument can measure 100 samples per hour, including urine color, whereas clarity is entered manually. The strip is dipped into the sample and placed on the tray. Test transport, measurement, and disposal are automatic. Individual programming of result ranges, grading, and units is available. Instrument cleaning is minimal and is performed once a day; calibration is required twice a month.

The Chemstrip Urine Analyzer meets the needs of a large urinalysis laboratory by processing 300 strips per hour. It analyzes test strips placed on a transport tray, allows full sample identification, correlates and manages sediment microscopy data, and prints out or transmits results to the laboratory computer system. Bar coding enables microscopic sediment results to be entered and linked to test strip findings and patient data for correlation and patient assessment. Default settings are used to monitor the quality of results. Minimal maintenance is required because the instrument contains a cleaning cycle function and disposable transport and waste trays. Calibration is performed every 2 weeks and printed for a permanent report.

The Chemstrip Super Automated Urine Analyzer is a fully automated "walk-away" urine chemistry instrument with the ability to process 300 samples per hour, thereby meeting the needs of a large urinalysis laboratory. Urine specimens are loaded in a 60-position carousel with 55 routine positions and 5 stat positions. Sample volumes are detected and adjusted, and automatically mixed. A sorter mechanism supplies a single test strip from the sorter drum to a sorter position. A gripping mechanism grasps the test strip and dips it into the urine specimen tube. A sensor attached to a mixing rod determines the volume of urine. The dipping mechanism lifts the test strip out of the sample tube while removing excess urine by dragging the strip along the inside of the specimen tube. The dipping mechanism then transfers the test strip to the reflectance photometer position. A transport plate positions the test strip at the reflectance photometer recording head where the specimen is measured at three different wavelengths (555, 620, 660 nm) at 48 seconds and/or 120 seconds after dipping. The result is converted to a concentration value and printed or transferred to a laboratory computer. An optional built-in bar-code reader is available for patient identification. The instrument is calibrated with a special calibration strip once every 2 weeks. This instrument also is incorporated in the IRIS 939UDx workstation.

The Behring Rapimat II/T is a semiautomated urine chemistry instrument that also corrects for urine color using a blanking pad. Its unique feature is selective thermostatic heating of the leukocyte esterase test pad to enhance the enzymatic reaction. The Rapimat II/T includes a measure of ascorbic acid content to check for possible reaction interference. Strips are placed on a conveyer belt to be taken into the instrument. Results are printed with the physical description and microscopic findings. Abnormal results are flagged as determined by the user. It does have bar-code availability and can store 300 sample results. Maintenance requires weekly cleaning; calibration is required every 1000 tests and is printed for a permanent record.

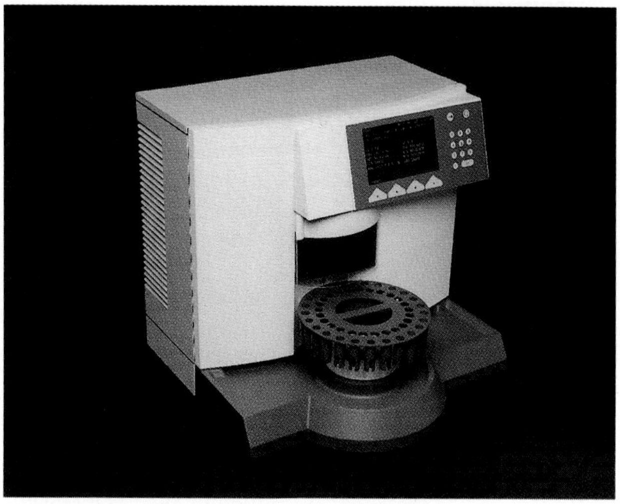

FIGURE A–3 Clinitek Atlas Automated Urine Chemistry Analyzer. (Courtesy of Bayer Diagnostics, Elkhart, IN.)

Automated Microscopy

In a routine urinalysis, a test strip determines the chemical analytes and the formed elements are determined by microscopy. Manual microscopy is not easily standardized because of the high variation among operators even in the same institution. Intensive specimen processing affects accuracy as rare elements such as casts or crystals may be lost during handling. Results are not quantitative because they must be reported in ranges or averages. Overall, manual microscopy is not cost effective because of the poor use of personnel in-batch processing and poor turn-around-time for stats. The development of urinalysis workstations capable of performing microscopic urinalysis has provided a solution to these problems for laboratories with a high volume of urinalysis. The IRIS/Sysmex UF-100 Urine Cell Analyzer is dedicated to microscopic analysis, whereas the Yellow IRIS and its successors, the Model 300 and 500 Workstations and the 939UDx Urine Pathology System (Chatsworth, CA) are designed to perform chemical and microscopic urinalysis.

The IRIS/Sysmex UF-100 Urine Cell Analyzer is designed for large urinalysis laboratories with predominantly normal microscopic results and can process 100 samples per hour. The UF-100 uses laser-based flow cytometry along with impedance detection, light scatter, and fluorescence to identify the individual characteristics and count stained urine sediment particles in a flowing stream. The instrument is easy to operate by placing a 10-position linear rack on the instrument and initiating the autoanalysis with a touch of the screen. Uncentrifuged urine is aspirated into the instrument and the conductivity is measured. The sample is stained with two dyes that radiate an orange and green fluorescence. The DNA within the cells is stained by the orange dye, phenathridine; the nuclear membranes, mitochondria, and negatively charged cell membranes are stained with a green dye, carbocyanine. The stained sample is passed through the flow cell where it is hydrodynamically focused and presented to a laser light beam (488 nm) that produces fluorescence and light scatter. Particles are identified by measuring the change in impedance of the sediment elements as well as the height and width of the fluorescent and light scatter signals, which are presented in scattergrams and histograms. The width of the fluorescent signal measures cellular inclusions and the width of forward light scatter measures the length of cells. Values are presented in a numerical quantitation (cells per microliter) and abnormal results are "flagged" for confirmatory review. An internal quality control system monitors performance. One thousand patient results including scattergrams, histograms, and specimen characteristics are stored. A bidirectional interface is provided to download and report results.

The Models 300 and 500 workstations are self-contained, operator-attended workstations capable of performing specific gravity, routine chemical analysis, and slideless microscopic analysis from an uncentrifuged specimen (Figure A–4). On Models 300 and 500, chemical analysis is performed using Boehringer Mannheim Chemstrip reagent strips and a CHEMSTRIP reflectance photometer. For testing, 6 mL of room temperature urine is required. The patient identification or specimen number is manually entered using a keypad or optional bar-code reader. Color and clarity must be entered or "yellow" and "clear" will automatically be reported. Urine is poured over the strip as it is poured into the instrument for the specific gravity and microscopic, excess urine is blotted by the operator, and the strip is placed on a platform tray and manually transferred to a built-in reflectance reader. Results of the reflectance readings are displayed and reviewed on a video monitor and integrated into the analyzer unit. Urine entering the instrument is divided into two portions for the specific gravity (2 mL) using an IRIS Mass Gravity Meter and to the mixing vessel for the IRIS Slideless Microscope (4 mL). Specific gravity is determined by harmonic oscillation. A standard volume of urine is maintained in a U-shaped tube, and a sound wave of fixed frequency is transmitted into one end of the tube. The change in frequency recorded as the sound wave exits the other end of the tube is directly related to the specific gravity. For microscopic analysis, a stained well-mixed urine specimen is forced in a moving stream through a sheath of envelope fluid into the microscope flow cell at a constant rate (Figure A–5). A process known as hydroplanar positioning forces all particles to flow in a single plane as they pass the optical path of the microscope (Figure A–6). Multiple freeze-frame pictures are taken as a particle passes the microscope and as a high-intensity strobe light flashes; data from these are analyzed by a computer processor as to size and number. Particles are placed into three low-power (100×) and five high-power (400×) groups based on their size, and the low-power and high-power digitized images are presented to the operator on a color monitor. The operator then makes the final identification by touching an appropriate area or category on the monitor screen (Figure A–7). Touch buttons allow any corrections to be made to the computer classification of any particles. When all results are confirmed, the operator touches a button that sends a complete report to the laboratory information system or printer, including patient

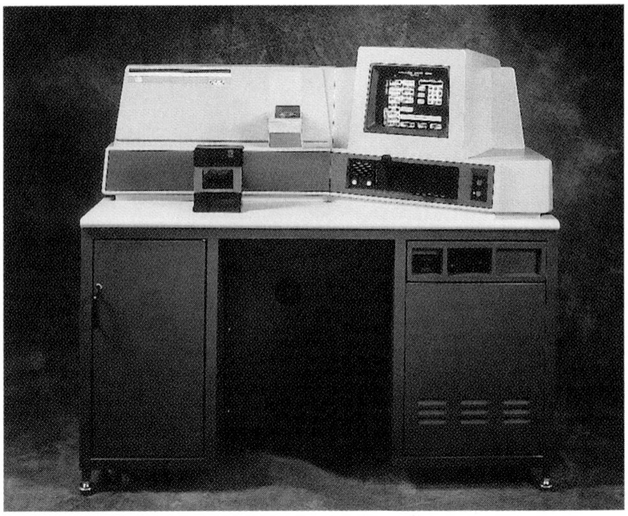

FIGURE A–4 Model 500 Workstation. (Courtesy of International Remote Imaging Systems, Chatsworth, CA.)

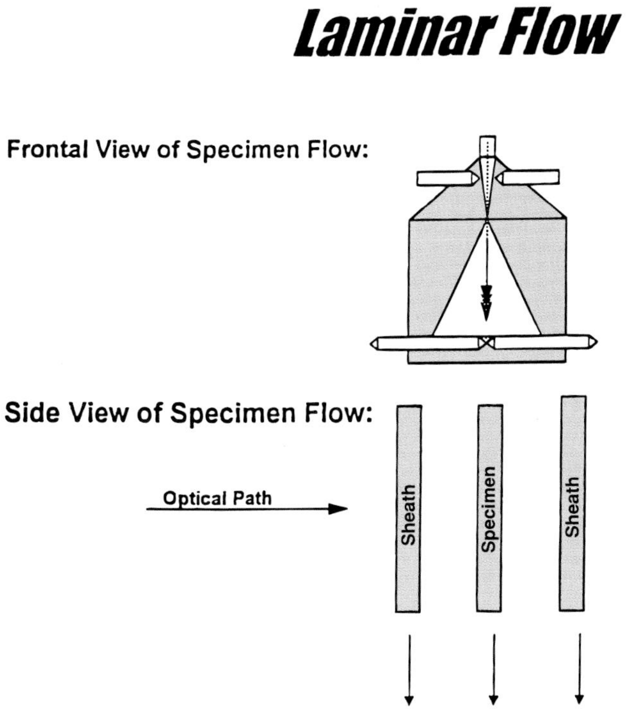

FIGURE A–5 Diagram of laminar flow. (Courtesy of International Remote Imaging Systems, Chatsworth, CA.)

identification, all chemistry results, specific gravity, color, clarity, and microscopic data. Each urine specimen is processed and reported before the next sample may be introduced. Normal samples are complete in 1 minute and abnormal samples with a variety of particles take 2 to 5 minutes. The Model 500 workstation contains a body fluid package to include cerebrospinal, pleural, peritoneal, pericardial, peritoneal lavage, peritoneal dialysate, seminal, and synovial fluids. Calibration is performed daily with calibration strips. Computer capabilities provide the ability to customize reporting units, screen routine samples, report the microscopic examination as negative, perform more extensive microscopic searching on specified patients, store images on floppy disks for later analysis, correct for dilutions, and perform counting and microscopic analysis of other body fluids.

The most sophisticated urinalysis instrument with complete routine urinalysis automation is the 939UDx NNA (neural net automation) Urine Pathology System. Designed for medium to large urinalysis laboratories, the 939UDx is the only automated analyzer that can automatically perform, classify, and report all aspects of a complete urinalysis. The system consists of three components to perform fully automated chemistry test strip results, specific gravity, color and clarity, and microscopic sampling from bar-coded sample tubes on uncentrifuged urine by loading the sample carousel only once. The three components are the Roche-Boehringer Mannheim Chemstrip Super Urin-

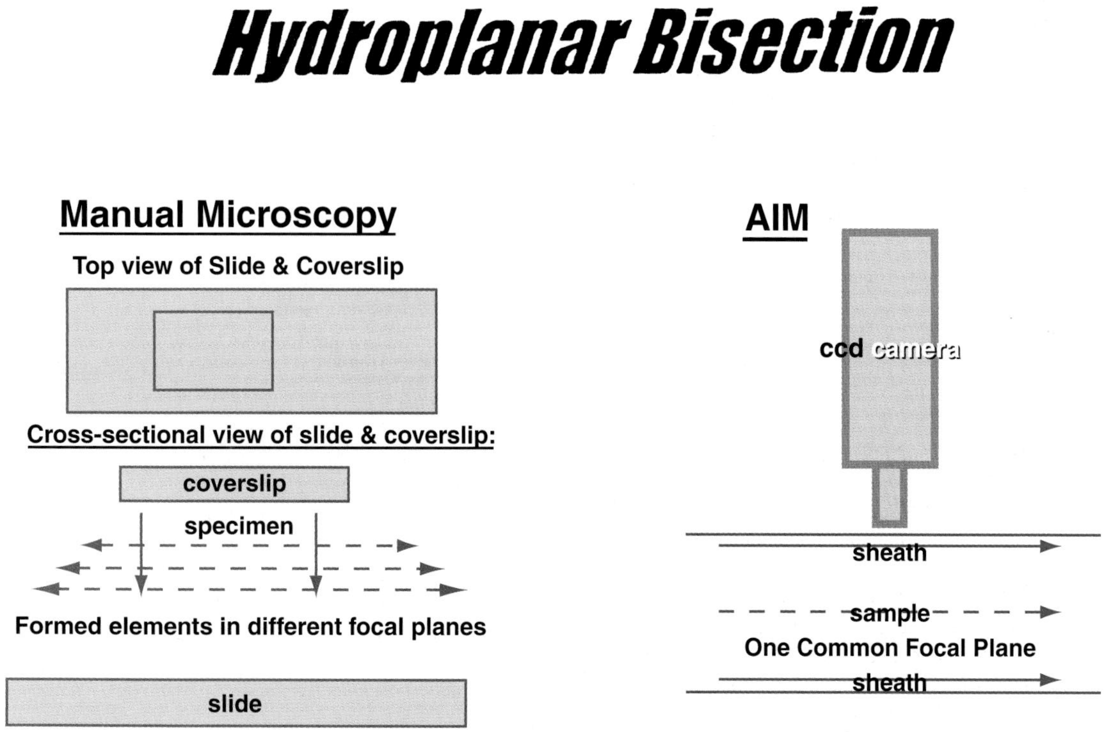

FIGURE A–6 Diagram of hydroplanar positioning. (Courtesy of International Remote Imaging Systems, Chatsworth, CA.)

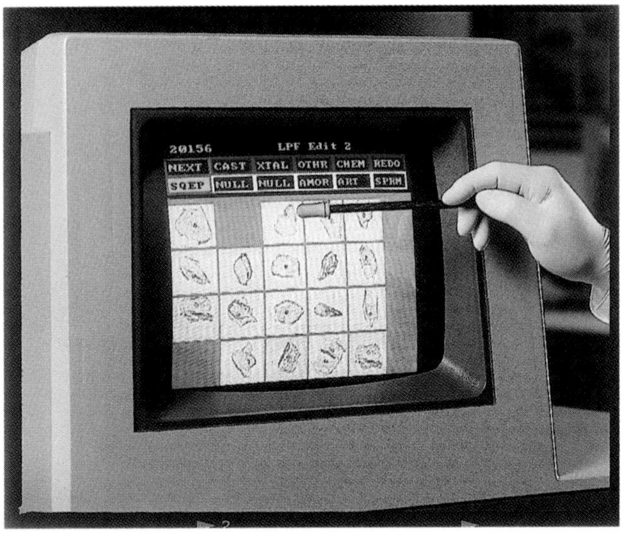

FIGURE A–7 Operator editing workstation screen. (Courtesy of International Remote Imaging Systems, Chatsworth, CA.)

alysis Analyzer, the IRIS Flow Microscope Analyzer, and the IRIS ViewStation, all interlinked to provide a complete urinalysis (Figure A–8).

Neural net automation software included in the instrument automatically counts and classifies particles as RBCs, WBCs, bacteria, squamous epithelial cells, nonsquamous epithelial cells, hyaline casts, nonhyaline casts, yeast, crystals, sperm, mucus, WBC clumps, and amorphous. Constituents must meet a predefined minimum concentration to be included in the autoclassification. Laboratories can program the neural net software to block autoreporting of results based on both concentration and types of constituents present.

The instrument can process batches of up to 55 urine samples and process up to 250 specimens without microscopics per hour. The minimum amount of urine required is 7 mL; of this specimen, 3 mL is transported to the Mass Gravity Meter for specific gravity determination and the remaining 4 mL is transported to the sample chamber for staining prior to microscopic imaging. Plastic, glass, or KOVA-style tubes are used. Special pediatric tubes are available for specimens of 3.5 to 6.5 mL. Specimens less than 3.5 mL cannot be run. Uncentrifuged urine specimens are placed in bar-coded tubes and placed into any position of a sample disk carousel with the bar code placed correctly toward the periphery of the carousel. The carousel is placed into the autosampler of the Super UA (Super Urinalysis Analyzer).

With the touch of a button, the Super Urinalysis Analyzer automatically processes test strips and can complete a disk cycle in 12 minutes. As each tube bar code is scanned, a mixing rod mixes the urine and a test strip is dipped into each tube for wetting and placed in the photometer. As each measurement is complete, the result is sent to the ViewStation. After completion of testing for the batch, the carousel is removed from the Super Urinalysis Analyzer and transferred to the Flow Microscope autosampler. After aspiration by the autosampler, the specimen goes to the vacuum chamber where color and clarity are measured; then the sample is delivered into the sample chamber, where it is mixed automatically with stain as the specimen is prepared for microscopy. The stained sample and sheath fluid enter the flow cell at the same rate, then pass into the

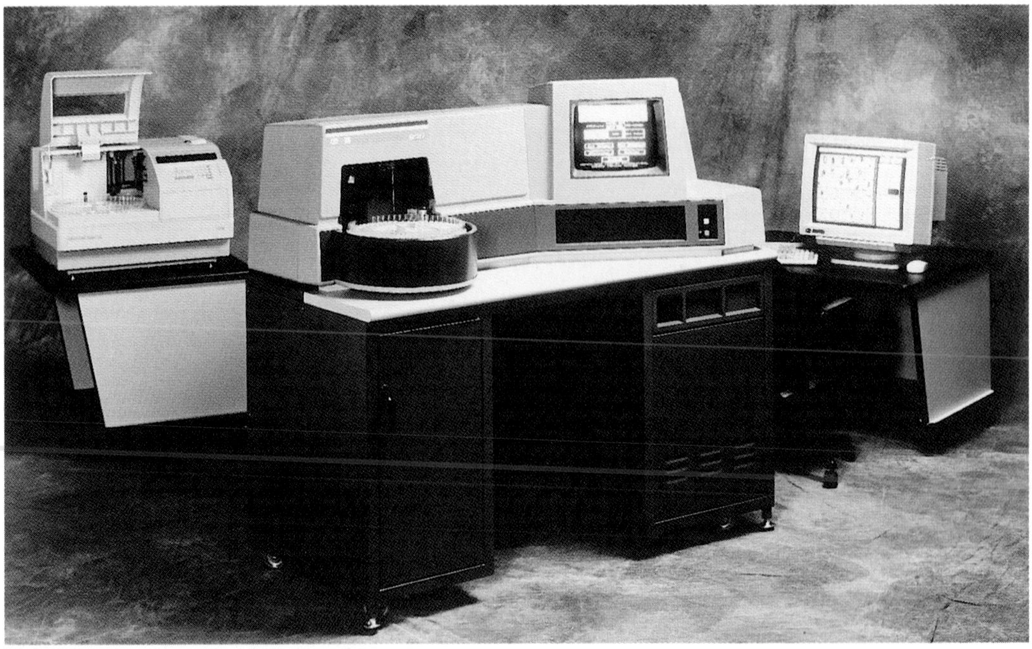

FIGURE A–8 Model 939UDx Urine Pathology System. (Courtesy of International Remote Imaging Systems, Chatsworth, CA.)

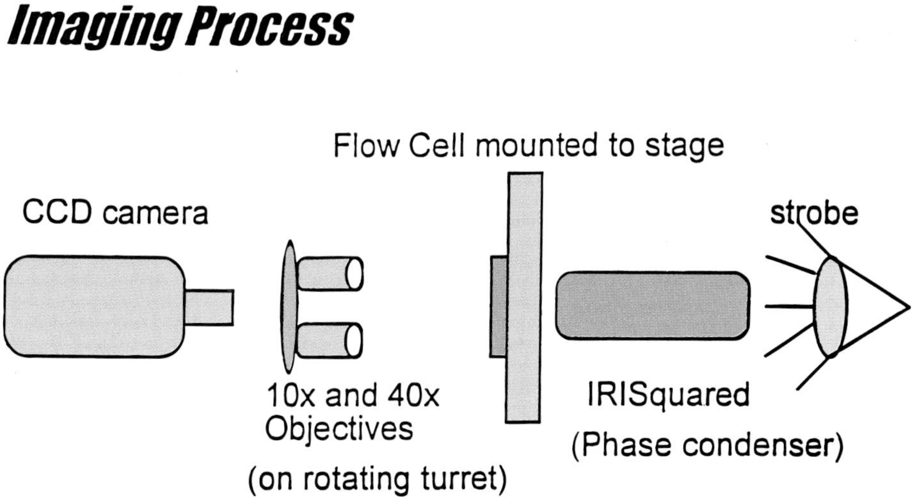

FIGURE A–9 Low-power and high-power imaging process. (Courtesy of International Remote Imaging Systems, Chatsworth, CA.)

IRIS Slideless Microscope, where analytes are oriented and imaged by a video camera. The composition of the sheath fluid and the pressure within the system aids in the hydrodynamic orientation of the sample to obtain maximum exposure of particles to the IRIS Slideless Microscope. As the sheath fluid envelopes the sample, a laminar flow is created that causes the widest cross-section of the particles to face the optical path. As these particles are transported through the flow chamber, the maximum area is bisected by the optical path, creating a planar view on one focal plane. The sample is illuminated with a strobe lamp and viewed with the video camera. As the stream of specimen is illuminated by the strobe lamp, the flashing of the strobe lamp freezes the motion of urine particles. The stop motion pictures are viewed by the 10× and 40× objectives and captured by the video camera as images (Figure A–9). Low-power and high-power examinations are used in the same manner as traditional microscopic procedures.

The particles captured by the video camera are analyzed by the image processor and sorted into groups or ranks, based on particle size. The image data are digitized and sent to the ViewStation computer, where image processing and classifying are finalized and presorted images are displayed for operator review. The image data are logged into the specimen records in the database in hard disk memory. The ViewStation database assembles and consolidates all result

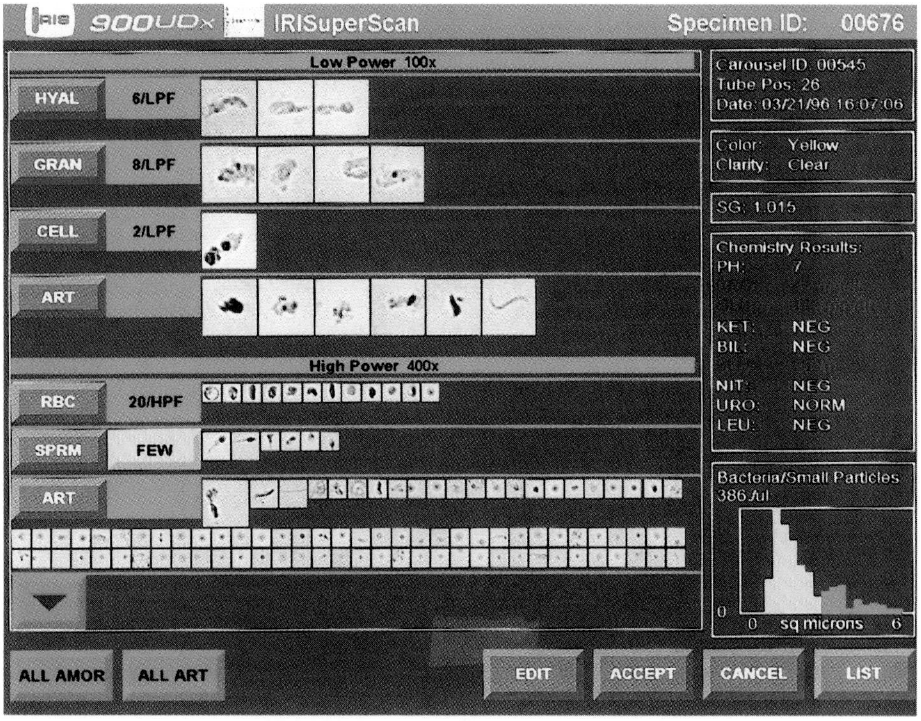

FIGURE A–10 Model 939UDx viewing screen. (Courtesy of International Remote Imaging Systems, Chatsworth, CA.)

information for each specimen from the Super UA and the FlowMicroscope, and displays all the relevant information on the touch screen monitor. Microscopic images, color and clarity, specific gravity chemistry results, and the bacteria histograms are presented to the operator for visual review and editing. Small-particle histograms are a graphic display of size distribution of any small sediment particles (ranging from 1 to 6 μm^2) found during the microscopic examination. The histograms help to decide whether bacteria are present in these small size ranges or if the detected particles are small crystals or amorphous. Results are quantitated as a numerical result or as a graded result with the exception of bacteria. The operator interacts with the monitor to review and confirm analyte images and can edit results at any time (Figure A–10). Abnormal results are flagged according to laboratory specifications. The printer generates a final report. Manual confirmation is needed to identify the types of inclusion casts, nonsquamous epithelial cells and crystals, to verify motility and the flagella of *Trichomonas*, and to confirm fat globules.

The ViewStation software includes specimen tracking, editing, quality control, display configuration, flagging, and archiving/backup features. The Intel Pentium ViewStation computer offers "off-line" result review and release, so that operators in different locations can access each module of the 939UDx.

Calibration on the Super Urinalysis Analyzer is performed every 2 weeks using a calibration strip. The Flow Microscope, specific gravity, color and clarity subsystems are factory calibrated and monitored by the "self test" program. Maintenance is minimal and automatically performed with the start-up self-test procedures.

Additional Information Sources

Bayer Diagnostics: http://www.bayerdiag.com/products.

International Remote Imaging Systems: http://www.proiris.com/irisbus/products/urinalysis.

Roche-Boehringer Mannheim Diagnostics: http://www.boehringer-mannheim.com/rapid/urinalysis.

Answer Keys

Answers to Study Questions

CHAPTER 1

1. **Biologic hazards:** infectious microorganisms; **sharp hazards:** needles, lancets, broken glass; **chemical hazards:** reagents, preservatives; **radioactive hazards:** radioisotopes; **electrical hazards:** instrumentation; **fire/explosive hazards:** Bunsen burners, organic chemicals; **physical hazards:** wet floors, heavy objects.
2. **Source:** urine specimen; **mode of transmission:** spills, ungloved hands, failure to wash hands, uncapped centrifuge tubes; **host:** laboratory worker.
3. To protect health-care workers from exposure to blood-borne pathogens.
4. Universal Precautions; only specimens containing visible blood are covered.
5. OSHA
6. Yes. The worker may have developed an allergy to latex, which could result in an anaphylactic reaction.
7. Protection of laboratory workers from possible urine splashes and aerosols.
8. Drying the hands and turning off the water.
9. Urine
10. Towels are discarded in a biohazard container and the counter is cleaned with sodium hypochlorite diluted 1:5 or 1:10.
11. In a puncture-resistant container.
12. Immediately flush the area with water.
13. Hydrochloric acid is added to water to prevent possible splashing.
14. Consult the MSDS.
15. The MSDS and Chemical Hygiene Plan are on file in the workplace; NFPA symbols are placed on doors, cabinets, and containers.
16. Extremely dangerous to health, extremely flammable, may deteriorate, avoid use of water.
17. When the worker is pregnant.
18. Turn off the circuit breaker, unplug the source, move the source using glass or wood.
19. Rescue, alarm, contain, and extinguish.
20. Class A: wood, paper, cloth.

CHAPTER 2

1. Tubular reabsorption and secretion.
2. Filtration is controlled only by particle size.
3. The glomerular endothelial cells contain pores.
4. When blood pressure decreases, renin is produced to stimulate the retention of sodium.
5. A solution containing the same concentration of low-molecular-weight substances as plasma.
6. **Active transport:** glucose, amino acids, sodium, chloride, phosphorus, calcium; **passive transport**: water, urea.
7. When the blood level of that substance reaches its renal threshold.
8. Water is passively reabsorbed from the descending loop and sodium and chloride are actively reabsorbed from the ascending loop; the walls of the ascending loop are impermeable to water, which maintains the osmotic gradient of the medulla.
9. The permeability of the walls of the collecting duct to water is controlled by ADH in response to body hydration.
10. Increased
11. Tubular secretion.
12. Hydrogen
13. Secretion of hydrogen ions facilitates the reabsorption of bicarbonate ions.
14. The pH is consistently alkaline.
15. **Endogenous substances:** urea, creatinine, $beta_2$ microglobulin; **exogenous substances:** inulin, radionucleotides.
16. Creatinine clearance results are lowered.
17. 100 mL/min
18. The results must be corrected for body size.

19. Healthy glomeruli are capable of increasing their filtering capacity in response to a decrease in functional glomeruli.
20. Renal concentration is regulated by body hydration.
21. Osmolarity represents the number of particles present and is not influenced by particle size and density.
22. Freezing point and vapor pressure depression.
23. Vapor pressure osmometer.
24. Normal
25. C_{osm} = 0.5 mL/min; C_{H_2O} = + 1.5 mL/min and excretion of excess water.
26. Adequate renal blood flow must be present for nonfiltered substances to reach the capillaries for secretion.
27. 600 mL/min
28. Approximately 8 percent of the renal blood flow does not come in contact with functional renal tissue.
29. The inability to produce an acid urine in the presence of metabolic acidosis.
30. Increased

CHAPTER 3

1. Urine is easily collected and testing methods are relatively inexpensive.
2. Water
3. Urea
4. Test the fluid for a high concentration of urea or creatinine.
5. Anuria, oliguria, polyuria.
6. Diabetes mellitus.
7. Disposable containers are less likely to be contaminated and a 50-mL capacity provides the appropriate size for adequate specimen volume and for specimen mixing.
8. Labeling two specimens at the same time and mixing up the labels.
9. Unlabeled specimen; specimen and accompanying requisition do not match; contaminated specimen or container; insufficient quantity; improper transportation or preservation.
10. Turbidity; pH; nitrite.
11. Increased bacteria; decreased red blood cells; decreased casts.
12. Increased bacterial growth and metabolism.
13. Protein; bilirubin, urobilinogen, leukocyte esterase.
14. Refrigeration inhibits bacterial growth, and no chemical preservatives are required.
15. Boric acid only affects pH.
16. No. The sodium fluoride preservative in the gray-top tube will interfere with the reagent strip glucose reaction.
17. A first morning specimen is the most concentrated, resulting in better detection of abnormal constituents.
18. Falsely elevated
19. Midstream clean-catch; catheterized; suprapubic aspiration.
20. The COC form documents that the specimen collected by the patient is the same one that is analyzed and reported.

CHAPTER 4

1. Urochrome is produced and excreted at a constant rate, so its concentration is affected only by the amount of water present in the urine.
2. **Yellow foam:** bilirubin; **white foam:** protein.
3. The thick yellow-orange pigment in phenazopyridine masks reagent strip color reactions.
4. The urine contains increased RBCs.
5. Myoglobin is more rapidly cleared from the plasma than is hemoglobin.
6. Urine containing porphyrins that has been exposed to air.
7. The specimen contains hemoglobin that has been oxidized to methemoglobin. This may be seen in old specimens or in fresh specimens as a result of glomerular bleeding.
8. Oxidation of melanogen to melanin produces a black urine; homogentisic acid turns black in alkaline urine.
9. Urinary and intestinal tract infections may produce blue or green urine. Breath deodorizers (Clorets), methocarbamol (Robaxin), amitriptyline (Elavil), and methylene blue may produce blue or green urine.
10. Amorphous phosphates produce a white precipitate and amorphous urates produce a pink precipitate; the precipitation is pH dependent.
11. To dissolve amorphous urates.
12. The specimen will contain fewer contaminating structures, and clarity will better represent the actual urine.
13. When a chemical test(s) for protein, RBCs, orWBCs, or bacteria is positive.
14. Microscopic
15. The density of a solution compared with the density of a similar volume of distilled water.
16. Yes. Because substances not dissolved in the urine do not contribute to the specific gravity.

17. Significant pathologic constituents may not be detected in a dilute specimen.
18. Specific gravity is influenced by the size of the molecules, such as urea, glucose, and protein that are not significant in renal concentration.
19. Requires a large volume of urine; requires temperature correction; user interpretation is subjective.
20. The refractometer reading of distilled water is adjusted to 1.000 using the set screw and calibration is checked with 5 percent sodium chloride or 9 percent sucrose for readings of 1.022 and 1.034 ± .001, respectively.
21. The specimen is not urine.
22. 1.020 − (.006 + .008) = 1.006. A higher specific gravity would be expected on a first morning specimen.
23. Reagent strip and repeat refractometry on a diluted specimen.
24. Radiographic dye is present. High-molecular-weight plasma expanders are present.
25. **Pathologic:** infection by urea-splitting organisms; **nonpathologic:** old specimen.

CHAPTER 5

1. a. Reagents will leach from the strip, causing false-negative results.
   b. Runover among pads will invalidate results.
   c. False-negative results (particularly LE) because of insufficient reaction time.
   d. Inability to correctly correlate reaction colors because of differences in reagent strips.
2. Results will be falsely decreased; enzymatic reactions are temperature dependent.
3. a. Dessicant in the container and tightly closing the container after removing strips.
   b. Tightly closing containers and avoiding using strips in the presence of fumes.
   c. Opaque containers.
   d. Storing at temperatures below 30°C.
4. The last date the strips can be guaranteed to produce accurate results.
5. At least once every 24 hours; a new bottle is opened; questionable results are obtained; there is concern over reagent strip integrity.
6. Urine pH (acid or alkaline) determines the type of crystals and calculi formed.
7. The specimen has remained unpreserved at room temperature for too long (a new specimen should be collected).
8. The pH range needed is too broad for one indicator to measure.
9. a. 2, b. 1, c. 2, d. 3, e. 1, f. 2, g. 3.
10. Bence Jones protein precipitates at 40°C to 60°C and dissolves at 100°C.
11. Glomerular proteinuria occurs when protein (primarily albumin) passes through the glomerulus, whereas tubular proteinuria represents defects in the tubular reabsorption of low-molecular-weight proteins usually filtered and reabsorbed.
12. The patient requires better stabilization of blood glucose levels.
13. When the pH remains constant, certain indicators change color in the presence of protein; highly alkaline urine will override the reagent strip pH buffer producing a color change related to pH not protein.
14. Multiple myeloma.
15. Blood glucose levels greater than the renal threshold for glucose produce glucose concentrations in the filtrate that exceed the maximum reabsorptive capacity of the tubules.
16. The hormone thyroxin opposes the action of insulin by breaking down glycogen to glucose; epinephrine inhibits insulin secretion.
17. Renal tubular dysfunction.
18. Glucose oxidase catalyzes a reaction between glucose and room air to form hydrogen peroxide, which is then broken down by peroxidase to produce oxygen that oxidizes a chromogen producing a color.
19. Old specimens; glycolysis.
20. Reducing substances that reduce cupric ions to cuprous ions releasing oxygen to produce an oxidized colored substance.
21. A strongly positive result will be reported as negative.
22. Screening for galactosuria in children.
23. Reagent strips are more sensitive than Clinitest; contamination of containers by strong oxidizing agents.
24. Inadequate metabolism or intake of carbohydrates and increased loss of carbohydrate.
25. Acetoacetic acid. Glycine enhances detection of acetone.
26. Reaction color from interfering substances fades after standing, whereas color from ketones increases.
27. a. **Red blood cells:** glomerular damage, trauma.
    b. **Hemoglobin:** intravascular hemolysis.
    c. **Myoglobin:** muscle destruction.

28. Myoglobin is more rapidly cleared from the plasma.
29. Denaturation of hemoglobin to ferritin by the renal tubular epithelial cells producing hemosiderin granules.
30. Myoglobin is present.
31. To detect hemoglobin peroxidase.
32. Intact red blood cells are present.
33. Ascorbic acid is a strong reducing agent that can inhibit oxidation of the color-producing chromogens.
34. Unconjugated bilirubin; conjugated bilirubin; urobilinogen.
35. **Bilirubinuria:** bile-duct obstruction, liver damage; **jaundice without bilirubinuria:** hemolytic disorders.
36. Ictotest is more sensitive and less affected by interfering substances.
37. Old specimens exposed to light.
38. A portion of the urobilinogen produced in the intestine is reabsorbed into the blood and passes through the kidneys as it recirculates to the liver.
39. Hemolytic anemia results in increased bilirubin passing into the intestine; therefore, production of urobilinogen and its reabsorption into the blood are increased causing elevated urine levels. Biliary obstruction prevents passage of bilirubin into the intestine resulting in no production of urobilinogen to be excreted in the urine.
40. Multistix uses Ehrlich's reagent, which detects urobilinogen, porphobilinogen, sulfonamides, indican, *p*-amino salicylic acid, methyldopa, procaine, and chloropromazine. Chemstrip uses a diazo reaction that is specific for urobilinogen.
41. **Urobilinogen:** soluble in chloroform and butanol; **porphobilinogen:** insoluble in chloroform and butanol; **Ehrlich reactive compounds:** insoluble in chloroform, soluble in butanol.
42. Add two drops of urine to 2 mL of Hoesch reagent and observe for a red color.
43. Detection of UTI.
44. Automated strip readers may detect an atypical color reaction and report a positive report.
45. Non-nitrate reducing bacteria are present; nitrite has been further reduced to nitrogen; lack of dietary nitrate; antibiotic administration; presence of large amounts of ascorbic acid; high specific gravity.
46. Yes. Because if the specimen is fresh, in vitro bacterial multiplication will not have occurred.
47. The LE reaction will detect esterase released from lysed leukocytes.
48. Inflammation of renal tissue, fungal and parasitic infections.
49. These are diazo reactions and ascorbic acid will combine with the diazonium salt and prevent the desired reaction.
50. Hydrogen ions are released from the polyelectrolyte in proportion to specimen concentration.
51. Reagent strips are not affected by nonionizing high-molecular-weight substances.
52. The alkaline pH of the urine requires additional hydrogen ions to be released from the polyelectrolytes to produce a color change; therefore, the true concentration is not represented.

CHAPTER 6

1. Cost-effective; some abnormalities may not be detected.
2. Color, clarity, protein, glucose, blood, nitrite, leukocyte esterase; glucose is included to detect possible yeast infection.
3. Centrifuged specimens do not have to be transferred to a slide.
4. Old, unpreserved specimen; amorphous precipitation; failure to mix the specimen.
5. The normal values stated by the laboratory are based on a particular volume. The laboratory can correct the report of a low-volume specimen by multiplying by the appropriate factor or report the volume used for the physician to interpret the results.
6. Relative centrifugal force corrects for diameter of the centrifuge head.
7. Disrupting the sediment by using the manual brake; centrifuging uncapped tubes causing aerosol production.
8. Sediment concentration factor equals 30 and will be 15 if 1 mL of sediment is used.
9. Failure to mix the specimen and vigorously agitating the sediment.
10. A consistent volume of sediment is examined; factors for calculation of cellular elements per milliliter are supplied; heavy structures, such as casts, are uniformly spaced throughout the examination area.
11. Magnification 100× is used for overall evaluation of the sediment and detection and quantitation of casts. Magnification 400× is used for identification of sediment constituents and quantitation of cells.
12. Failure to examine the sediment under reduced light; focusing in the wrong plane; failure to use the fine adjustment.

13. Casts are reported as the average per 10 lpfs; RBCs and WBCs are reported as the average per 10 hpfs.
14. 185,185 RBCs/mL
15. Crystal violet and safranin O.
16. **Nuclear detail:** toluidine blue, 2 percent acetic acid; **lipids:** Sudan III, Oil Red O, polarization.
17. To stain urinary eosinophils.
18. Permanent slides are prepared by cytocentrifugation, stained with Papanicolaou's stain, and examined by cytologists and pathologists.
19. 400×; RBCs, WBCs, RTE cells, casts, crystals, bacteria.
20. Polarizing microscopy.
21. Phase-contrast objective and phase rings; adjustment of the phase-contrast rings to a concentric position.
22. Interference-contrast microscopy.
23. False
24. **Hyposthenuria:** large ghost cells; **hypersthenuria:** crenated, shrunken, irregular.
25. Oil droplets and air bubbles are highly refractile; yeast cells exhibit budding.
26. **Macroscopic:** coagulation disorders, advanced glomerular disease, and acute infection; **microscopic:** renal calculi and malignancy.
27. Varying size, hypochromic, fragmented, cellular protrusions; passage of RBCs through the glomerulus.
28. Neutrophil; acute interstitial nephritis.
29. Large WBCs in which the granules exhibit Brownian movement; They are seen in hypotonic urine.
30. Size and nuclear characteristics.
31. **Squamous:** large, irregular cells from the linings of the vagina and urethras; **transitional:** spherical, polyhedral, or caudate with a central nucleus from the linings of the urethra, bladder, ureters, renal calyces, and pelvis; **renal tubular:** cuboidal or columnar with an eccentric nucleus from the linings of the renal tubules and collecting ducts.
32. Clue cells are squamous epithelial cells covered with *Gardnerella vaginalis* bacteria.
33. **Pathologic:** malignancy; **nonpathologic:** invasive procedures.
34. Tubular destruction is indicated; substances in the urinary filtrate are reabsorbed by RTE cells.
35. RTE cells absorbing filtered lipids.
36. Yes; it contains triglycerides and neutral fats and no cholesterol.
37. An old specimen.
38. Yeast infections are associated with urine containing glucose.
39. The size of the renal tubules or collecting ducts and elements in the urinary filtrate determine the size and composition of the casts; Tamm-Horsfall protein.
40. Stasis of urine flow.
41. RBC and WBC casts indicate the cells are present in the nephron, whereas free RBCs and WBCs may originate throughout the urinary tract.
42. Pyelonephritis; WBCs and WBC casts.
43. Disintegration of cellular casts and excretion of lysosomes by tubular cells.
44. Stasis of urine flow resulting from dehydration produces casts, particularly hyaline and also granular casts that contain lysosomes from increased cellular metabolism; RBCs may be forced through the glomerular membrane; the sediment returns to normal following rest.
45. Extreme stasis of urine flow.
46. Low temperature, increased concentration, and pH affect chemical solubility.
47. Polarizing microscopy and solubility characteristics.
48. a. 5, b. 1, c. 2, d. 4.
49. a. 2, b. 5, c. 1, d. 6, e. 4.
50. a. 5, b. 4, c. 6, d. 1, e. 2, f. 3, g. 7.

CHAPTER 7

1. QC guarantees accurate analytic testing results and QA includes quality of specimens and patient care.
2. A procedure manual.
3. Annually and when changes are made.
4. 2, 1, 2, 3, 2, 1.
5. Yes. The error producing the inaccurate result can be made consistently.
6. Conditions identical to those of patient sample testing.
7. Shift
8. Check the integrity and expiration date and lot numbers of the control and reagent strips; run a new control; open a new bottle of reagent strips.
9. The date and the laboratory worker's initials.
10. The lot number and expiration date of the control and the test results.
11. Positive and negative controls.
12. Waived, provider-performed microscopy; moderate complexity; and high complexity.
13. **Waived:** reagent strip urinalysis, urine pregnancy test; **PPM:** urine microscopic; **moderate complexity:** automated urinalysis using the Clinitek 200; **high complexity:** urine culture and sensitivity.

14. PPM, moderate, and high complexity.
15. Procedural training.
16. Twice the first year and then annually.
17. QA maintains established levels of quality, whereas TQM and CQI develop methods to improve quality and customer satisfaction.
18. Availability, timeliness, effectiveness, efficiency, safety of services, continuity of care, respect and care by personnel.
19. Patients, health-care providers, personnel in other departments, patient's family and friends.
20. Improved patient outcomes.
21. **Flow charts:** breakdown a process into steps; **cause and effect diagrams:** identify factors that contribute to a problem; **Pareto charts:** identify the major contributors to a problem; **run charts:** determine cyclic and seasonal differences compared to an average.
22. **Plan:** process of making a change by identifying customer expectations and identifying methods for improvement; **Do:** testing the improvement processes designed in the Plan step; **Check:** evaluating the results and effects of the changes made; **Act:** implementing the change in a standardized format throughout the institution.
23. Improving organizational performance.
24. Plan, design, measure, assess, and improve.

CHAPTER 9

1. Inherited and metabolic.
2. Color and odor.
3. PKU, tyrosinuria, alkaptonuria, and melanuria.
4. With early detection of PKU and implementation of dietary restrictions, mental retardation can be prevented.
5. Blood levels of phenylalanine rise more quickly than detectable urine levels of phenylpyruvic acid.
6. Phenylalanine hydroxylase
7. No. Increased phenylalanine counteracts the inhibitory effect of beta-2-thienylalanine on *Bacillus subtilis* growth.
8. Monitoring of diagnosed cases.
9. Underdevelopment of the liver in premature infants, acquired severe liver disease, and failure to inherit essential metabolic enzymes; underdeveloped liver function is the least serious.
10. A positive reaction requiring further testing.
11. Homogentisic acid turns black in the presence of alkali.
12. Homogentisic acid is a reducing agent.
13. The specimen may contain melanin and indicate the presence of a malignant melanoma.
14. Positive reactions are PKU—permanent blue-green, tyrosyluria—transient green, alkaptonuria—transient blue, and melanuria—gray-black.
15. The color, consistency, and odor of the urine resemble that of maple syrup.
16. Ketones
17. Isovaleric acidemia; methylmalonic acidemia.
18. Intestinal disorders cause increased amounts of tryptophan to be converted to indole that is reabsorbed and recirculated to the liver, where it is converted to indican and excreted in the urine and subsequently oxidized to indigo blue. A blue diaper indicates the inherited disorder Hartnup disease; in contrast, blue urine in an adult represents an acquired intestinal disorder.
19. The urine may contain 5-HIAA. False positive reactions are caused by serotonin-containing food (bananas, pineapple, or tomatoes) or phenothiazines and acetanilids.
20. Cystinosis is caused by failure to inherit the gene needed to completely metabolize cystine, whereas in cystinuria, cystine can be metabolized, but an inherited disorder prevents its tubular reabsorption from the urinary filtrate.
21. Cystine is less soluble than lysine.
22. The cyanide-nitroprusside test is positive for both substances and the silver-nitroprusside test is only positive for homocystine.
23. **Urine:** ALA, porphobilinogen, uroporphyrin; **feces or bile:** coproporphyrin and protoporphyrin; **blood:** protoporphyrin.
24. **Neurologic:** acute intermittent porphyria; **photosensitivity:** porphyria cutanea tarda, congenital erythropoietic porphyria, erythropoietic protoporphria; **neurologic and photosensitivity:** variegate porphyria.
25. Lead poisoning
26. α-Aminolevulinic acid, coproporphyrin, and protoporphyrin.
27. The Watson-Schwartz test result will be positive for porphobilinogen, but not uroporphyrin.
28. Mucopolysaccharidoses is present.
29. Markedly increased uric acid crystals.
30. The presence of galactosuria.

CHAPTER 10

1. Supply nutrients to the nervous tissue, remove metabolic wastes, and cushion the nervous tissue against trauma.
2. CSF is produced by filtration in the choroid plexuses, flows through the subarachnoid space, and is reabsorbed in the arachnoid villi.
3. a. The tube may be contaminated with skin flora.
   b. The tube may be contaminated with blood cells introduced during the puncture.
   c. The glucose concentration will be markedly decreased.
   d. RBCs and WBCs will have disintegrated.
4. Pink xanthochromia indicates the presence of fresh oxyhemoglobin, whereas yellow xanthochromia occurs when oxyhemoglobin has been converted to bilirubin.
5. T, H, H, T, H.
6. Possible tubercular meningitis.
7. Yes. A clear specimen could contain as many as 200 WBCs/μL or 500 RBCs/μL.
8. 500 cells/μL
9. Saline; acetic acid containing methylene blue.
10. To correct for cells and protein introduced into the specimen by a traumatic tap.
11. Concentrated using sedimentation, filtration, centrifugation, or cytocentrifugation.
12. Albumin increases cellular yield and decreases cellular distortion.
13. Meningitis
14. Lymphocytes; ependymal, choroid plexus, and spindle-shaped cells; eosinophils; lymphocytes; macrophages/RBCs.
15. Bone marrow contamination.
16. Choroid plexus cells have distinct cytoplasmic borders and uniform appearance of the nucleii and cytoplasm.
17. Primary CNS tumors; lung, breast, renal, and gastrointestinal metastases; melanoma; leukemias; and lymphomas.
18. The filtration across the blood-brain barrier is selective.
19. False
20. Prealbumin is the second most prevalent protein fraction in CSF.
21. Damage to the blood-brain barrier, CNS production of immunoglobulins, decreased clearance of protein from the CSF, and degeneration of neural tissue.
22. Trichloroacetic acid precipitates both albumin and globulin. Coomassie blue binds to albumin and other proteins.
23. The CSF/serum albumin index measures blood-brain barrier integrity, and the IgG index measures immunoglobulin synthesis within the CNS.
24. To determine whether the proteins forming the bands are being produced exclusively in the CNS; multiple sclerosis.
25. By determining whether the fluid contains the tau isoform of transferrin.
26. The pressure of myelin basic protein indicates recent myelin sheath destruction.
27. The normal range for CSF glucose is defined as 60 percent to 70 percent that of the blood glucose.
28. A change in the transport of glucose across the blood-brain barrier and increased use of glucose by brain cells.
29. Glutamine is produced from ammonia and α-ketoglutarate to detoxify ammonia; therefore, when ammonia is increased, glutamine production is increased.
30. Centrifuge the fluid.
31. **False-negative:** a small number of organisms are present and are overlooked; **false-positive:** stain precipitation or debris.
32. *Cryptococcus neoformans* is an opportunistic infection associated with AIDS.
33. *Escherichia coli*, because it is gram negative.
34. Rheumatoid factor.
35. Active syphilis is not present within the CNS. Active syphilis is present within the CNS and the result is most probably not positive because of blood contamination.

CHAPTER 11

1. Sperm are produced in the seminiferous tubules in the testes and mature in the epididymis.
2. Testes and epididymis—sperm; seminal vessels—seminal fluid; prostate—proteolytic enzymes, acid phosphatase, zinc, and citric acid; bulbourethral glands—mucus.
3. The count will be falsely decreased.
4. Collect another sample in 2 weeks.
5. To provide a baseline for determining the time required for liquifaction.
6. No, many condoms contain spermicidal agents.

7. Standard Precautions to prevent exposure to hepatitis virus and HIV.
8. Red—blood; yellow—urine, medications, and prolonged abstinence; white and turbid—WBCs.
9. The sperm concentration and count because the majority of the sperm are contained in the first part of the ejaculation, which may not have been collected.
10. No, droplets indicate appropriate viscosity.
11. Increased prostatic fluid.
12. Sperm concentration = 81,000,000/mL; sperm count = 243,000,000 per ejaculate
13. Sperm concentration = 405,000/mL; sperm count = 1,215,000 per ejaculate
14. Normal—No. 12; Abnormal—No. 13
15. Immobilize the sperm; preserve and stain the sperm depending on the diluting fluid used.
16. Speed and direction.
17. Slow forward motion with noticeable lateral movement.
18. Objective measurement of sperm velocity and direction.
19. The acrosomal cap is located at the tip of the sperm head and contains enzymes necessary for ovum penetration.
20. Head abnormalities affect ovum penetration and tail abnormalities affect motility.
21. Kruger strict criteria include measurement of head, neck, tail, and acrosome size and detection of vacuoles.
22. Three million neutrophils is abnormal and indicates an infection.
23. The concentration is normal, but contains abnormally decreased viable sperm and, therefore, decreased motility and fertility.
24. Vasectomy reversal, trauma, and infection.
25. If antibodies are attached to the sperm, the bivalent AHG will bind to both the sperm and the coated RBCs, producing microscopically visible clumps.
26. The immunobead test detects IgG, IgM, and IgA antibodies and demonstrates the specific areas of the sperm being affected.
27. Acid phosphatase is found in high concentrations only in semen.
28. The only concern is the presence or absence of sperm.
29. Hypoosmotic swelling test.
30. Standardized procedures developed by the World Health Organization, proficiency testing from the College of American Pathologists and American Association of Bioanalysts, and commercial controls.

CHAPTER 12

1. Lubrication, nutrition, and cushioning of joints.
2. Noninflammatory—degeneration; inflammatory—rheumatoid arthritis, lupus, gout, and pseudogout; septic—infection; hemorrhagic—trauma and coagulation disorders.
3. WBC count and differential—noninflammatory, inflammatory, and septic; Gram stain and culture—septic; polarizing microscopy—crystal-induced inflammation.
4. Arthrocentesis
5. To avoid contamination with possible polarizing artifacts.
6. **Dark-yellow:** inflammation; **milky:** crystals; **blood streaked:** traumatic tap; **green:** infection.
7. To provide viscosity for joint lubrication. Addition of acetic acid causes clot formation in the presence of hyaluronic acid.
8. Normal, hypotonic, or saponin-containing saline is used as a WBC diluent, because acetic acid diluting fluid would cause clot formation.
9. **Increased neutrophils:** infection; **increased lymphocytes:** nonseptic inflammation; **ragocytes:** rheumatoid arthritis.
10. **MSU:** gout; **CPPD:** pseudogout.
11. **Calcium oxalate:** renal dialysis; **corticosteroid crystals:** injection of anti-inflammatory medications.
12. Unstained, wet preparation.
13. MSU. CPPD
14. MSU crystals because the fast ray runs perpendicular to the grain.
15. Blue
16. Glucose is included in the synovial fluid ultrafiltrate of plasma, and protein is not filtered.
17. Septic arthritis.
18. *Hemophilus sp.* and *Neisseria gonorrheae* are common causes of septic arthritis, and they require chocolate agar for growth.
19. Rheumatoid arthritis and systemic lupus erythematosus.
20. Lyme disease

CHAPTER 13

1. To provide lubrication between the parietal and visceral serous membranes.

2. **Congestive heart failure:** decreased hydrostatic pressure; **hypoproteinemia:** decreased oncotic pressure; **inflammation:** increased capillary permeability or infection; **lymphatic tumor:** obstruction.
3. Pleural fluid; peritoneal or ascitic fluid.
4. Differentiation can narrow the cause of the effusion down to being either a systemic disorder or a disorder affecting the serous membranes.
5. **Transudate:** congestive heart failure, nephrotic syndrome, cirrhosis; **exudate:** infection (pneumonia, tuberculosis, peritonitis) or malignancy.
6. **Appearance:** clear, pale yellow; **fluid to serum protein ratio:** <0.5; **fluid to serum LD:** <0.6; **cell count:** $<1000/\mu L$. The fluid–to–serum protein and LD ratios are most significant.
7. Blood from a hemothorax will have a hematocrit similar to that of blood; a hemorrhagic effusion will have a much lower hematocrit.
8. An effusion caused by thoracic duct leakage will contain chylous material with a high concentration of triglycerides that will stain with Sudan III.
9. **Neutrophils:** pneumonia, pancreatitis, pulmonary infarction; **lymphocytes:** tuberculosis, viral infection, autoimmune disorders, malignancy; **eosinophils:** trauma introducing air or blood, allergic reactions, parasitic infections; **plasma cells:** tuberculosis.
10. Mesothelial cells are normal cells lining the serous membranes.
11. Decreased mesothelial cells are associated with tuberculosis.
12. Nuclear and cytoplasmic irregularities; cytoplasmic molding; hyperchromatic nucleoli; abnormal nuclear–to–cytoplasmic ratios.
13. Yes, because serous fluid is an ultrafiltrate of plasma.
14. The rupture causes an influx of acidic gastric fluid.
15. Increased neutrophils indicating bacterial endocarditis and malignant cells.
16. Ascites is the abnormal accumulation of fluid in the peritoneal cavity.
17. To determine the presence of intra-abdominal bleeding.
18. The serum-ascites albumin gradient is 0.7 indicating an exudate that contains increased albumin as compared to a transudate.
19. The ascitic fluid effusion may be caused by ovarian malignancy.
20. Aerobically and anaerobically.

CHAPTER 14

1. To provide protection for the fetus and allow movement of the fetus.
2. Production of fetal urine.
3. Increased amniotic fluid accumulates when the fetus fails to begin swallowing. Increased fetal swallowing, urinary tract defects, and membrane leakage cause decreased amniotic fluid.
4. To determine possible accidental puncture of the maternal bladder during amniocentesis.
5. To prevent photo-oxidation of bilirubin to biliverdin.
6. Specimens are delivered on ice and refrigerated.
7. To prolong cell viability and integrity.
8. Centrifugation
9. **Dark green:** presence of meconium; **colorless:** normal; **yellow:** presence of bilirubin; **red-brown:** fetal death.
10. Bilirubin is present; oxyhemoglobin is present.
11. To determine the severity of hemolytic disease of the newborn.
12. Failure of the skin to close exposes neural tissue and capillaries to the amniotic fluid, allowing increased diffusion of AFP into the fluid.
13. Multiples of the laboratory's reference level for AFP at a particular week of gestation.
14. When severe HDN is present, the physician must determine whether the fetal lungs are mature enough to withstand a premature delivery.
15. Lecithin is the primary surfactant that stabilizes the alveoli in the lungs and must have been produced in adequate amounts to provide stabilization of the fetal lung post delivery.
16. Less than 1.6 because lecithin production does not increase until approximately 35 weeks of gestation.
17. Amniostat-FLM detects the presence of phosphatidylglycerol and is a rapid test that does not require performance of thin-layer chromatography.
18. Decreased lecithin; the presence of phospholipid is required to reduce the surface tension of the solution and counteract the alcohol in the solution, which is an antifoaming agent.
19. The L/S ratio uses sphingomyelin as an internal standard on which to base a rise in lecithin concentration and the microviscosity test uses albumin as the internal standard for the same purpose.
20. No, an L/S ratio of 2.0 indicates FLM, whereas a microviscosity ratio of 70 or

greater is the recommended value for FLM.

21. Lamellar bodies contain phospholipid and increase the OD of the fluid; therefore, the number of lamellar bodies present and the OD of the fluid are directly related to FLM.
22. The Amniostat-FLM, because it is an immunologic reaction and is specific for phosphatidylglycerol.

CHAPTER 15

1. Small intestine.
2. Reabsorption of water.
3. **Secretory diarrhea:** fecal neutrophils; **osmotic diarrhea:** fecal fats, Clinitest, muscle fibers.
4. Disposable container; physician's glove; occult blood collection kit.
5. Bowel habits vary and passage of food through the digestive tract may take up to 72 hours.
6. The gas that has accumulated in the container must be slowly released.
7. Stools appear pale and frothy because the passage of bilirubin and bile into the intestine is blocked. Urobilinogen, the precursor of color-producing urobilin, is not present, resulting in the pale color. Bile salts that aid in the digestion of fat are absent, producing the bulky, frothy stool.
8. A black, tarry stool indicates upper gastrointestinal bleeding, and a bloody stool is associated with lower gastrointestinal bleeding.
9. No, the antibiotic may be oxidizing bilirubin to biliverdin.
10. **Pathologic:** colitis, dysentery, malignancy; **nonpathologic:** excessive straining.
11. More water is reabsorbed from the fecal material while it remains in the colon.
12. Damage to the intestinal mucosa.
13. **Rotavirus:** no; ***Salmonella:*** yes.
14. Use a lactoferrin immunoassay.
15. At least 10 fibers containing both vertical and horizontal striations will be seen; qualitative fecal fats examination.
16. Triglycerides stain directly with Sudan III; to detect fatty acids, the specimen must be mixed with acetic acid and heated prior to staining.
17. A slide positive for neutral fats contains more than 60 large orange-red droplets per hpf; a slide positive for fatty acids contains more than 100 orange-red droplets that measure 6 to 75 μm in size.
18. Guaiac reagent is less likely to produce false-positive results caused by normal fecal constituents; the test detects the pseudoperoxidase activity of hemoglobin.
19. At least two samples taken from different parts of three stools should be tested; samples should be taken from the center portions of the stool to avoid false-positive results from external contamination.
20. The Hemoquant test detects both hemoglobin and porphyrin and the FlexSure FOBT is specific for human hemoglobin. Hemoquant is more sensitive because it detects porphyrin, which can form as a degradation product of hemoglobin as it passes from the upper gastrointestinal tract.
21. Increased fat in the stool; yes; the normal coefficient of fat retention is at least 95 percent; therefore, a value of 85 percent indicates steatorrhea.
22. Fetal hemoglobin is present.
23. Yes. Trypsin normally produced by the pancreas is not present in the feces; analyze the specimen for the presence of chymotrypsin or elastase I.
24. Increased bacterial use of fecal carbohydrates.
25. Malabsorption or maldigestion of carbohydrates.

Answers to Case Studies and Clinical Situations

CHAPTER 2

1. a. 160 to 180 mg/dL
   b. Renal tubular reabsorption is impaired.
   c. 1.010
   d. The presence of high-density protein molecules.
   e. Measuring urine-to-serum osmolarity.
2. a. Juxtaglomerular apparatus → Renin $\xrightarrow{\text{Angiotensinogen}}$ Angiotensin I → Angiotensin II = Vasoconstriction, increased sodium reabsorption, increased aldosterone to retain sodium.
   b. Increased sodium content in the plasma retains water to increase blood volume and pressure.
   c. Production of renin decreases and, therefore, the actions of the renin-angiotensin-aldosterone system.
3. a. The physician can calculate the approximate creatinine clearance using the Cockcroft-Gault formula.

b. Yes, the calculated creatinine clearance is 80 mL/min.

4. a. Serum from the midnight specimen is not being separated from the clot and refrigerated in a timely manner.
   b. Yes, lactic acid affects both cryoscopic and vapor pressure osmolarity readings.
   c. If the laboratory is using a cryoscopic osmometer, results will be affected by alcohol ingestion; vapor pressure results would not be affected and could be used as a comparison.
5. a. Diabetes insipidus.
   b. Decreased production of ADH.
   c. Lack of tubular response to ADH.

CHAPTER 3

1. a. No, the specimen should be analyzed and the volume reported. Persons with decreased glomerular filtration rates may also exhibit oliguria.
   b. Failure to collect a complete specimen will result in a low clearance rate not related to renal function.
2. a. The specimen is a dilute random specimen that has remained more than 2 hours at room temperature prior to being tested.
   b. Collect a 2-hour postprandial specimen.
3. a. A prostatic infection cannot be determined because the patient has a urinary tract infection.
   b. White blood cells present following prostate massage only need to be compared with one premassage specimen.
   c. A prostate infection is present.
4. a. The specimen temperature was measured.
   b. The temperature was too low.
   c. The specimen analyzed did not belong to the defendant.
   d. By maintaining a thoroughly documented COC form.

CHAPTER 4

1. a. No, because red blood cells would produce a hazy-cloudy specimen.
   b. Hemoglobin from intravascular hemolysis and myoglobin from muscle-tissue damage.
   c. Yes, the red blood cells may have hemolyzed.
   d. Dietary intake, exercise, and medications.
2. a. Yes, the specimen may contain melanin or homogentisic acid.
   b. Homogentisic acid.
   c. Melanin.
   d. Breakdown of red blood cells followed by oxidation of hemoglobin to methemoglobin.
3. a. Radiographic dye.
   b. 1.060
   c. Add 3 mL of water to 1 mL of urine and mix.
   d. Reagent strip
4. a. Beets
   b. Yes, beets produce a red color in alkaline urine, and the fresh specimen may have an acid pH or she hasn't recently eaten beets.
5. a. **Support:** the specimen may be old and bilirubin has oxidized to biliverdin and glycolysis may have occurred.
   b. **Disagree:** The specimen is concentrated and the white foam is from protein that will be detected by reagent strip.
   c. **Support:** The specimen may be old.
   d. **Disagree:** The specimen can be accurately analyzed by reagent strip.

CHAPTER 5

1. a. The patient's blood glucose level exceeds the renal threshold for glucose, causing glucosuria.
   b. Diabetes mellitus.
   c. Diabetic nephropathy.
   d. Better stabilization of the blood glucose levels.
   e. Tubular dysfunction
2. a. Yellow foam
   b. Ictotest
   c. Possible biliary-duct obstruction preventing bilirubin from entering the intestine.
   d. Icteric
   e. Specimens must be protected from light.
3. a. Hemoglobinuria
   b. Increased hemoglobin presented to the liver results in increased bilirubin entering the intestine for conversion to urobilinogen.
   c. The circulating bilirubin is unconjugated.
   d. Perform a Watson-Schwartz test; retest the specimen using a Chemstrip.
4. a. Negative chemical reactions for blood and nitrite. Ascorbic acid interference for both reactions. Random specimen or further

reduction of nitrite could cause the negative nitrite.
   b. Glucose, bilirubin, LE.
   c. The dark yellow color may be caused by beta-carotene instead of specimen concentration.
   d. Non-nitrite–reducing microorganisms; lack of dietary nitrate; antibiotic administration.
5. a. To check for possible exercise-induced abnormal results.
   b. Negative protein and blood, possible changes in color and specific gravity.
   c. Renal
6. a. No, the specimen is clear.
   b. Myoglobinuria
   c. Muscle damage from the accident (rhabdomyolysis).
   d. Yes, myoglobin is toxic to the renal tubules.
7. a. Laboratory personnel are not tightly capping the reagent strip containers in a timely manner.
   b. Personnel performing the CLIA-waived reagent strip test are not waiting 2 minutes to read the LE reaction.
   c. The student is not mixing the specimen.
   d. The automated reagent strip reader is reporting atypical color reactions and the strips are not being visually examined.

CHAPTER 6

1. a. Yeast grows best at a low pH with an increased concentration of glucose.
   b. Yes, this exceeds the renal threshold.
   c. No, yeast is not capable of reducing nitrate to nitrite.
   d. Moderate blood with no RBCs.
   e. Myoglobin is the cause of the positive chemical test result for blood.
2. a. The large objects are in a different plane than the urinary constituents.
   b. Contamination by artifacts.
   c. No, because they are in a different plane.
   d. Polarizing microscopy.
3. a. Renal tubules.
   b. Yes, viral infections can cause tubular damage.
   c. RTE cells absorb urinary filtrate and squamous cells do not.
   d. Liver damage inhibits processing of reabsorbed urobilinogen.
   e. Disorders producing intravascular hemolysis.
4. a. The patient is taking a pigmented medication, such as phenazopyridine.
   b. Yes
   c. An Ictotest could be run, but is not indicated by the patient's symptoms.
   d. Ask what medications the patient is taking.
   e. Phenazopyridine
   f. Ampicillin
5. a. Calcium oxalate.
   b. Monohydrate and dihydrate calcium oxalate.
   c. **Oval:** monohydrate; **envelope:** dihydrate.
   d. Monohydrate.
6. a. Microscopic results do not match the chemical tests for blood, nitrite, and leukocyte esterase.
   b. The specimen has been unpreserved at room temperature for too long, the cells have disintegrated, and the bacteria have converted the nitrite to nitrogen.
   c. The pH.
   d. Ask the clinic personnel to instruct the patient to collect a midstream clean-catch specimen and have the specimen delivered immediately to the laboratory.
7. a. No, because they are associated with strenuous exercise.
   b. The positive blood reaction is from hemoglobinuria or myoglobinuria resulting from participating in a contact sport. The protein is orthostatic.
   c. Increased excretion of RTE cell lysosomes in the presence of dehydration.
8. a. Yes, the waxy casts are probably an artifact, such as a diaper fiber. Waxy casts are not associated with negative urine protein.
   b. No, this is normal following an invasive procedure.
   c. Yes, tyrosine crystals are seen in severe liver disease; therefore, the bilirubin should be positive. The crystals may be an artifact.
   d. Yes, uric acid crystals have been mistaken for cystine crystals.
   e. Yes, radiographic dye crystals associated with a high specific gravity resemble cholesterol crystals.
   f. No, *Trichomonas* is carried asymptomatically by men.
   g. Yes, calcium carbonate crystals are found in alkaline urine; therefore, clumps of amorphous urates may be present.

CHAPTER 7

1. a. Review of the procedure by a designated authority has not been documented.
   b. Instructions and training are not being provided to personnel performing collections.
   c. A safety statement about the heat produced by the reaction is not in the procedure manual.
   d. The bottles have not been dated and initialed.
2. a. Yes, provided you comply with the proficiency testing, patient test management, and QC and QA requirements for moderate complexity testing.
   b. The CLIA status will be moderate complexity, proficiency testing will be required, and inspections will be conducted.
3. a. The PDCA strategy.
   b. Analyze the problems, using flow charts, cause and effect and/or Pareto charts and discuss theories to correct the problems. Test the recommended changes, analyze the results of these tests, and implement effective changes.
4. a. Correct; proficiency survey tests should be rotated among personnel performing the tests.
   b. Accept; QC on the Clinitest tablets must only be performed when they are used to perform a test.
   c. Correct; documentation of technical competency should be performed on all personnel working in the section and educational qualifications assessed.

CHAPTER 8

1. a. Acute glomerulonephritis.
   b. M protein in the cell wall of the group A streptococcus.
   c. Glomerular bleeding.
   d. No, they are also passing through the damaged glomerulus.
   e. Good prognosis with appropriate management of secondary complications.
   f. Henoch-Schönlein purpura.
2. a. IgA nephropathy/Berger's disease
   b. Serum IgA level
   c. Chronic glomerulonephritis/end-stage renal disease.
   d. Impaired renal tubular function associated with end-stage renal disease.
   e. The specific gravity is the same as that of the ultrafiltrate, indicating a lack of tubular concentration.
   f. The presence of extreme urinary stasis.
3. a. Nephrotic syndrome.
   b. Nephrotic syndrome may be caused by sudden, severe hypotension.
   c. Changes in the electrical charges in the glomerular membrane produce increased membrane permeability.
   d. Decreased plasma albumin lowers the capillary oncotic pressure causing fluid to enter the interstitial tissue.
   e. Reabsorption of filtered lipids by the RTE cells.
   f. Staining with Sudan III and observation under polarized light.
4. a. Minimal change disease.
   b. Nephrotic syndrome, focal segmental glomerulosclerosis.
   c. Good prognosis with complete remission.
5. a. Goodpasture's syndrome.
   b. The autoantibody attaches to the glomerular capillaries, causing complement activation and destruction of the capillaries.
   c. Wegener's granulomatosis.
   d. Antineutrophilic cytoplasmic antibody.
   e. Granuloma formation resulting from autoantibodies binding to neutrophils in the vascular walls and initiating an immune response.
6. a. Cystitis, UTI.
   b. The specimen is very dilute.
   c. Irritation of the urinary tract will cause a small amount of bleeding. The cells and bacteria may cause a trace protein or it may be a false positive due to the high pH.
   d. Yes, glitter cells are seen in hypotonic urine.
   e. Female children.
   f. Pyelonephritis.
7. a. Intravenous pyelogram.
   b. Chronic pyelonephritis.
   c. WBC cast.
   d. Reflux nephropathy.
   e. Performing a Gram stain.
   f. Radiographic dye.
   g. Permanent tubular damage and progression to chronic, end-stage renal disease.
8. a. Abnormal
   b. Acute interstitial nephritis.
   c. This disorder is an inflammation not an infection.

d. Discontinue the medication because it is causing the allergic reaction.

9. a. Acute renal failure.
   b. The prerenal sudden decrease in blood flow to the kidneys.
   c. Lack of renal concentrating ability.
   d. Tubular damage.
   e. The increased diameter of the damaged distal convoluted tubule and extreme urinary stasis allowing casts to form in the collecting ducts.
10. a. Renal lithiasis.
   b. The high specific gravity.
   c. Yes, the dark yellow color and high specific gravity indicate a concentrated urine, which induces the formation of renal calculi.
   d. Calcium oxalate.
   e. Increased hydration and dietary changes.
11. a. Renal lithiasis.
   b. Wegener's granulomatosis.
   c. FSGS.
   d. Rapidly progressive glomerulonephritis.
   e. Membranous glomerulonephritis.
   f. Fanconi's syndrome.
   g. Acute renal failure.

CHAPTER 9

1. a. Underdevelopment of the liver.
   b. It will produce a transient green color.
   c. Yes, with severe acquired liver disease.
   d. Tyrosine crystals; leucine crystals, bilirubin crystals.
   e. Protect the specimen from light.
2. a. DNPH test.
   b. Isovaleric acidemia.
   c. Maple syrup urine disease.
   d. *p*-nitroaniline test. Methylmalonic acidemia is present.
   e. Yes, this reaction is associated with maple syrup urine disease.
   f. Amino acid chromatography.
3. a. Renal lithiasis.
   b. Impaired renal tubular reabsorption of cystine.
   c. Lysine, arginine, ornithine.
   d. They are more soluble than cystine.
   e. Cyanide-nitroprusside test.
   f. The disorder is inherited.
4. a. Yes.
   b. Yes, uric acid crystals accumulating on the surface of the diaper could have an orange color.
   c. Lesch-Nyhan disease.
   d. Yes, the disease is inherited as a sex-linked recessive.
   e. Hypoxanthine guanine phosphoribosyltransferase.
5. a. Yes, the urine may contain homogentisic acid or melanin.
   b. A transient blue reaction with homogentisic acid or a gray-black reaction with melanin.
   c. Gray-black reaction.
   d. Yes, melanin will react with sodium nitroprusside.
6. a. Yes, the purple color could indicate the presence of indican in the urine.
   b. Ferric chloride with chloroform extraction and amino acid chromatography.
   c. Hartnup disease.
   d. Good with proper dietary supplements.
7. a. Porphyria.
   b. No, the Watson-Schwartz test will only detect porphobilinogen, and the blockage in the heme pathway may be at another location, producing a product requiring fluorescent testing.
   c. Yes, if the accumulated ALA is first converted to porphobilinogen using acetylacetone.
8. a. Fructose.
   b. Parenteral feeding.

CHAPTER 10

1. a. Cerebral hemorrhage because of the presence of erythrophagocytosis, even distribution of blood, and patient's history.
   b. No, they would be consistent with peripheral blood entering the CSF.
   c. No, they are consistent with the percentages seen in peripheral blood.
   d. CK BB
   e. A traumatic tap
   f. Glutamine level
2. a. India Ink preparation.
   b. *Cryptococcus meningitis*.
   c. Immunologic testing for *Cryptococcus*.
   d. Rheumatoid factor.
   e. Acid-fast staining and culture.
   f. Noticeable oligoclonal bands in both the CSF and serum.
3. a. CSF/serum albumin index = 8.6
   b. Yes
   c. IgG index = 3.1
   d. Immunoglobulin synthesis within the CNS.
   e. Multiple sclerosis.
   f. Oligoclonal banding only in the CSF.
   g. Myelin basic protein
4. a. Bacterial meningitis.

b. No, there is at least a 10 percent chance that the Gram stain will be negative.
c. Bacterial antigen immunoassay or limulus lysate
d. Yes, a CSF lactate level greater than 35 mg/dL would aid in confirming bacterial meningitis.

5. a. Stain precipitate is being confused with gram-positive cocci.
b. Differentials are being reported from the counting chamber.
c. The albumin is contaminated.
d. The specimens are not being promptly delivered to the laboratory.

CHAPTER 11

1. a. Sperm concentration, motility, and morphology.
b. 21,000,000; no
c. Fructose level to determine if there is sufficient fructose in the seminal fluid to support the sperm metabolism.
d. Add 50 mg of resorcinol to 33 mL of concentrated hydrochloric acid, pour the hydrochloric acid mixture into approximately 50 mL of distilled water in a volumetric flask, allow solution to cool, and then dilute to 100 mL.
2. a. Male antisperm antibodies may form following vasovasectomy procedures.
b. The MAR test and the immunobead test.
c. Penetration of the cervical mucosa or ovum by head-directed antibodies; movement through the cervical mucosa by tail-directed and neck-directed antibodies.
d. Hamster egg penetration assay by head-directed antibodies; cervical mucus penetration test by head-directed, neck-directed, or tail-directed antibodies.
3. The specimen contains urine, which is toxic to sperm, therefore, decreasing viability.
4. The specimen was improperly collected and the first part of the ejaculation was lost.
5. a. Yes, there is insufficient prostatic fluid present.
b. Zinc, citrate, and acid phosphatase.
c. Sperm motility is severely affected.

CHAPTER 12

1. a. Sterile, heparinized tube, liquid EDTA tube, nonanticoagulated tube.
b. MSU crystals seen in gout.
c. Highly birefringent, needle-shaped crystals under polarized light that turn yellow when aligned with the slow vibration of compensated polarized light.
d. Infection is frequently a complication of severe inflammation.
2. a. WBC diluting fluid containing acetic acid was used.
b. Normal, hypotonic, or saponin-containing saline should be used.
c. Blockage of the apertures by viscous fluid can be prevented by incubating the fluid with hyaluronidase. Detection of tissue cells and debris included in the count can be made by analyzing the scattergram.
3. a. Noninflammatory.
b. Hydroxyapatite crystals.
c. The normal glucose result is consistent with noninflammatory arthritis.
d. Yes, these results indicate a degenerative joint disorder.

CHAPTER 13

1. a. Pleural fluid.
b. Transudate, because all the test results are consistent with those of a transudate.
c. Pleural fluid to serum ratios of cholesterol and bilirubin.
2. a. Pneumonia.
b. Chest tube drainage.
3. Acid-fast staining and culture and adenosine deaminase measurement.
4. a. To differentiate between cirrhosis and peritonitis; cirrhosis.
b. Pancreatitis or gastrointestinal perforation; alkaline phosphatase.
c. Rupture or accidental puncture of the bladder.
5. The patient has been a victim of blunt trauma and the physician wants to determine if abdominal bleeding is occurring; abdominal bleeding.
6. Thyroid profile; CA 125

CHAPTER 14

1. a. Yes.
b. FLM
c. The level of phosphatidylglycerol present in the fetal lungs.
d. Phosphatidylglycerol is essential for FLM, and levels do not always parallel lecithin levels in fetuses of diabetic mothers.
2. a. A neural tube disorder, such as spina bifida or anencephaly.

   b. An acetylcholinesterase level.
   c. The amniotic fluid specimen contains blood.
3. Increased, because lecithin bound to dye decreases polarization.
4. The results may be falsely decreased because some of the phospholipids may be sedimented.
5. a. False-positive result.
   b. False-positive result.
   c. No effect.
   d. False-positive result.
6. a. False-positive result.
   b. False-positive result.
   c. False-postive or test interference.
   d. No effect.

CHAPTER 15

1. a. Secretory diarrhea.
   b. Stool culture.
   c. **Probable:** *Salmonella*, *Shigella*, *Campylobacter*, *Yersinia*, *E. coli*; **Improbable:** *Staphylococcus*, *Vibrio*.
   d. Osmotic diarrhea.
2. a. Microscopic examination for fecal fats.
   b. Neutral fats stain directly and appear as large, orange-red droplets; soaps and fatty acids appear as smaller orange-red droplets after pretreatment of the specimen with heat and acetic acid.
   c. Quantitative fecal fat test.
   d. Bulky and frothy.
   e. Muscle fiber screening and the gelatin test for trypsin.
   f. **Muscle fiber:** failure to include red meat in the diet; **gelatin test:** intestinal degradation of trypsin or the presence of trypsin inhibitors.
   g. Chymotrypsin or elastase I.
3. a. **Patient #1:** gastric reflux medication containing bismuth may produce black stools; **patient #2:** medications such as aspirin and other nonsteroidal anti-inflammatory agents may cause gastric bleeding; **patient #3:** red meat was not avoided for 3 days prior to sample collection.
   b. Provide dietary and medication instructions to patients.
   c. The HemeSelect or FlexSure OBT immunologic procedure.
4. a. The Apt test cannot be performed because the hemoglobin is already denatured.
   b. The pH will be low because increased carbohydrates are available for bacterial metabolism.
   c. The infant had ingested maternal blood.
   d. Yes, adequate carbohydrates are not present, and fats are being metabolized for energy.

Abbreviations

AAB American Association of Bioanalysis
AChE Acetylcholinesterase
ADH Antidiuretic hormone
AER Albumin excretion rate
AFP Alpha-fetoprotein
AGN Acute glomerulonephritis
AHG Antihuman globulin
AIDS Acquired immunodeficiency syndrome
AIN Acute interstitial nephritis
ALA α-Aminolevulinic acid
ANA Antinuclear antibody
ANCA Antineutrophilic cytoplasmic antibody
ARF Acute renal failure
ART Assisted reproductive technology
ASO Antistreptolysin O
ATN Acute tubular necrosis

BAT Bacterial antigen test
BSI Body substance isolation
BUN Blood urea nitrogen

CAP College of American Pathologists
CASA Computer-assisted semen analysis
CDC Centers for Disease Control and Prevention
CEA Carcinoembryonic antigen
CHP Chemical Hygiene Plan
CLIA '88 Clinical Laboratory Improvement Amendments
CNS Central nervous system
COC Chain of custody
COLA Commision on Laboratory Assessment
CPPD Calcium pyrophosphate
CQI Continuous quality improvement
CSF Cerebrospinal fluid
CTAB Cetyltrimethylammonium bromide
CV Coefficient of variation

DNPH 2,4-dinitrophenylhydrazine

EDTA Ethylenediaminetetracetic acid
ELISA Enzyme-linked immunoabsorbent assay
EU Ehrlich unit

FEP Free erythrocyte protoporphyrin
FLM Fetal lung maturity
FOBT Fecal occult blood testing
FSGS Focal segmental glomerulosclerosis

GTT Glucose tolerance test

H^+ Titratable acid/Hydrogen ion
HBV Hepatitis B virus
HCFA Health Care Financing Administration
HCO_3^- Bicarbonate ion
HDN Hemolytic disease of the newborn
5-HIAA 5-Hydroxyindoleacetic acid
HIV Human immunodeficiency virus
hpf High-power field

IEF Isoelectric focusing
IFE Immunofixation electrophoresis
IgA Immunoglobulin A
IOP Improving organizational performance
IVF In vitro fertilization

JCAHO Joint Commission on Accreditation of Healthcare Organizations

LD Lactate dehydrogenase
LE Leukocyte esterase
LED Light-emitting diode
LIS Laboratory information system
lpf Low-power field
L/S Lecithin-sphingomyelin ratio

MAR Mixed agglutination reaction
MBP Myelin basic protein
MoM Multiples of the median
mOsm Milliosmole
MPGN Membranoproliferative glomerulonephritis
MSDS Material Safety Data Sheet
MSU Monosodium urate (uric acid)

NaCl Sodium chloride
NCCLS National Committee for Clinical Laboratory Standards
NFPA National Fire Protection Association
NH_4^+ Ammonium ion

OD Optical density
OSHA Occupational Safety and Health Administration

PAH *p*-aminohippuric acid
PDCA Plan-Do-Check-Act
PKU Phenylketonuria
PM Preventive maintenance
PPE Personal protective equipment
PPM Provider-performed-microscopy
PSP Phenolsulfonphthalein

QA Quality assurance
QC Quality control

RBC Red blood cell
RCF Relative centrifugal force

RF	Rheumatoid factor
RPGN	Rapidly progressive (or crescentic) glomerulonephritis
RPM	Revolutions per minute
RPR	Rapid plasma reagin
RTE	Renal tubular epithelial (cells)
SD	Standard deviation
SSA	Sulfosalicylic acid
TAT	Turn-around-time
Tm	Maximal reabsorptive capacity/Tubular reabsorptive maximum
TQM	Total quality management
UP	Universal Precautions
UTI	Urinary tract infection
WBC	White blood cell
WHO	World Health Organization

Glossary

accreditation The process by which a program or institution documents meeting established guidelines
accuracy Closeness of the measured result to the true value
acrosomal cap Tip of a spermatozoa head containing enzymes for entry into an ovum
active transport Movement of a substance across cell membranes into the bloodstream by electrochemical energy
acute phase reactants Low-molecular-weight plasma proteins associated with infection and inflammation
aerosol Fine suspension of particles in air
afferent arteriole A small branch of the renal artery through which blood flows to the glomerulus of the kidney
albinism An inherited condition marked by decreased production of melanin
albuminuria Protein (albumin) in the urine
aldosterone A hormone that regulates reabsorption of sodium in the distal convoluted tubule
alimentary tract The digestive tract, including structures between the mouth and the anus
alkaptonuria Homogentistic acid in the urine caused by a failure to inherit the gene to produce homogentisic acid oxidase
aminoacidurias Disorders in which increased amino acids are present in the urine
amniocentesis Transabdominal puncture of the uterus and amnion to obtain amniotic fluid
amnion The membranous sac containing the fetus and amniotic fluid
amyloid material A starchlike protein-carbohydrate complex that is deposited abnormally in tissue in some chronic disease states
andrology The study of diseases of the male reproductive organs
antiglomerular basement membrane antibody Autoantibody against alveolar and glomerular capillary basement membranes found in Goodpasture's syndrome
anuria Complete stoppage of urine flow
arachnoid villi Projections on the arachnoid membrane of the brain through which cerebrospinal fluid is reabsorbed
arthritis Inflammation of the synovial joints
arthrocentesis The puncture of a joint to obtain synovial fluid
ascites Abnormal accumulation of peritoneal fluid
azotemia Increased nitrogenous waste products in the blood

bacterial endocarditis Inflammation of the endocardial membrane of the heart caused by bacterial infection
bacteriuria Bacteria in the urine
beta$_2$ microglobulin A subunit of the class I major compatibility antigens that enters the blood at a constant rate
bilirubin A bright yellow pigment produced in the degradation of heme
biohazardous Pertaining to a hazard caused by infectious organisms
birefringence The ability to refract light in two directions
blood-brain barrier The barrier between the brain tissue and capillary blood through which substances are selectively filtered
body substance isolation A guideline stating that all moist body substances are capable of transmitting disease
Bowman's capsule Part of the nephron containing the glomerulus
bright-field microscopy A procedure by which magnified images appear dark against a bright background

carcinogenic Capable of causing cancer
casts Elements excreted in the urine in the shape of renal tubules
catheterized specimen A urine specimen collected by passing a sterile tube into the bladder
chain of custody Step-by-step documentation of the handling and testing of legal specimens
chain of infection A continuous link transmitting harmful microorganisms between a source and a susceptible host
chemical hygiene plan Protocol established for the identification, handling, storage, and disposal of all hazardous chemicals
chemical sieving Macroscopic screening of urine to determine the need for a microscopic examination
choroid plexuses A network of capillaries in the ventricle of the brain that produces cerebrospinal fluid
chylous material A milky lymphatic fluid containing triglycerides and chylomicrons
clarity Transparency of urine ranging from clear to turbid
coefficient of variation Standard deviation expressed as a percentage of the mean
collecting duct Part of the nephron where the final concentration of urine takes place through the reabsorption of water
constipation Infrequent production of feces resulting in small, hard stools
continuous quality improvement An institutional program that focuses on customer satisfaction and expectations
control mean Average of all data points
control range Limit in which expected control values lie, usually plus or minus two standard deviations
countercurrent mechanism A selective urine concentration process in the ascending and descending loops of Henle
creatinine A substance formed by the breakdown of creatine during muscle metabolism
creatinine clearance A test used to measure the glomerular filtration rate
crenated Shrunken and irregularly shaped or notched
cylindruria The presence of urinary casts
cystinosis An inherited recessive disorder disrupting the metabolism of cystine
cystinuria Cystine in the urine as a result of a defect in the renal tubular reabsorption of amino acids

cystitis An inflammation of the bladder
cytogenetic analysis An analysis of cellular chromosomes

D-dimer A product of fibrinolysis
demyelination The destruction of the myelin sheath that protects a nerve
density Concentration of solutes present per volume of solution
diarrhea Watery stools
diarthroses Freely movable joints
disinfectant A substance that destroys microorganisms that is used on surfaces rather than the skin
distal convoluted tubule Part of the nephron between the ascending loop of Henle and the collecting duct where the final concentration of urinary filtrate begins
dysentery An inflammation of the intestines caused by microorganisms resulting in diarrhea
dysmorphic Irregularly shaped
dyspnea Difficulty breathing

edema An accumulation of fluid in the tissues
efferent arteriole The small renal artery branch through which blood flows away from the glomerulus
effusion An accumulation of fluid between the serous membranes
endogenous procedure A test using a substance originating within the body
erythrophagocytosis Engulfment of red blood cells by macrophages
exogenous procedure A test that requires a substance to be infused into the body
external quality control An evaluation using preanalyzed materials received from an agency outside the laboratory
exudate Serous fluid effusion caused by conditions producing damage to the serous membranes

Fanconi's syndrome A group of disorders marked by renal tubular dysfunction associated with some inherited and acquired conditions
fasting specimen The second voided urine specimen collected after fasting
ferritin A major storage form of iron found in the liver, spleen, and bone marrow
fetal lung maturity The presence of a sufficient amount of surfactant lipoproteins to maintain alveolar stability
first morning specimen The first voided urine specimen collected immediately upon arising; recommended screening specimen
flatus Gas expelled from the anus
free water clearance A test to determine the ability of the kidney to respond to the state of body hydration
fructosuria The presence of fructose in the urine

galactosuria The presence of galactose in the urine
gastrocolic fistula Abnormal passageway between the stomach and the colon
ghost cells Red blood cells that have lost their hemoglobin, leaving only the cell membrane; appearing in hyposthenuric urine
glans The glandlike body at the tip of the penis
glomerular filtration rate The volume of plasma that is filtered by the glomerulus in a specified time
glomerulonephritis An inflammation of the glomerulus resulting in impaired glomerular filtration
glomerulosclerosis The destruction of glomeruli by scarring and fibrin deposition
glomerulus Tuft of capillary blood vessels located in Bowman's capsule where filtration occurs
glucose tolerance specimens Fractional collection specimens; urine specimens are collected at the same time as blood samples are drawn to compare the levels of glucose in blood and urine
glycogenesis The conversion of glucose to glycogen
glycogenolysis The conversion of glycogen to glucose
glycosuria Glucose in the urine (glucosuria)
granuloma Modular accumulation of inflammatory cells

harmonic oscillation densitometry A method of measuring specific gravity using the change in the frequency of a sound wave after it enters a solution
Hartnup disease A recessive inherited disorder marked by intestinal absorption abnormalities and renal aminoaciduria
hematuria Blood in the urine
hemoglobinuria Hemoglobin in the urine
hemolytic disease of the newborn Rh incompatibility between mother and fetus that can cause hemolysis of the fetal red blood cells
hemoptysis Blood in the sputum
hemosiderin An insoluble form of storage iron; a product of red blood cell hemolysis
hemothorax The accumulation of blood in the pleural cavity
homocystinuria The presence of homocystine in the urine caused by an inherited autosomal recessive disorder
2-hour postprandial specimen Fractional collection specimen; urine specimen collected 2 hours after eating
hyaluronic acid Glycosaminoglycan found in synovial fluid that provides lubrication to the joints
hydramnios Excess amniotic fluid
hydrostatic pressure Pressure exerted by a liquid
hyperglycemia Elevated glucose levels in the blood
hypernatremia Elevated blood sodium levels
hypersthenuric Pertaining to urine specific gravity greater than the 1.010 of the glomerular filtrate
hyponatremia Decreased blood sodium levels
hyposthenuric Pertaining to urine specific gravity lower than the 1.010 of the glomerular filtrate
hypoxia Lack of oxygen

iatrogenic Pertaining to a condition caused by treatment, medications, or diagnostic procedures
immune complexes Antigen-antibody combinations
inborn error of metabolism Failure to inherit the gene to produce a particular enzyme
indicanuria The presence of indican in the urine
infertility The inability to conceive
interference-contrast microscopy A procedure by which three-dimensional images of a specimen are obtained
internal quality control The preparation and evaluation of control materials within the laboratory
interstitial Pertaining to spaces between tissue cells
inulin A fructose-derived substance that is filtered by the kidney and not reabsorbed or secreted and that can be used to measure the glomerular filtration rate
ischemia Deficiency of blood to a body area
isosthenuric Pertaining to urine specific gravity the same as the 1.010 of the glomerular filtrate

jaundice Yellow appearance of skin, mucous membranes, and eye sclera due to increased amounts of bilirubin in the blood
juxtaglomerular apparatus Specialized cells located on the afferent arteriole that regulate secretion of renin

ketonuria Ketones in the urine

labia The outer folds of the vagina

lactosuria The presence of lactose in the urine
lamellar body Organelle produced by type II pneumonocytes in the fetal lung that contain lung surfacants
lecithin-sphingomyelin ratio A comparison of lung surfactants that is performed to determine fetal lung maturity
Lesch-Nyhan disease An inherited sex-linked recessive purine metabolism disorder marked by excess uric acid crystals in the urine
leukocyturia Leukocytes (white blood cells) in the urine
liquefaction The conversion of solid or coagulated material to a liquid form
lithiasis The formation of renal calculi (kidney stones)
lithotripsy A procedure using ultrasonic waves to crush renal calculi
loop of Henle The U-shaped part of the renal tubule consisting of a thin descending limb and a thick ascending limb

macula densa Specialized cells located on the distal convoluted tubule that interact with the juxtaglomerular cells
malabsorption Impaired absorption of nutrients by the intestine
maldigestion Impaired digestion of foodstuffs
maple syrup urine disease An autosomal recessive trait causing increased levels of the branched chain amino acids, leucine, isoleucine, valine, and their ketone acids in the urine
Material Safety Data Sheet A document provided by the vendor or manufacturer of a chemical substance describing the chemical's characteristics
maximal reabsorptive capacity The maximum reabsorption ability for a solute by renal tubules
meconium The dark-green mucus containing stool formed by a fetus
medullary interstitium Spaces between the cells in the medulla of the kidney that contain highly concentrated fluid
melanoma A tumor of the melanogen-producing cells, which is frequently malignant
melanuria Increased melanin in the urine
melituria Increased urinary sugar
meninges Protective membranes around the brain and spinal cord
meningitis Inflammation of the meninges, frequently caused by microbial infection
metabolic acidosis A decrease in the blood pH caused by a metabolic increase in acidic elements
microalbuminuria Low levels of urine protein not detected by reagent strips
midstream clean-catch specimen Specimen collected in a sterile container after cleansing the glans penis or urinary meatus; the first portion of urine is voided into the toilet, the midportion is collected, and the remaining portion is voided into the toilet
mucopolysaccharides Glycosaminoglycans consisting of a protein core with polysaccharide branches
mucopolysaccharidoses A group of genetic disorders marked by excess mucopolysaccharides in blood and urine
myoglobinuria Myoglobin in the urine

necrosis Death of cells
nephron A functional unit of the kidney that forms urine
nephropathy Disease of the kidneys
nephrotic syndrome A renal disorder marked by massive proteinuria, lipiduria, and edema caused by disruption of the glomerular membrane
nocturia Excessive urination during the night

occult blood Blood that is not visible to the naked eye
Occupational Safety and Health Administration The government agency created to protect employees from potential health hazards in the workplace through the development and monitoring of regulations
oligohydramnios Decreased amniotic fluid
oligoclonal bands Electrophoretic bands migrating in the gamma region that are present in cerebrospinal fluid and serum
oliguria A marked decrease in urine flow
oncotic pressure The osmotic pressure of a substance in solution caused by the presence of colloids
organic acidemias The accumulation of organic acids in the blood, mainly isovalaric, propionic, and methylmalonic acids
orthostatic proteinuria Increased protein in urine only when an individual is in an upright position
osmolar clearance The amount of plasma filtered each minute to produce a urine with the same osmolarity as plasma
osmolarity The osmotic pressure of a solution expressed in milliosmols per kilogram; it is affected only by the number of particles present
osmotic diarrhea An increased retention of water and solutes in the large intestine associated with malabsorption and maldigestion
osmotic gradient The difference in the concentration of substances on either side of a membrane
outcomes Results of the process to improve customer satisfaction

pancreatic insufficiency The decreased ability of the pancreas to secrete digestive enzymes
paracentesis Surgical puncture into the abdominal cavity to obtain peritoneal fluid
parietal membrane Serous membrane lining the walls of the pleural, pericardial, and peritoneal cavities
passive transport Movement of molecules across a membrane by diffusion because of a physical gradient
pentosuria The presence of pentose sugars in the urine
pericardiocentesis Surgical puncture into the pericardial cavity
pericarditis An inflammation of the membranes enclosing the heart
peritoneal lavage Introduction and subsequent removal of fluid into the peritoneal cavity to detect the presence of abnormal substances
peritonitis An inflammation of the membranes lining the peritoneal cavity
peritubular capillaries The capillaries surrounding the renal tubules
personal protective equipment Items used to protect the body from infectious agents
phase-contrast microscopy Procedure in which magnified images show varied intensities of light and dark and are surrounded by haloes
phenylketonuria The presence of abnormal phenylalanine metabolites in the urine
pigmented villonodular synovitis Proliferation of synovial cells forming brown nodules, resulting in inflammation, pain, and hemorrhagic effusions
pleocytosis Increased numbers of normal cells in the cerebrospinal fluid
podocytes Epithelial cells of the inner lining of Bowman's capsule that contain footlike processes
polarizing microscopy A procedure in which magnified birefringent images appear bright or colored against a black background
polydipsia Excessive thirst
polyuria Marked increase in urine flow
porphobilinogen Immediate precursor of the porphyrins involved in the synthesis of heme
porphyrias Disorders of porphyrin metabolism that are inherited or acquired

porphyrins Intermediate compounds in the synthesis of heme
porphyrinuria The presence of porphyrins in the urine
postrenal proteinuria Increased protein in the urine caused by infections/inflammation that add protein to the urine after its formation
precision Reproducibility of a test result
prerenal proteinuria Increased protein in the urine caused by factors affecting the plasma before it reaches the kidney
preventive maintenance Checks on instruments and equipment on a regular schedule
process System of what is done to the patient
proficiency testing Performance of tests on specimens provided by an external monitoring agency
protein error of indicators Indicators change color in the presence of protein at a constant pH
proteinuria Protein in the urine (albuminuria)
proximal convoluted tubule The nearest tubule to the glomerulus where reabsorption of essential substances begins
pseudochylous material Milky appearing effusion that does not contain chylomicrons
purpura Small capillary hemorrhages
pyelonephritis Infection of the renal tubules

quality assurance Methods used to guarantee quality patient care
quality control Methods used to monitor the accuracy of procedures

radioisotope A substance that emits radiant energy
ragocytes Neutrophils containing ingested clumps of IgG
random specimen Urine collected at any time without prior patient preparation
refractometry Measurement of the light-bending capability of solutions
Reiter cells Vacuolated macrophages containing ingested neutrophils associated with nonspecific arthritic inflammation
reliability The ability to maintain both precision and accuracy
renal plasma flow The volume of plasma passing through the kidneys per minute
renal proteinuria Protein in the urine caused by impaired renal function
renal threshold Plasma concentration of a substance at which active transport stops and increased amounts are excreted in the urine
renal tubular acidosis The inability to produce an acid urine in the presence of metabolic acidosis
renin Proteolytic enzyme produced by the kidney that reacts with angiotensinogen to produce angiotensin to increase blood pressure
renin-angiotensin-aldosterone system Regulates flow of blood to and within the kidneys by responding to changes in blood pressure and plasma sodium content
resolution The ability to separate fine structures for visualization of detail
rhabdomyolysis Muscle destruction

secretory diarrhea The increased secretion of water and electrolytes into the large intestine caused by bacterial enterotoxins
semen Fluid containing spermatozoa
serous fluid Fluid formed as a plasma ultrafiltrate that provides lubrication between the parietal and visceral serous membranes
shift Abrupt change in the mean
Sjögren's syndrome An autoimmune disorder associated with a defect in glandular production of moisture
specific gravity The density of a solution compared with that of a similar volume of distilled water, influenced by both the number and size of the particles present
spermatids Immature spermatozoa
spermatozoa Sperm cells
standard deviation Measurement statistic that indicates the average distance each data point is from the mean
Standard Precautions Guideline describing personnel protective practices
steatorrhea Excess fat in the feces
stools Fecal material discharged from the large intestine
subarachnoid space The area between the arachnoid and pia mater membranes
suprapubic aspiration The technique to obtain sterile urine specimens for bacterial culture or cytologic examination by introducing a sterile needle through the abdomen into the bladder
surfactants Phospholipids secreted by type II pneumocytes to maintain alveolar integrity
syncytia A group of cells continuous with adjoining cells
synovial fluid Plasma ultrafiltrate containing hyaluronic acid that provides lubrication of the joints
synoviocytes Cells in the synovial membrane that secrete hyaluronic acid
systemic lupus erythematosus Autoimmune disorder affecting the connective tissue resulting in damage to organs, particularly the kidney and joints

Tamm-Horsfall protein Mucoprotein found in the matrix of renal tubular casts
thoracentesis Surgical puncture into the thoracic cavity to collect pleural fluid
three-glass collection Urine specimen collected in three separate sterile containers; used to determine prostatic infection
thrombosis Formation of a blood clot
timed specimen Urine specimen collected over an interval of time for a quantitative analysis of a urine chemical, usually a 24-hour collection
titratable acidity Hydrogen ions in the urine that can be quantitated by titration with a base to a pH of 7.4
total quality management Institutional policy to provide customer satisfaction
transudate Serous effusion produced as a result of disruption of fluid production and regulation between the serous membranes
traumatic tap Surgical puncture contaminated with capillary blood
trend Gradual change in one direction of the mean of a control substance
tubular reabsorption Substances moved from the tubular filtrate into the blood by active or passive transport
tubular secretion The passage of substances from the blood in the peritubular capillaries to the tubular filtrate
tubulointerstitial disease Renal disease affecting both the renal tubules and renal interstitium
turnaround-time Time from ordering a test through analysis in the laboratory to the charting of the report
tyrosinuria The presence of tyrosine in the urine

Universal Precautions Guideline stating that all patients are capable of transmitting blood-borne disease
urinary meatus The external urinary opening
urinometry An imprecise method for measuring urine specific gravity using a weighted float

urobilin The oxidized form of urobilinogen that provides the brown color to feces
urobilinogen A compound formed in the intestines by the bacterial reduction of bilirubin
urochrome Yellow pigment produced by endogenous metabolism that imparts the yellow color to urine
uroerythrin Pink pigment in urine derived from melanin metabolism that attaches to urates in the sediment

vasa recta A network of capillaries surrounding the loop of Henle
vasectomy Surgical removal of all or part of the vas deferens for the purpose of male sterilization
vasopressin Antidiuretic hormone that regulates reabsorption of water by the collecting ducts
vasovasostomy Repair of a severed vas deferens to restore fertility
visceral membrane The serous membrane covering the organs contained within a cavity
viscosity The amount of resistance to flow in a liquid
visicoureteral reflux Urine in the bladder passing back into the uterers

xanthochromia Yellowish discoloration of the cerebrospinal fluid

Index

Page numbers followed by f indicate figures; page numbers followed by t indicate tables.